AF668435

Ultrasound in Subfertility

Routine Applications and Diagnostic Challenges

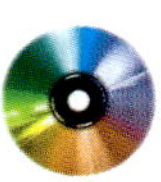

System requirement:

- Operating System – Windows Vista or above
- Recommended Web Browser – Google Chrome & Mozilla Firefox
- Essential plugins – Java & Flash player
  - Facing problems in viewing content – it may be your system does not have java enabled.
  - If Videos don't show up – it may be the system requires Flash player or need to manage flash setting. To learn more about flash setting click on the link in the help section.
  - You can test java and flash by using the links from the help section of the CD/DVD.

Accompanying CD/DVD Rom is playable only in Computer and not in DVD player.

CD/DVD has Autorun function – it may take few seconds to load on your computer. If it does not work for you then follow the steps below to access the contents manually:

- Click on my computer
- Select the **CD/DVD** drive and click open/explore – this will show list of files in the CD/DVD
- Find and double click file – "launch.html"

For more information about troubleshoot of Autorun click on: http://support.microsoft.com/kb/330135

Ultrasound in Subfertility

Routine Applications and Diagnostic Challenges

SECOND EDITION

Editors

K Jayaprakasan MD DNB MRCOG PhD
Subspecialist and Honorary Associate Professor
Reproductive Medicine and Surgery
Consultant Gynecologist
Royal Derby Hospital, Derby
University of Nottingham
Nottingham, UK

Sonal Panchal MD
Consultant Radiologist
Dr Nagori's Institute for Infertility and IVF
Ahmedabad, Gujarat, India
Professor
Dubrovnik International University
Croatia

Foreword
Roy Homburg

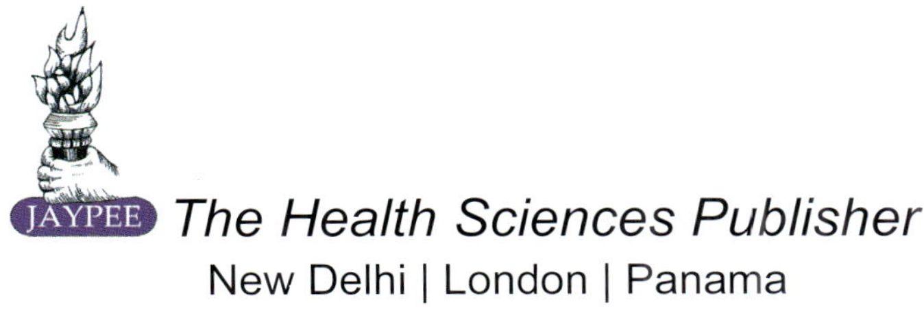

The Health Sciences Publisher
New Delhi | London | Panama

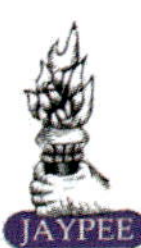

Jaypee Brothers Medical Publishers (P) Ltd

Headquarters
Jaypee Brothers Medical Publishers (P) Ltd.
4838/24, Ansari Road, Daryaganj
New Delhi 110 002, India
Phone: +91-11-43574357
Fax: +91-11-43574314
E-mail: jaypee@jaypeebrothers.com

Overseas Offices
JP Medical Ltd.
83, Victoria Street, London
SW1H 0HW (UK)
Phone: +44-20 3170 8910
Fax: +44(0)20 3008 6180
E-mail: info@jpmedpub.com

Jaypee-Highlights Medical Publishers Inc.
City of Knowledge, Bld. 235, 2nd Floor, Clayton
Panama City, Panama
Phone: +1 507-301-0496
Fax: +1 507-301-0499
E-mail: cservice@jphmedical.com

Jaypee Brothers Medical Publishers (P) Ltd.
17/1-B, Babar Road, Block-B, Shyamoli
Mohammadpur, Dhaka-1207
Bangladesh
Mobile: +08801912003485
E-mail: jaypeedhaka@gmail.com

Jaypee Brothers Medical Publishers (P) Ltd.
Bhotahity, Kathmandu, Nepal
Phone: +977-9741283608
E-mail: kathmandu@jaypeebrothers.com

Website: www.jaypeebrothers.com
Website: www.jaypeedigital.com

Inquiries for bulk sales may be solicited at: jaypee@jaypeebrothers.com

Ultrasound in Subfertility: Routine Applications and Diagnostic Challenges

First Edition: 2014
***Second Edition:* 2019**

ISBN: 978-93-5270-507-8

Printed at: Ajanta Offset & Packagings Ltd., Faridabad, Haryana.

Contributors

Ashok Khurana MD
Consultant in Reproductive Ultrasound
The Ultrasound Laboratory
Defence Colony, New Delhi, India

Chaitanya Nagori MD
Consultant in Reproductive
Medicine and Gynecological Endocrinology
Dr Nagori's Institute for Infertility and IVF
Ahmedabad, Gujarat, India

G Swapna DMRD
Consultant Radiologist
Sonoscan-Ultrasonic Scan Center
Coimbatore, Tamil Nadu, India

Giuseppina Lamanna MD
IVF Consultant
London Women's Clinic, London, UK

Jaideep Malhotra MD FRCOG FRCPI
Managing Director ART Rainbow IVF, India

Jane Stewart MD FRCOG
Subspecialist in Reproductive Medicine and Surgery
Consultant Gynecologist
Newcastle Fertility Center, Biomedicine West Wing
International Center for Life, Newcastle upon Tyne, UK

Janine Elson MD FRCOG
Subspecialist in Reproductive Medicine and Surgery
Consultant Gynecologist
CARE Fertility, Nottingham, UK

Kamal Ojha MD MRCOG
Consultant in Obstetrics
Gynecology and Reproductive Medicine
St Georges Hospital NHS Trust, London, UK

K Jayaprakasan MD DNB MRCOG PhD
Subspecialist and Honorary Associate Professor
Reproductive Medicine and Surgery
Consultant Gynecologist
Royal Derby Hospital, Derby
University of Nottingham, Nottingham, UK

Lil Valentin MD PhD FRCOG
Professor
Department of Obstetrics and Gynecology
Skåne University Hospital
Malmö, Sweden

Lukasz Polanski MBBS
Specialty Doctor, Addenbrookes Hospital
Cambridge, UK

Miriam Baumgarten MD
Consultant in Reproductive Medicine
Addenbrookes Hospital, Cambridge, UK

Narendra Malhotra MD FRCOG
Managing Director
Global Rainbow Healthcare, India

Nick Raine-Fenning MBChB MRCOG PhD
Reader and Associate Professor
Reproductive Medicine and Surgery
Nottingham University Research and
Treatment Unit in Reproduction (NURTURE)
Division of Obstetrics and Gynecology
School of Clinical Sciences
University of Nottingham
Nottingham, UK

Ouma Pillai MRCOG
Consultant in Obstetrics and Gynecology
St Georges Hospital NHS Trust
London, UK

S Boopathy Vijayaraghavan MD DMRD
Consultant Radiologist
Sonoscan-Ultrasonic Scan Center
Coimbatore, Tamil Nadu, India

Sonal Panchal MD
Consultant Radiologist
Dr Nagori's Institute for Infertility and IVF
Ahmedabad, Gujarat, India
Professor
Dubrovnik International University, Croatia

Foreword

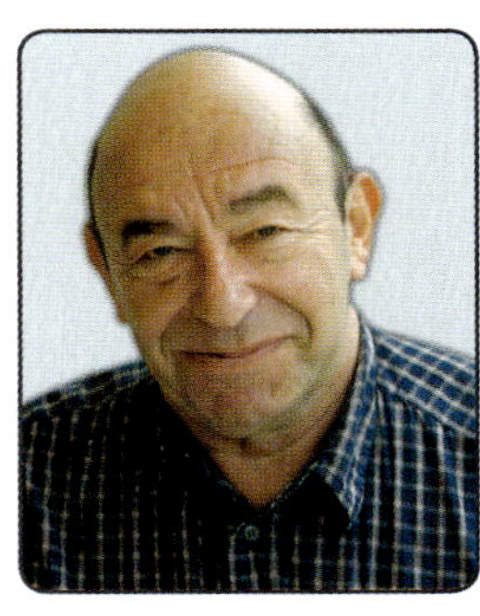

It is, probably, true to say that none of the medical subspecialties has progressed and developed in the last 40 years more than the fascinating field of infertility. From the time I was a medical student in the early 1960s up to the present moment, I have been privileged to witness one of the most amazing evolutions in modern medical practice. During my student days, a consultation for an infertile couple usually consisted of some wise and understanding nodding of the head, an explanation of the frequency and timing of intercourse and a standard manual vaginal examination of the pelvic organs. Clomiphene citrate and human menopausal gonadotropins were just being introduced and the foresight, brilliance and stubbornness of Edwards and Steptoe saw the advent of IVF and their first success in 1978. Intracytoplasmic sperm injection (ICSI) then gave hope to those suffering from sperm deficiencies.

In the 1970s, I saw my first demonstration of an ovarian follicle on ultrasound examination using a B-scan or gray scale machine. To my untrained eyes, these pictures looked like a snowstorm in Siberia! These machines were soon destined to become museum pieces with the rapidly advancing technology of ultrasound detection. Today, nothing in the pelvis can evade detection and refinement has followed refinement, not only producing amazing resolution but also introducing the possibility of techniques based on ultrasound, invaluable in our everyday practice.

This beautifully produced book elegantly presents us with an update of exactly where we are today. The editors, Kannamannadiar Jayaprakasan and Sonal Panchal are to be congratulated in gathering expert contributors and producing a book of outstanding quality. It starts with a remarkably understandable explanation of ultrasound principles, applications and examination techniques with important tips on how to get the best from the machine and with suggestions that ultrasound examination may well replace invasive techniques of diagnostic hysteroscopy and laparoscopy. The detailed examination of the uterus that is then described, leaves no related pathology hidden and the following chapters deal with the investigation of female infertility with excellent illustrations of how to assess the uterine cavity, tubes and antral follicle count. These chapters introduce us to three-dimensional and color Doppler applications before moving on to ovarian pathology and pelvic endometriosis. The use of ultrasound is now irreplaceable for assisted reproduction treatment and the chapters on monitoring of treatment cycles and ultrasound-guided procedures are valuable contributions to our knowledge. The assessment of the complications of treatment and the application of ultrasound for male infertility are elegantly dealt with and the book concludes with an amazing description of three-dimensional techniques.

With contributions from the UK, India and Sweden, this is not merely a book on ultrasound but witnesses the progress that has been made in our field with a bang up-to-date report and all credit is due to the contributors and editors for providing us with such a valuable document.

Roy Homburg MBBS FRCOG
Professor and Head of Research
Fertility Center, Homerton University Hospital
London, UK

Preface

Ultrasound is an essential tool in the assessment and management of subfertile couples undergoing fertility treatment. Ultrasound allows a noninvasive, direct assessment of the pelvic organs. The role of ultrasound has been proved beyond doubt for the pretreatment evaluation of the subfertile female, for treatment planning and monitoring, as well as for evaluation of the subfertile male. Invention of new modalities and softwares like Doppler, 3D-4D ultrasound, automated volume calculations, global vascular assessments, various render modes, all have contribution in this assessment. It has therefore become essential for every consultant, practicing or wishing to practice infertility, to learn and do ultrasound systematically.

We have tried to bring together a group of international experts to make each chapter as a guide for both inexperienced and experienced ultrasound practitioners to perform a high-quality ultrasound. We have taken utmost effort to provide plenty of ultrasound images and videos relevant to each clinical scenario to ease the learning process. We have adopted a systematic approach beginning with basic ultrasound principles, taking through correct examination techniques during a pelvic assessment, ultrasound screening of various uterine and adnexal pathologies, evaluation of tubal and ovarian function and application of ultrasound in monitoring treatment response, in assessing complications of fertility treatment and in guiding assisted reproduction treatment procedures. Special chapters are dedicated to provide an overview on the role of ultrasound in managing male infertility and also on 3D ultrasound techniques and its applications in subfertility.

We are thankful to the readers of this book for their support that lead to the release of the Second edition of this book. We are extremely grateful to all the authors, who have submitted chapters for this book. We appreciate their valuable time and effort that they put in to provide such excellent contributions despite them being quite busy in their professional life. Further, we are so privileged and honored that Prof Roy Homburg has written Foreword for the book, after going through all the draft chapters. We are ever so grateful to him for his invaluable support.

K Jayaprakasan
Sonal Panchal

Contents

DVD Contents

Chapter 1
Gain Settings: Correct Settings are Essential for Accurate B-mode Assessment

Chapter 2
Transabdominal Scan to Assess Pelvic Organs
Systematic Way of Doing a Transvaginal Scan
Transvaginal Scan with Different Image Orientation
Standardized Methods for Taking Uterine and Ovarian Measurements

Chapter 3
Lateral Subserous Fibroid
Submucous Fibroid
Leiomyoma with Power Doppler
Calcified Fibroid
Adenomyosis on Gray Scale
Adenomyosis on Power Doppler
Longitudinal Scan of the Uterus Showing Duplication Abnormality
Transverse Scan of Uterus Showing Duplication Abnormality
Arcuate Uterus on B-mode and 3D US
Complete Septate Uterus on B-mode
Septate Uterus on 3D Scan

Chapter 4
Endometrial Polyp
Endometrial Polyp on Saline Infusion Sonography
Broad-based Polyp on Saline Infusion Sonography

Chapter 5
Saline Infusion Salpingography on B-mode
Saline Infusion Salpingography on Color Doppler
HyCoSy with Contrast Mode on 2D US
HyCoSy with Contrast Mode on 2D US—Whole Tube not Seen in a Single Plane
HyCoSy Volume Reconstruction on 3D

Chapter 6
Antral Follicle Count Assessment Using 2D Ultrasound
Antral Follicle Count Assessment from Stored 3D Data Set
Antral Follicle Count Assessment Using SonoAVC—Technique
Antral Follicle Count Assessment Using SonoAVC—Output
Low Ovarian Reserve as Indicated by Only a Few Antral Follicles and Small Ovaries
Ovarian Volume Measured Using VOCAL from 3D Data Set
3D Power Doppler Ovarian Blood Flow Measurement

Chapter 1

Ultrasound: Principles and Applications

Ashok Khurana

Chapter Outline

INTRODUCTION

While a basic knowledge of the principles of physics of ultrasound for the everyday practice of ultrasound is essential, a deep understanding may not be necessary. This is equally relevant to ultrasound in subfertility as well. What is more pertinent is a working knowledge of how the machine acquires, processes, and displays an image, and how the knobs and software improve the image. The aim is to obtain an image that quickly and reliably helps to answer the questions that are sought from the examination.

GETTING STARTED

In order to rapidly obtain optimal images on a daily basis, a three-step training strategy is what is often useful. This requires no knowledge or understanding of physics or the principles of ultrasound, and is an empirical approach to a quick start. The first step is an all-important and efficient shortcut of a hands-on demonstration of each knob and menu of the unit by an applications expert from the manufacturer. This should be followed by a hands-on routine on the patient with the applications expert standing by for a few days. The third step is working with the unit independently. As a final follow-up, it is wise, efficient, and inexpensive to recall the applications expert for 1 day on every 3 weeks or so for a few months, so that the technology in the unit is then optimally utilized. Follow-up exposure at workshops that demonstrate newer equipment and techniques by experts is useful for refining technique on an ongoing basis and learning newer applications. At this stage, a working knowledge of applied physics and applied mathematics becomes indispensable.

This chapter is a practical treatise of applied physics in the perspective of obtaining an optimal image. Pure physics has been dispensed with, since it would occupy unnecessary space in this book!

PHYSICS OF TRANSDUCER CHOICE

The choice of transducers in evaluating subfertile and indeed, all gynecological patients is based on the understanding of two equations in physics. The first is the relationship of frequency (f) and wavelength (l). Velocity (n) is a product of wavelength and frequency ($n = lf$). The second equation relates to ultrasound beam geometry. The depth (d) at which the transition of the beam takes place from the near field to the far field is given by the equation $d = r^2/l$, where r is the diameter of the circular transducer.

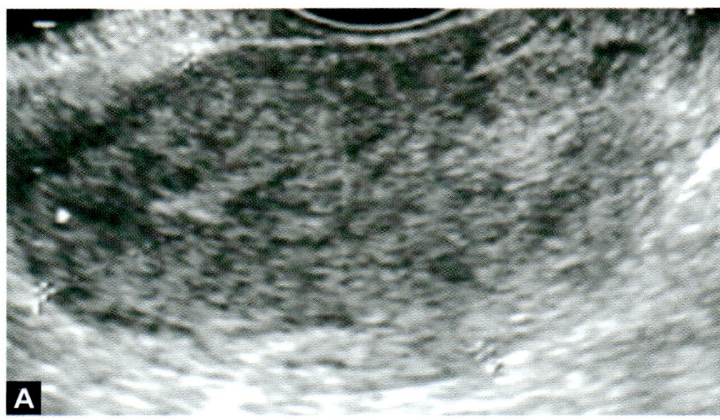

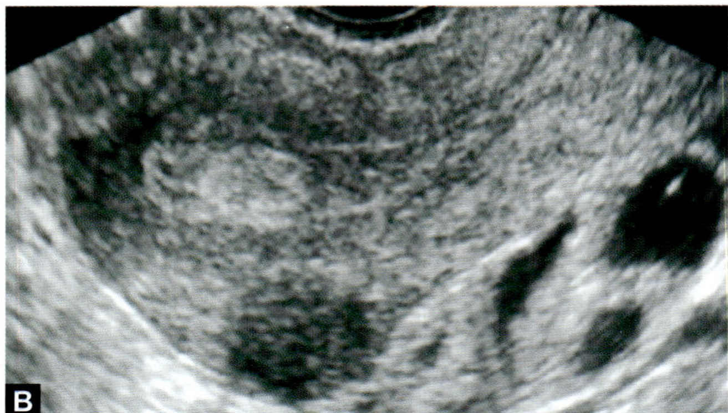

Figs. 1.1A and B: Images from the same patient using a (A) 5 MHz and a (B) 12 MHz transducer frequency. The inhomogeneous endometrium translates into an echogenic polyp. The indistinct posterior uterine wall on a higher frequency reveals an intramural fibroid. Thick-walled fluid loculi are evident posterior to the uterus on a high-frequency study.

Information from these relationships yields guidelines for tailoring transducer use.

The velocity with which a sound wave makes its way through any material is dependent on the density of the medium and is 330 m/s in air, 1,480 m/s in water, 1,589 m/s in muscle, and 3,500 m/s in bone.[1] Ultrasound machines are now standardized and calibrated to use 1,540 m/s as the speed of sound in human tissue. Since the velocity is a product of wavelength and frequency ($n = lf$), the higher the frequency the shorter the wavelength. Frequency refers to the degree of highness or lowness of a tone. The loudness of a tone is referred to as intensity.

Low-frequency sound, such as the human voice, spread all over a room. High-frequency sound behaves like light and moves like a beam along a straight line. High-frequency ultrasound moves through tissue as a narrow beam and can be focused by acoustic lenses. This is possible in the nearer relatively narrow part of the beam. The depth equation ($d = r^2 l$) implies that the wider the transducer face and the longer the wavelength (i.e. low frequency) the greater the depth. Resolution, however, depends on frequency; therefore, the higher the frequency the better the resolution.

The vast majority of scans in fertility patients are transvaginal scans. Since the transducer is closer to the region of interest than with transabdominal scans, a higher transducer frequency can be used. This greatly enhances resolution. Currently available transducers employ frequencies of up to 12 MHz, and the difference in resolution is remarkable (Figs. 1.1A and B). The trade-off with higher frequencies is of course, depth penetration of the beam, and these higher-frequency transducers have a limited resolution beyond a certain distance from the transducer. This limitation can be overcome by using a multifrequency transducer. Console keys permit a choice of low, middle, and high frequencies with the same transducer, enabling a great combination of resolution and depth. Transabdominal transducers have an advantage of a more panoramic field of view and a greater depth of penetration. These are therefore useful for identifying extraovarian adnexal structures and ovaries located at the pelvic brim. They are also indispensable for the assessment of associated abdominal lymph node disease, the suprarenal glands, kidneys, liver, abdominal peritoneal disease, and the pleura.

Transvaginal transducers are either mechanical or electronic array transducers. Mechanical transducers have one or more crystals that rotate or oscillate. Electronic transducers either have an array of crystals that are fired sequentially (phased array) or a set of crystals shaped to produce the sector image.[2] A large number of variations on these three types are commercially available and the user is warned to sift through the hyperbole and mystique of pseudophysics in making a choice! In general, mechanical transducers are less expensive. They have a wide field of view but have poorer resolution in the near field. Focal zones are fixed. Electronic array transducers cost more but have the advantage of good near-field resolution and multiple focal zones.

RESOLUTION

Technically, resolution refers to the ability of the ultrasound unit to differentiate two different adjacent structures as two discrete different structures and not fuse them into a single structure. High resolution refers to a very short distance between these two structures, and low resolution refers to a larger distance between these structures.

Axial resolution refers to the resolution along the path of the beam and is the most discerning resolution. This is also termed as the radial resolution or the range resolution. The shorter the pulse, i.e. the higher the frequency, the better the axial resolution.

Lateral resolution refers to resolution in the plane perpendicular to the plane of the beam. This is also called the azimuth plane. Beam quality and the size of side lobes determine lateral resolution. Side lobes are like skirts around the main lobe. "Main lobe" refers to the thin, round, and useful portion of the ultrasound beam. When such a beam passes through tissue and is reflected back, structures in the side-lobe zone are wrongly assigned to the main beam. These falsify and degrade the image. Lateral resolution can be improved by focusing the ultrasound beam. This is achieved by complex technology. From a practical viewpoint, arrows along the margin of the image indicate focused areas and these can be manually set to enhance the axial resolution at the depth of interest. This is a simple and extremely useful step in imaging but is largely neglected by most operators.

Axial resolution has a direct bearing on measurements. Since axial resolution is superior to lateral resolution, measurements are more accurate in the axial direction.

Elevation plane resolution refers to resolution in the slice thickness perpendicular to the axial plane. Good elevation plane resolution prevents superimposition of solid echoes over cystic areas in the slice thickness. This aspect of resolution is not electronically enhanceable and is achieved by a fixed acoustic lens. Limitations in this plane can be overcome only by operator's knowledge, skill, and vigilance.

HOW AND WHY KNOBS THAT SHOULD BE USED OFTEN, SHOULD BE USED

Depth, Magnification, and Zoom

Depth refers to the depth of tissues on display. It is wise to commence with a deeper region of interest to ensure that deeply located lesions are not missed. The depth is then reduced to a level that includes the region of interest. Typically, the depth should be adjusted so that the main area of interest ultimately occupies two-thirds of the screen.[3] Reducing depth increases magnification in the near field and this improves resolution. All available pixels are used to form the image, and the image therefore improves.[4] When the depth is too large it takes much longer for the transducer to receive echoes that return from deeper structures. This reduces the frame rate adversely. The zoom function allows magnification of one area on the monitor.[3] The image appears larger. The resolution of the magnified area does not change. Zoom allows a better study of small areas of interest. Beyond a point in zoom mode, the pixels become too few and the image becomes grainy. The structure to be assessed in detail should, therefore, be imaged at as shallow a depth as possible.

Zoom selects a square area that is sized in real time before it is activated. Depth should be adjusted before zoom is selected.

Gain

Adjusting gain alters how the transducer perceives returning echoes. Increasing the gain brightens the display of the returning echo information. Gain may be adjusted for the entire image (overall gain), or at depth, known as time-gain compensation (TGC).[3] Excessive gain makes the image too bright, and too little gain makes it dark (Figs. 1.2A and B). Excessive gain can make the picture bright with noise. This can obscure fluid echoes (Figs. 1.3A and B). Too little gain may create fluid echoes where no fluid exists (Figs. 1.4A and B). Many currently available medium- and high-end units now have a one-touch image optimization button that works automatically to fix the gain in an image.

Power Level

Power and gain are not the same. Power level refers to the amount of energy produced by the transducer.[4] Gain amplifies returning waves. Increasing the power helps to image deeper structures. It may, however, produce secondary vibrations in tissues. This can produce ring-down artifacts (Fig. 1.5). Some sound energy may bounce back and forth within a cyst, resulting in reverberation artifacts (Fig. 1.6). Power that is too low produces a faint image.[4] A weak signal gets mixed up with inherent noise in any equipment, and the result is a degraded image called snow[4] (Figs. 1.7A and B). Power should, therefore, be adjusted to ensure a balance between snow and artifacts.

Tissue Harmonic Imaging

While conventional ultrasound uses the same frequency bandwidth for both the transmitted and received signals, tissue harmonic imaging (THI) uses a low frequency for transmitted signal and a high frequency for the received signal. When echoes return after being reflected, they do so not only at the basic frequency but also at multiples of the

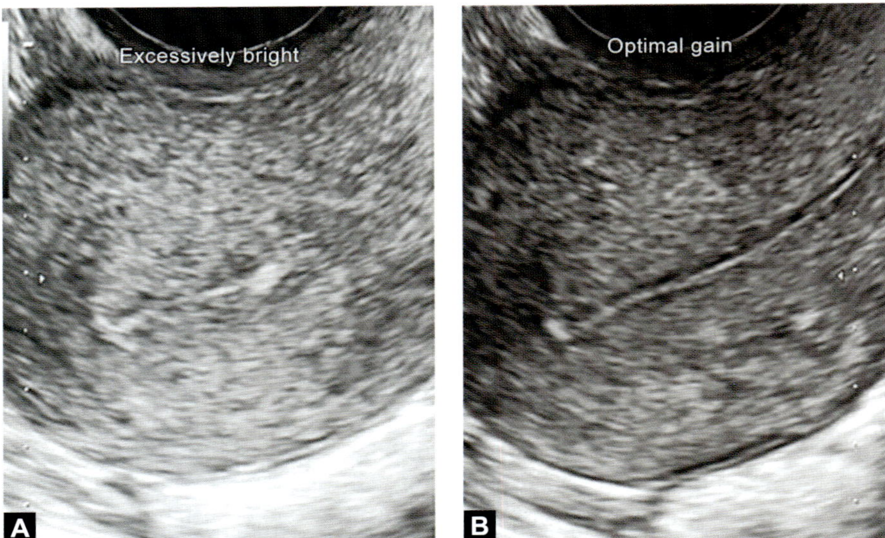

Figs. 1.2A and B: Excessive gain obscures textural detail. There is excessive gain in the image (A) and the texture and margins of the endometrium are indistinct. The image (B) has optimal gain. The triple-layered proliferative phase morphology is distinct and no focal lesion is evident.

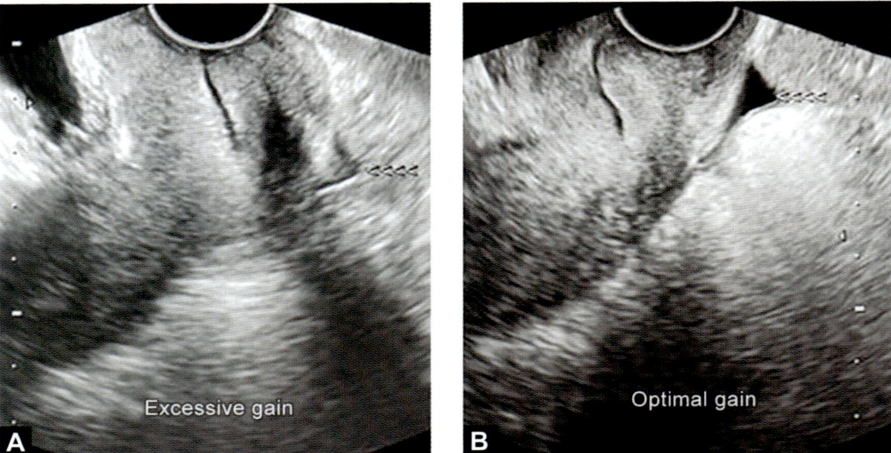

Figs. 1.3A and B: Excessive gain can obscure fluid echoes. The image (B) was obtained at optimal gain settings and shows a small quantity of free fluid (<<<<) in the pouch of Douglas. The image (A) was obtained at high-gain settings and the fluid (<<<<) is largely obscured.

basic frequency. These higher frequency waves experience less attenuation, less scatter, and less side-lobe artifact and may generate clearer images, particularly at the interface between fluid and tissue. The trade-off is a slightly longer processing time. This is now routinely available on most ultrasound machines.

Dynamic Range

A clear cyst is best assessed with a minimum of gray levels. A wider range of grays better assesses solid lesions. Dynamic range permits this variation of gray scale (Figs. 1.8A and B). Dynamic range is the range in acoustic power between the faintest and strongest signals. Dynamic range controls the image contrast with increasing the dynamic range produces a grayer image.

Focal Zones

While doing ultrasound scan, one should constantly check the position of focal zone/s to ensure that they are at the depth of interest. Multiple focal zones, which create a long

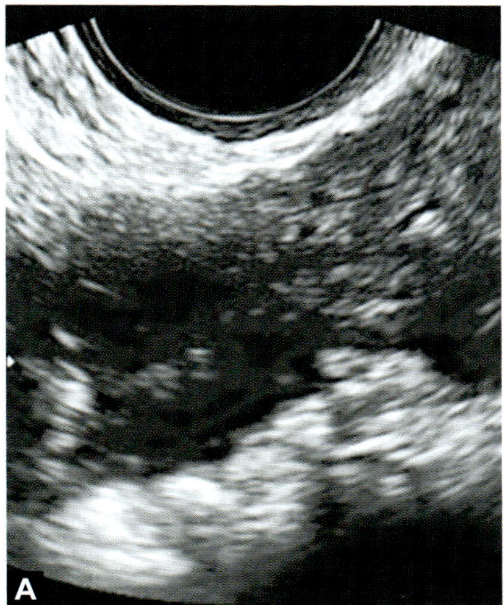

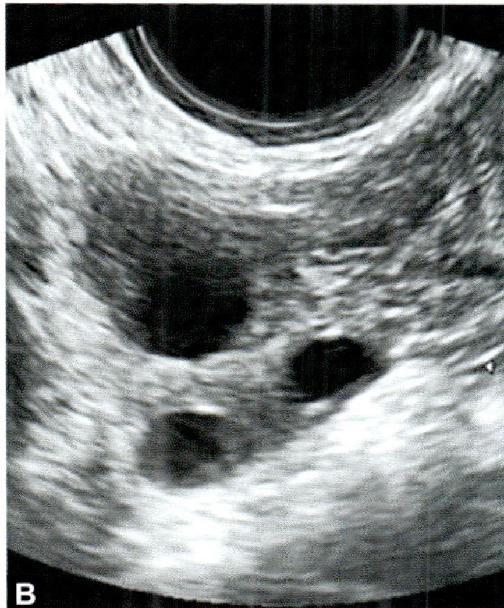

Figs. 1.4A and B: Inadequate gain can "create" fluid where none exists. In the image (A), a large fluid collection is evident in the right adnexa. Increasing the gain [image (B)] reveals an ovary with three antral follicles.

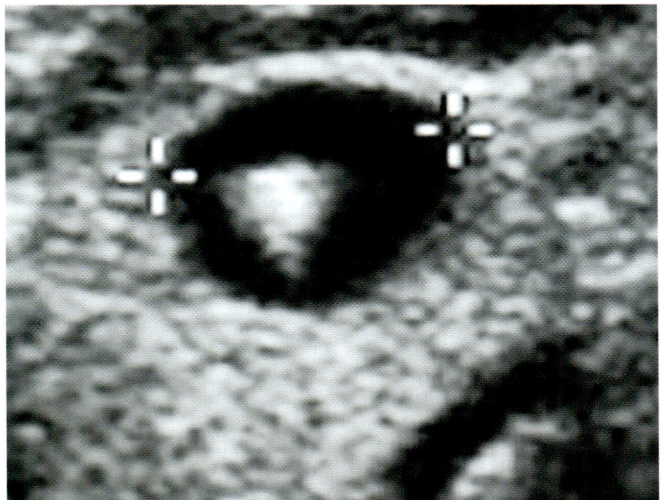

Fig. 1.5: Increasing the power in order to image deeper structures may produce secondary vibrations in tissues. This can produce ring-down artifacts.

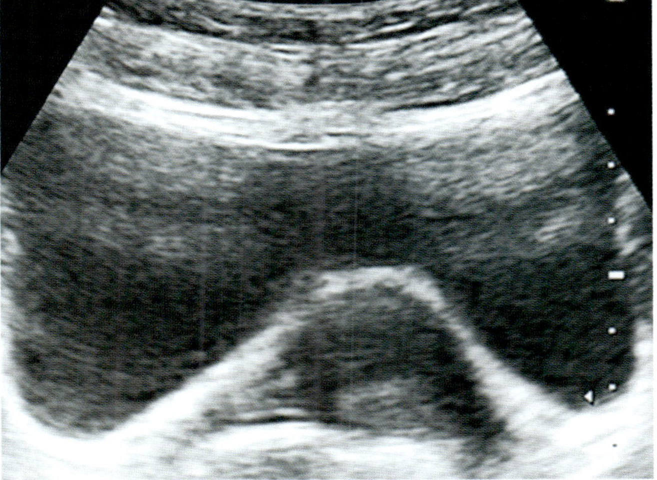

Fig. 1.6: Reverberation artifact. High-level echoes are seen in the anterior extent of the urinary bladder. These may obscure solid lesions and also render an entirely fluid lesion echogenic.

narrow beam, can be used to maximize lateral resolution over depth with the overall image quality will be improved throughout a static image. However, it is best to minimize the number of focal zones, when assessing moving structures as it may take more time to form a scan line and result in frame rate being reduced making the images disjointed.

Presets

Most current machines have settings that will adjust an image based on the anatomy being scanned. These presets are programmed to optimize images based on certain gain and power settings, focal zones, frame rates, and other settings.[3] It is imperative that the applications expert checks factory set presets.

DOPPLER STUDIES

The term "Doppler" is loosely used to indicate blood-flow information. It is based on the Doppler effect wherein the returning frequency of waves is altered by the movement of a target. The moving target is red blood cells in

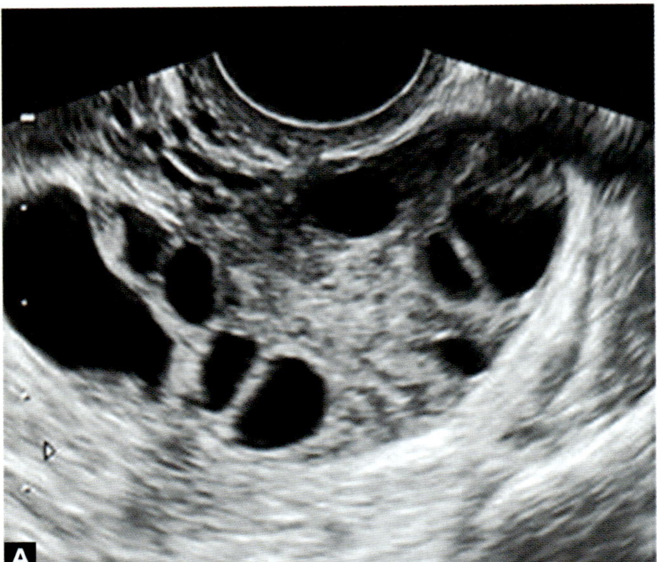

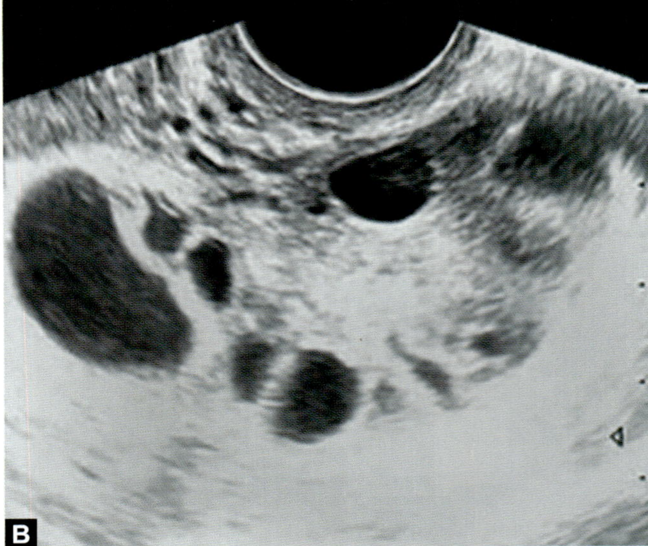

Figs. 1.7A and B: Inadequate power and excessive gain combine to create noise called snow (B). This creates medium-sized high-level echoes which obscure margins and fluid densities in the region of interest when comparing with the image obtained with optimum power and gain (A).

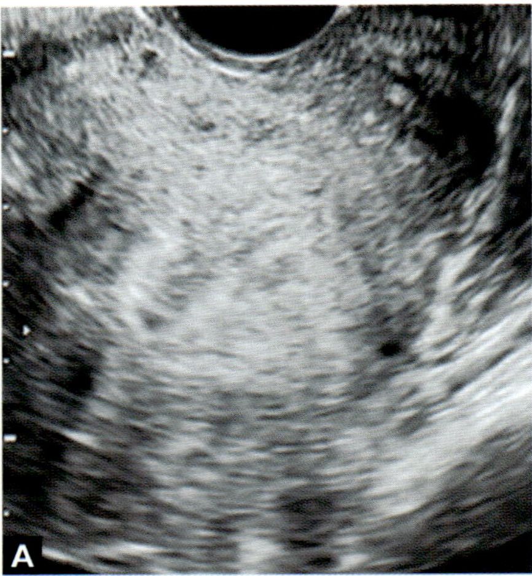

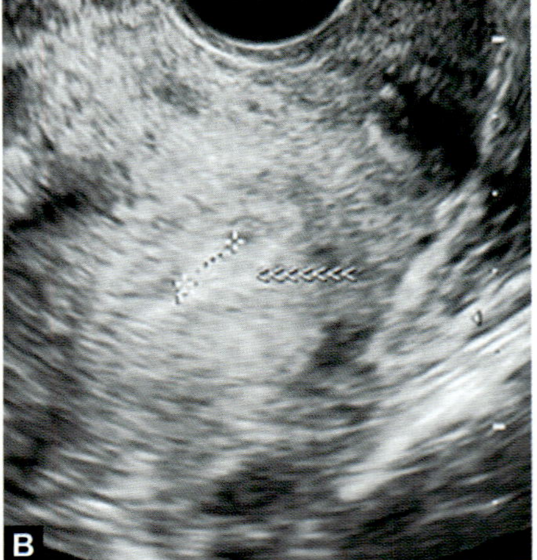

Figs. 1.8A and B: Solid organs and lesions are best studied by a wide dynamic range setting. The image (A) was done at fluid-level settings and failed to reveal an 8 mm echogenic polyp in the endometrium. The image (B) was optimized with a wide dynamic range and clearly (<<<<<<<) shows an echogenic endometrial polyp.

the blood vessels in the region of interest. The returning signal is mapped in two ways.[5] A map of the vessels can be obtained which can be superimposed on the gray-scale image. This is known as color flow mapping. This indicates direction and velocity of flow. The other method of mapping is known as the Doppler spectrum. This consists of a graph showing flow characteristics as a waveform (Fig. 1.9). These can then be quantified as velocities, ratios, and indices. The Doppler spectrum has an equivalent simultaneous audio signal as well which one learns to assess and analyze with increasing experience.[6]

Power Doppler is a newer form of flow imaging. It uses amplitude of scatter rather than a frequency shift to make a map of tissue flow. It is by its inherent nature far more sensitive to slow flow and therefore extremely useful in evaluating cyclical and pathologic changes in the female pelvis. Recent technical advances have made power Doppler directionality available as well. Doppler requires fine-tuning of sets as much as does gray scale.

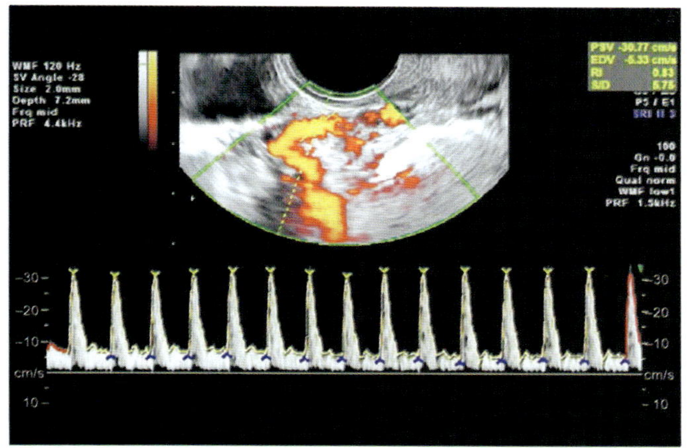

Fig. 1.9: Normal spectral Doppler image of a uterine artery with velocity-wave form.

Pulse Repetition Frequency or Scale

Adjusting the pulse repetition frequency (PRF) alters the sensitivity of Doppler for flow velocity (Figs. 1.10A to C). A lower PRF will result in a lower scale, more sensitive for slower flows, but may cause aliasing artifacts.[3] Pulse repetition frequency should be ideally kept low when assessing vessels with low-velocity blood flow (e.g. ovarian stromal arteries) and be kept high when assessing vessels with high-velocity blood flow (e.g. uterine arteries).

Doppler Gain

Similar to the basic B-mode or two-dimensional (2D) image, gain may be adjusted for Doppler. Increasing Doppler gain will amplify returning signals, resulting in more color or a stronger spectral signal (Figs. 1.11A to C and 1.12A to C). As in B-mode imaging, too much gain will

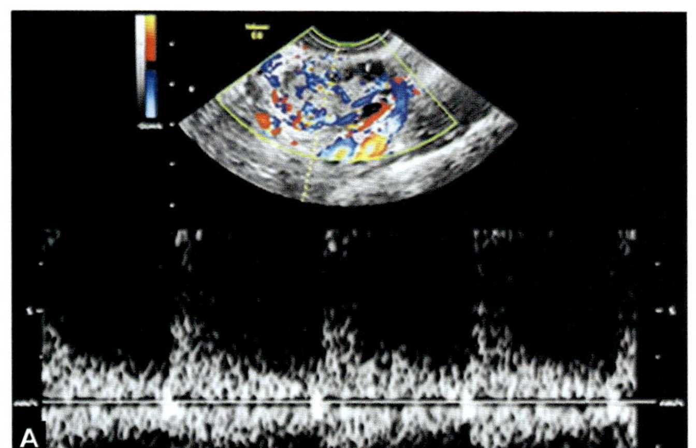

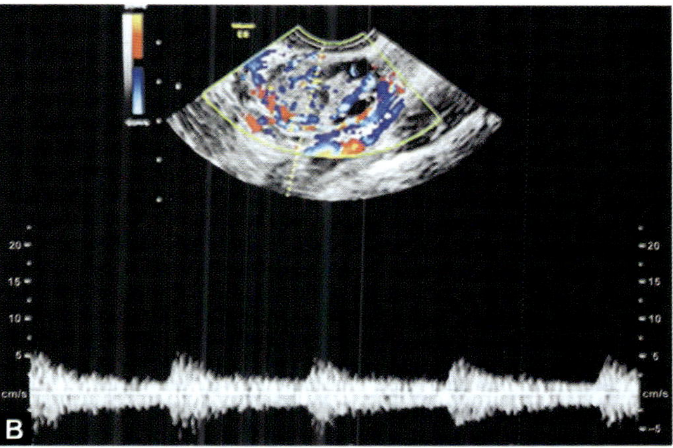

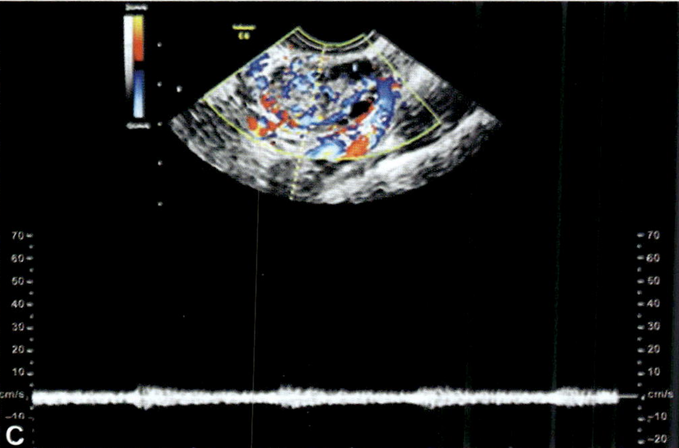

Figs. 1.10A to C: Doppler pulse repetition frequency (PRF) settings: PRF settings should be kept low for vessels with low-velocity blood flow and high for vessels with high-velocity blood flow. This figure demonstrates the effect of PRF on velocity-wave form on an ovarian stromal vessel. Pulse repetition frequency is kept low (A), optimum (B), and high (C).

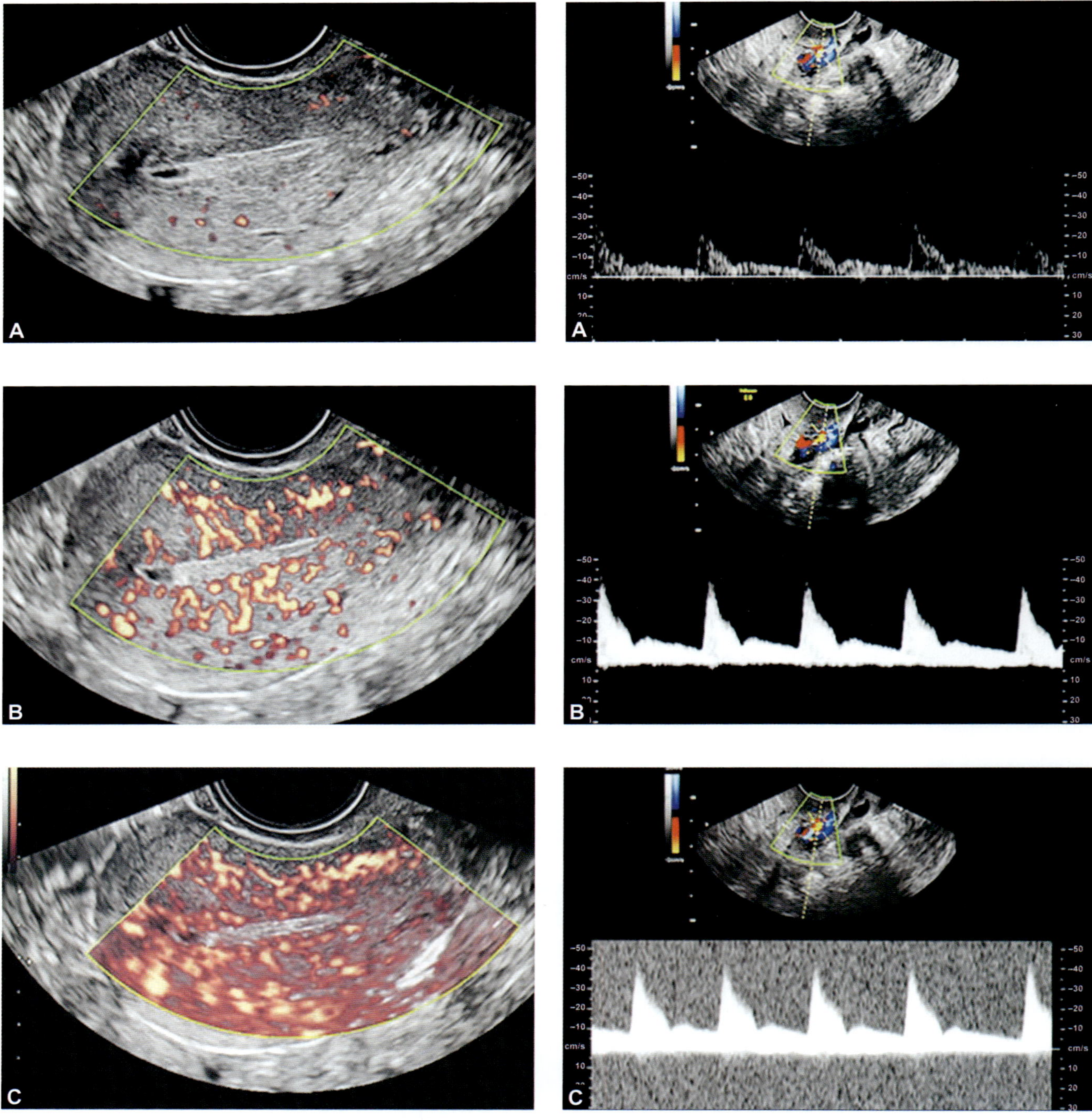

Figs. 1.11A to C: Doppler gain (Power Doppler): Increasing gain will amplify the returning signal resulting stronger Doppler signal. The gain is kept low (A), optimum (B), and high (C). Too much gain in (C) results in artifact signals.

Figs. 1.12A to C: Doppler gain (Pulse Wave): Increasing gain will amplify the returning signal resulting stronger Doppler signal. The gain is kept low (A), optimum (B), and high (C).

result in noise and artifact.[7] Doppler gain should be set so that the vessel lumen is filled with color but there is no spill outside.

Baseline

Doppler can display flow either toward or away from the probe. Typically for color or spectral Doppler, the "zero" is in the center of the scale (or Y-axis). If you want to look only at the positive or negative flow, you can adjust the baseline up or down.

Wall Motion Filter

Filter allows adjustment of the signal so that lower velocities up to a certain number will not be displayed. A higher filter will reduce artifact but may limit visualization of lower flow (Figs. 1.13 and 1.14).[3]

Probe Angle

When red blood cells move perpendicular to the ultrasound beam, the transducer fails to detect them.[4] Most machines, fortunately, will detect signals with even a minimal change beyond the perpendicular plane. When a vessel is anticipated to have slow flow, it should be imaged more vertically to the transducer.

Color Box Size

Large box sizes result in large amounts of data for processing. This slows the rate at which images are generated.

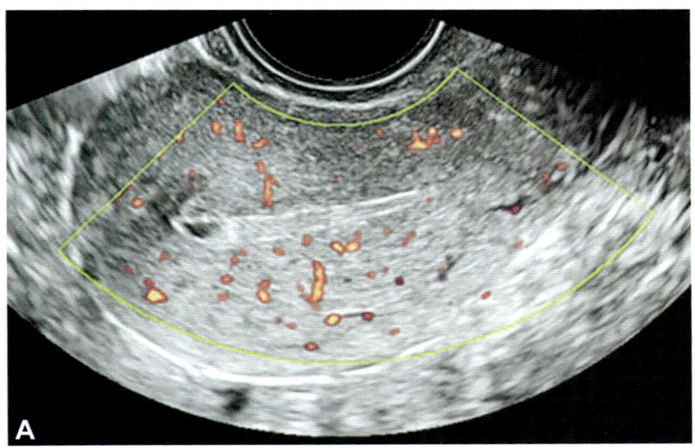

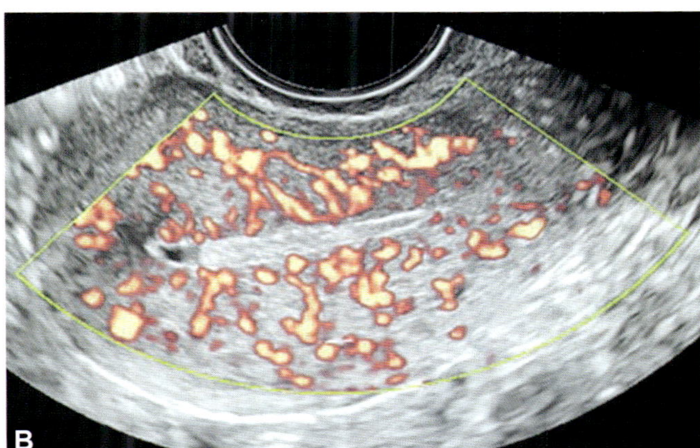

Figs. 1.13A and B: Wall motion filter (Power Doppler): A higher filter setting (A) limits artifacts, but limits visualization of lower flows, when compared with optimal setting (B).

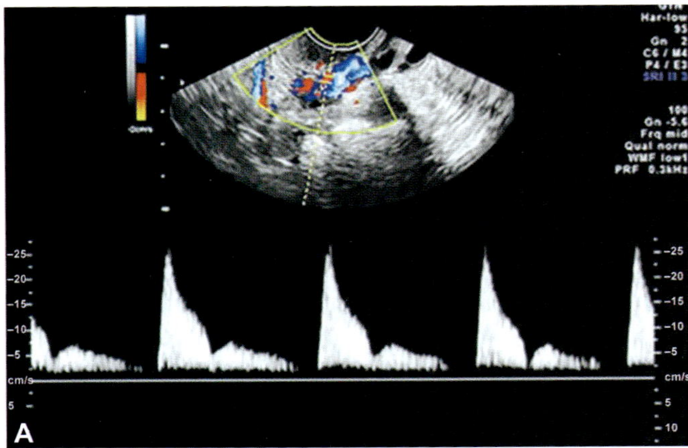

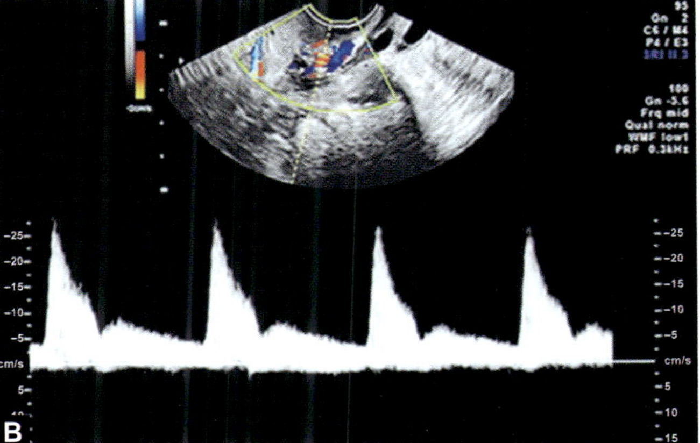

Figs. 1.14A and B: Wall motion filter (Pulse Wave Doppler): A higher filter setting (A) can affect pulse wave forms in comparison with optimal setting (B).

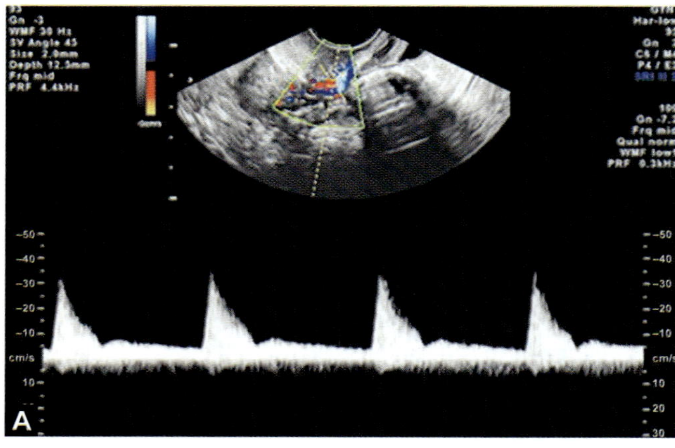

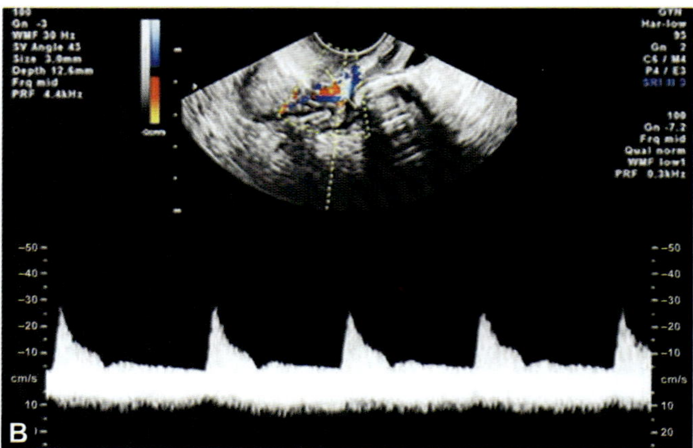

Figs. 1.15A and B: Doppler sample volume (Doppler gate) as well as size and location: The width of the Doppler gate is kept 2 mm (A) and 3 mm (B). In figure (B), the Doppler gate is wider than the diameter of the artery and is placed partly over an adjacent vein and therefore picking up both arterial and venous flow.

Even if the frame rate is increased, this delay in generating an image is not easily overcome. Until large computers get incorporated into machines, and this will happen only if computers get cheaper, small color boxes should be used.[4]

Sample Volume Size and Position

The precise location of sample volume may affect the appearance of the Doppler spectrum and therefore may affect the results of spectral Doppler measurements. The relationship between the size of the sampling box applied with pulsed-wave Doppler and the size of the vessel is another important consideration (Figs. 1.15A and B). The average flow velocity within the center of a small vessel may be double to that of the average velocity across its full width due to turbulence near the vessel wall. It follows therefore that too small a sample box placed centrally over a vessel may overestimate the true flow. Whilst the diameter of the ascending uterine artery ranges from 2 to 5 mm in the nonpregnant patient, the spiral arteries at the level of the endometrium measure 1–2 mm in diameter. The diameter of the ovarian stromal vessels is also around 1–2 mm. This leaves little room for placement error considering the smallest volume box usually starting at 1 mm. The width of the volume box (Doppler gate) should be adjusted to the inner diameter of the vessels to be evaluated.

Doppler Angle (Angle of Insonation)

The angle of insonation between the Doppler beam and the direction of vessel is generally calculated by the observer who rotates a line so that it lies parallel to the direction of blood flow (Figs. 1.16A to C). A 5° error in the orientation of this line leads to an error in the velocity measurement of less than 2%, but this increases to 5.4% if the real angle is 30° and 12% when it is 60°. In this respect, the most accurate velocity measurements are made when the angle of insonation is as close to zero as possible but this is not always possible as it is dependent on the position and direction of the blood vessel being studied.

3D AND 4D ULTRASOUND

In this era of rapidly evolving technology, three-dimensional (3D) and real-time three-dimensional (4D) ultrasound are emerging as necessary tools in the assessment of the pelvic viscera. As for other anatomical regions, freehand or automated devices may be used to acquire volume data for 3D evaluation of pelvic organs. In the freehand method, the transducer is manually moved through the region of interest and a position sensor registers the slice in space and time, or alternatively, image-based software may be built into the 3D package. The freehand method may be used on-line where the ultrasound unit manages all functions, or off-line where the analog video output is fed into a workstation. The transducer and attachments in the free-hand system are bulky and awkward to use particularly in the vagina. Most units currently in vogue are automated 3D probes. These are unit specific, more accurate, and easy to use. When these units are employed, an area of interest is chosen in the real-time 2D image, and the size and depth are outlined. A speed of acquisition is then selected and the acquisition activated. The transducer

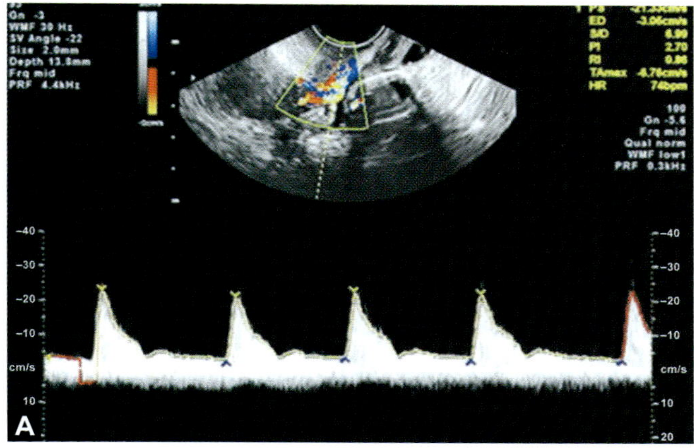

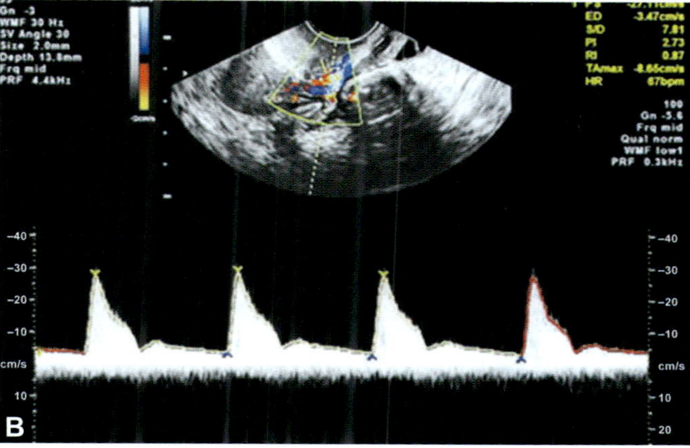

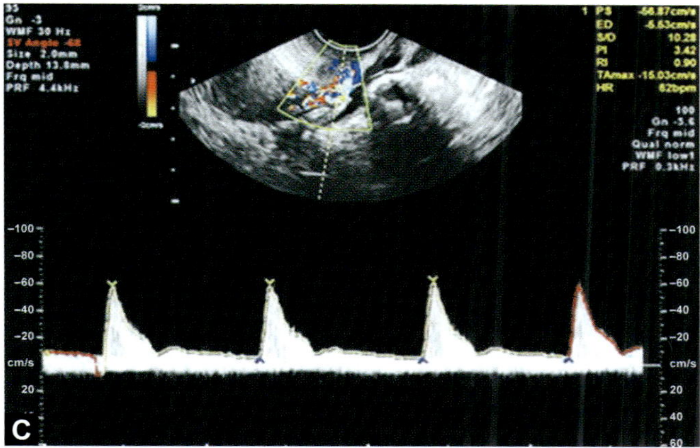

Figs. 1.16A to C: Doppler angle (angle of insonation): The angle of insonaton between the Doppler beam and the direction of vessel can affect the velocity measurements. At angles of insonation of 22° (A), 30° (B), and 68° (C), respectively, peak systolic velocity (PS) measurements from the same vessel were 21.33 cm/s, 27.11 cm/s, and 56.87 cm/s.

elements automatically sweep through the volume box chosen. The slower the speed of acquisition the higher the resolution. Resolution is highest in the plane of acquisition. The closer the plane of acquisition to the plane of study the better the resolution. The machine automatically receives and stores data from the region of interest and displays it in an orthogonal format. Images may then be rendered by various algorithms which rely on the difference between acoustic impedances at tissue interfaces and have been variably named by various manufacturers. In conventional ultrasound, the endometrium is visualized as a variably thick, linear, or ovoid structure in longitudinal, transverse, and oblique plane. The shape of the cavity is difficult to assess, as in the coronal plane. With 3D, the entire extent of the endometrium can be shown, including the corpus, fundus, cervix, and cornual areas.[8] Coronal, sagittal, and transverse planes can be simultaneously displayed to permit more exhaustive viewing (Fig. 1.17).

The images may be automatically zoomed in or out. Once acquired, the volume data can be reviewed by first rotating the planes to obtain standard anatomic orientations and then scrolling through the entire data to locate and characterize lesions, both focal and diffuse. Multiplanar orthogonal viewing offers virtually unlimited numbers of planes, and time constraints should not impede the endeavor to obtain information. In fact, the additional time spent on a 3D gynecologic scan is far less than on 3D obstetric scan because this time is spent not so much on data acquisition but in exploring the data obtained. The time factor would, of course, depend on the complexity of a case and on operator expertise. In experienced hands, the exercise takes no more than 3–10 minutes. Once identified in any one plane, the lesion can be marked by a center point, and this center point is automatically displayed in all three orthogonal planes. All or part of the studied volume can be automatically rendered and displayed as

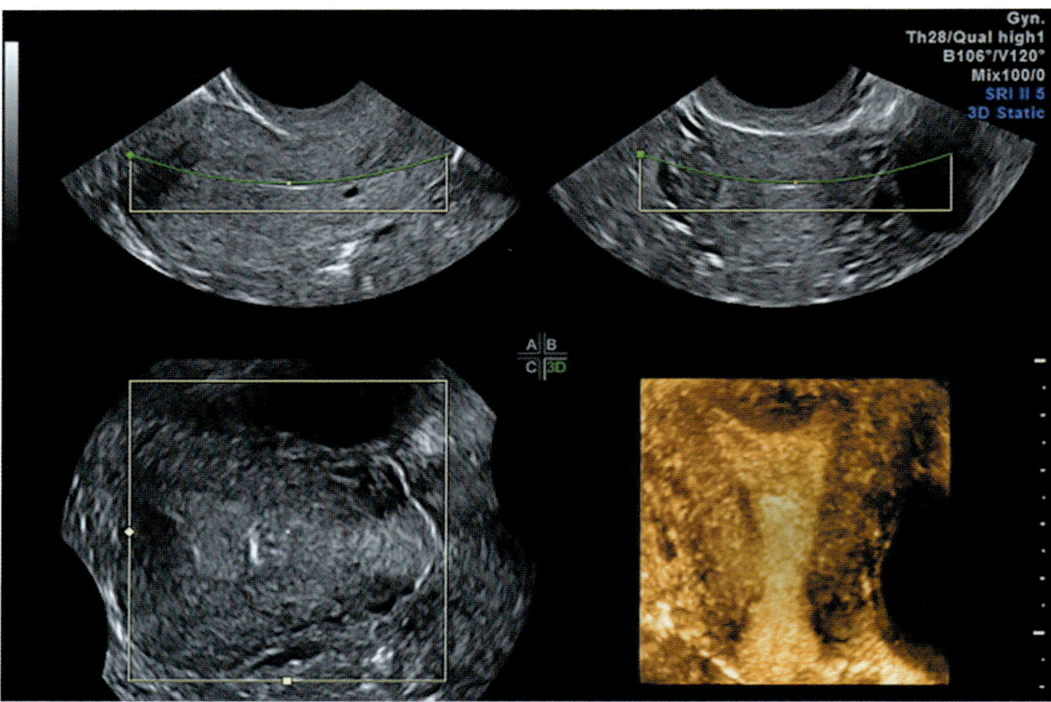

Fig. 1.17: Three-dimensional multiplanar view of a uterus showing longitudinal plane (upper left), transverse plane (upper right), coronal plane (lower left), and rendered view of transverse plane (lower right).

a single image or along with the orthogonal planes. The evaluation is enhanced by using volume measurements, niche mode studies, power Doppler studies, and a retrospective review of stored data. Unlike obstetric 3D, surface rendering is infrequently required in gynecologic 3D studies except in saline infusion sonohysterography where it often adds diagnostic information. The entire acquired data can be transmitted electronically to obtain second opinions, facilitate remote conferencing with experts, and can be efficiently stored for review and recall.

The sagittal plane is selected for volume measurements and the other two planes for ensuring that the entire pathology is included in the measured area. Surface rendering permits contoural evaluation. Niche mode studies permit a virtual tour of the entire lesion and surrounding tissue along with evaluation of vascular morphology. Three-dimensional power Doppler permits an unsurpassed view of vascularity and permits quantification of neovascularization. Three-dimensional saline infusion sonohysterography enhances the sensitivity in select situations. Real-time 3D (4D) is useful in saline infusion sonohysterography for storing data sets, excluding the need for reinstillation, permitting multiplanar analysis, and allowing magnification of stored data during re-evaluation.

In patients who have not been sexually active, 3D data acquisition via the rectum, using an intracavitary transducer, can greatly enhance delineation of pelvic lesions and developmental abnormalities when compared to transabdominal 3D studies.

Three-dimensional data are basically a sum total of 2D data sets, and, as a logical consequence, a 3D study does not replace a 2D study. It, in fact, extends the wealth of information obtainable from an ultrasound scan. Principles of 3D ultrasound and its application in subfertility are further detailed in Chapter 13.

SAFETY OF ULTRASOUND

The Bioeffects Committee of the American Institute of Ultrasound in Medicine has repeatedly established based on the available evidence that there are no confirmed biological effects on patients and their fetuses from the use of diagnostic ultrasound evaluation and that the benefits to patients exposed to the prudent use of this modality outweigh the risks if any.[1] It is wise, however, as for any medical test, to perform the examination only when clearly indicated. The operator performing the examination should exercise due care to use appropriate energies and keep a track of the duration of the study in order to comply with the "as low as reasonably achievable" (ALARA) principle. This principle simply states that the use of technicalities should be optimized to obtain quality images with frequencies, power, and duration.

CLEANING AND DISINFECTING THE PROBES

Why is It Required?

Bacterial contamination was observed on 98.8% of transvaginal probes. Microbial analysis revealed 36 different species of bacteria, including skin and environmental bacteria as well as pathogenic bacteria such as *Staphylococcus aureus*, enterobacteriaceae, and Pseudomonas spp.

CLEANING AND MAINTAINING THE PROBE

Cleaning means removing the visible contaminants from the probe. The probe must be cleaned, each time it is used. After every examination, ensure the acoustic coupling gel is completely wiped off the transducer. Transducers should not be left soaking in gel. Remove any transducer cover, biopsy guides, or protective devices from the transducer. When not in use it should be stowed in the relevant probe slot and should be covered to avoid its exposure to dust. Do not kink, tightly coil, or apply excessive force on the probe cable. Do not apply excessive bending or pulling force to the transducer cable. Do not let transducer cables dangle loosely from the ultrasound system where they might be caught in the casters while moving. Do not drop transducers into holders or disinfectant containers with lens face down.

Use a moistened soft cloth or wipe to remove any remaining contaminants that remain on the transducer or cable. Do not reuse cloths or wipes. Soap, detergents, or enzymatic cleaners should be used in accordance with the manufacturer's instructions. Use a lint-free soft and clean dry cloth or wipe to thoroughly dry the transducer and cable. Cleaning products should be as close to neutral pH as possible. Any gel, cleaning or disinfectant products containing surfactants, methanol, ethanol, benzyl or methyl alcohol, bleach, methyl or ethyl paraben, polyethylene glycol, mineral oil, lubricant oil, oil-based lotions, acetone, ammonia, anhydrous ammonia, iodine, iodine compounds, and acids with 5 pH or greater may damage or discolor your transducer. Though thus cleaning with the damp cloth or readily available wipes do not clean the probes actually. Not only the probe head, even the handle is a potential source of bacterial contamination.

Automated disinfection had a statistically significantly higher success rate of 91.4% (106/116) compared with 78.8% (89/113) for manual disinfection ($P = 0.009$).

The risk of contamination was increased by 2.9-fold when disinfection was performed manually [odds ratio, 2.9 (95%CI, 1.3–6.3)].[9]

DISINFECTING THE PROBE

When performing high-level disinfection of ultrasound probes with the (trophon® EPR) dedicated disinfectants supplied by the manufacturer, it is not necessary to disconnect the probe from the ultrasound system. However, the probe should be inactive (not selected) during the disinfection cycle. If rinsing is required, use caution not to expose the system connector to moisture or liquids. If the possibility of cross-contamination or exposure to unhealthy or nonintact skin exists, then high-level disinfection should be performed. Good hand-hygiene practice is highly recommended to help further reduce the risk of cross-contamination. A validated high-level disinfection process combined with the use of a sterile gel and a transducer cover is an accepted method of infection control for ultrasound transducers. Where possible, use of an automated system for disinfection of ultrasound transducers that is FDA-cleared and provides a consistent disinfection process and minimizes the risk of exposure to disinfectants is recommended. Do not immerse transducers deeper than permissible levels. Never immerse the connector or adapter into any liquid. The disinfection of the probe is essential when probe is used for any ultrasound-guided invasive procedures and also when the patients with vaginal infections have been examined.

CONCLUSION

A basic knowledge of ultrasound principles makes it simple to obtain optimal images in patients who have infertility.

KEY POINTS

- Electronic array transducers cost more but have the advantage of good near-field resolution and multiple focal zones

- Low frequency is good for penetration, and high frequency is good for resolution
- Resolution is ability to separate and define two different adjacent structures
- Axial resolution is superior to lateral resolution; measurements are more accurate in the axial direction
- Depth, magnification, and zoom should be often used to optimize images
- Power defines the energy produced by the transducer
- Gain refers to the amplitude of returning beam
- Dynamic range defines the number of gray shades and should be higher for examination of solid tissues
- Tissue harmonics improves resolution but reduces frame rate
- Power Doppler is more sensitive to low-velocity flows
  - For Doppler studies, low PRF for low-velocity vessels and high PRF for high-velocity vessels
  - Doppler gains should be so set that the vessel lumen is filled with color but there is no spill outside
  - Wall filter should be set not to cut down diastolic (low velocity) flows
  - When a vessel is anticipated to have slow flow, it should be imaged more vertically to the transducer
  - Small color boxes should be used
- 3D ultrasound: Coronal, sagittal, and transverse planes can be simultaneously displayed to permit more exhaustive viewing
  - Three-dimensional study does not replace a 2D study
  - Exercise due care to use appropriate energies and keep a track of the duration of the study in order to comply with the ALARA principle

REFERENCES

1. Eik-Nes SH. Physics and instrumentation. In: Wladimiroff JW, Eik-Nes SH (Eds). Ultrasound in Obstetris and Gynecology: European Practice in Gynaecology and Obstetrics, 1st edition. Philadelphia: Elsevier Limited; 2009. pp. 1-20.
2. Kennedy A, Peterson CM. Transvaginal sonography in reproductive endocrinology and infertility. In: Carrell DT, Peterson CM (Eds). Reproductive Endocrinology and Infertility: Integrating Modern Clinical and Laboratory Practice, 1st edition. New York: Springer; 2010. pp. 545-65.
3. Markowitz J. Probe selection, machine controls and equipment. In: Carmody KA, Moore CL, Feller-Kopman D (Eds). Handbook of Critical Care & Emergency Ultrasound, 1st edition. New York: McGraw Hill; 2011. pp. 25-38.
4. Peisner DB. Applied physics: selecting and adjusting the equipment. In: Timor-Tritsch IE, Goldstein SR (Eds). Ultrasound in Gynecology, 2nd edition. Philadelphia: Elsevier Limited; 2007. pp. 9-32.
5. Khurana A. Ultrasound in obstetrics. In: Misra R (Ed). Ian Donald's Practical Obstetric Problems, 6th edition. New Delhi: BI Publications Pvt. Ltd.; 2007. pp. 62-88.
6. Khurana A. Female genital system. In: Mani S (Ed). Textbook of Abdominal Ultrasound, 1st edition. New Delhi: Jaypee Brothers Medical Publishers; 2009. pp. 217-98.
7. Martin K. Properties, limitations and artefacts of B-mode images. In: Hoskins P, Martin K, Thrush A (Eds). Diagnostic Ultrasound: Physics and Equipment, 2nd edition. New York: Cambridge University Press; 2010. pp. 64-74.
8. Khurana A. The endometrium. In: Khurana A, Dahiya N (Eds). 3D and 4D Ultrasound: A Text and Atlas, 1st edition. New Delhi: Jaypee Brothers Medical Publishers; 2004. pp. 166-98.
9. Buescher DL, Möllers M, Falkenberg MK, Amler S, Kipp F, Burdach, Klockenbusch W, Schmitz R. Disinfection of transvaginal ultrasound probes in a clinical setting: comparative performance of automated and manual reprocessing methods. Ultrasound Obstet Gynecol. 2016;47:646-51.

Chapter

2

Pelvic Assessment: Examination Technique and Normal Anatomy

Lil Valentin

Chapter Outline

GYNECOLOGICAL ULTRASOUND EXAMINATION: OPTIMIZATION OF THE ULTRASOUND IMAGE, IMAGE ORIENTATION, AND EXAMINATION TECHNIQUE

A gynecological ultrasound examination can be performed transabdominally, transvaginally or—in exceptional cases—transrectally (using a transvaginal probe). Irrespective of the route of examination, it is important to optimize the image and to perform the examination in a systematic manner.

Optimizing the Image

The following functions of the ultrasound system need to be changed during every examination: image depth, magnification, focus, gain, and frequency. When searching for a particular organ or structure, use low magnification (large depth, wide scan angle, no zoom) to get an overview of the pelvis. When the organ or object of interest is seen, magnify the image to fill the ultrasound screen with that object. This can be achieved by decreasing the depth and diminishing the scan angle, or by activating the "true" zoom function (Figs. 2.1A and B). There are two types of zoom: (1) magnification zoom and (2) "true" zoom. There is no advantage of using a magnification zoom. If one uses the magnification zoom, ultrasound pixels get bigger and so image-quality deteriorates. However, when using a "true" zoom box, all ultrasound pixels and lines will be concentrated in the zoom box, and so image quality will improve. Place the focus at the level of the area of interest in order to achieve the best (lateral) resolution (Figs. 2.2A to C). One can use more than a single focus but then the frame rate will decrease (see the following text). Adjust the gain to make the image darker or lighter (Figs. 2.3A and B). Always choose the highest ultrasound frequency possible, because this results in the best (axial) resolution. However, if the object of interest is situated far away from the ultrasound transducer, one may need to reduce the frequency to optimize the image. This is because the depth of penetration is inversely related to the ultrasound frequency. The disadvantage of low frequency is a reduction in (axial) image resolution (Figs. 2.4A and B).

There are many other functions in an ultrasound system that can be used to change the appearance of the ultrasound image (e.g. preprocessing or edge enhancement, postprocessing, log compression or dynamic range,

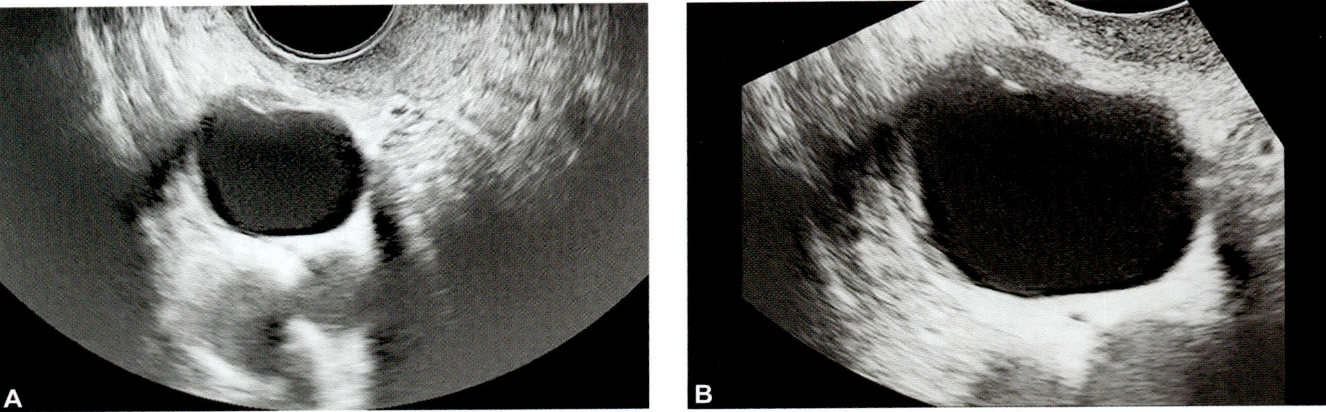

Figs. 2.1A and B: When searching for organs or lesions, use large depth and wide scan angle to get a good overview. To see more details, activate "the true" zoom function of the ultrasound system, alternatively decrease depth and use a smaller scan angle (A) adnexal cyst before zooming; (B) the same cyst after having activated the true zoom function.

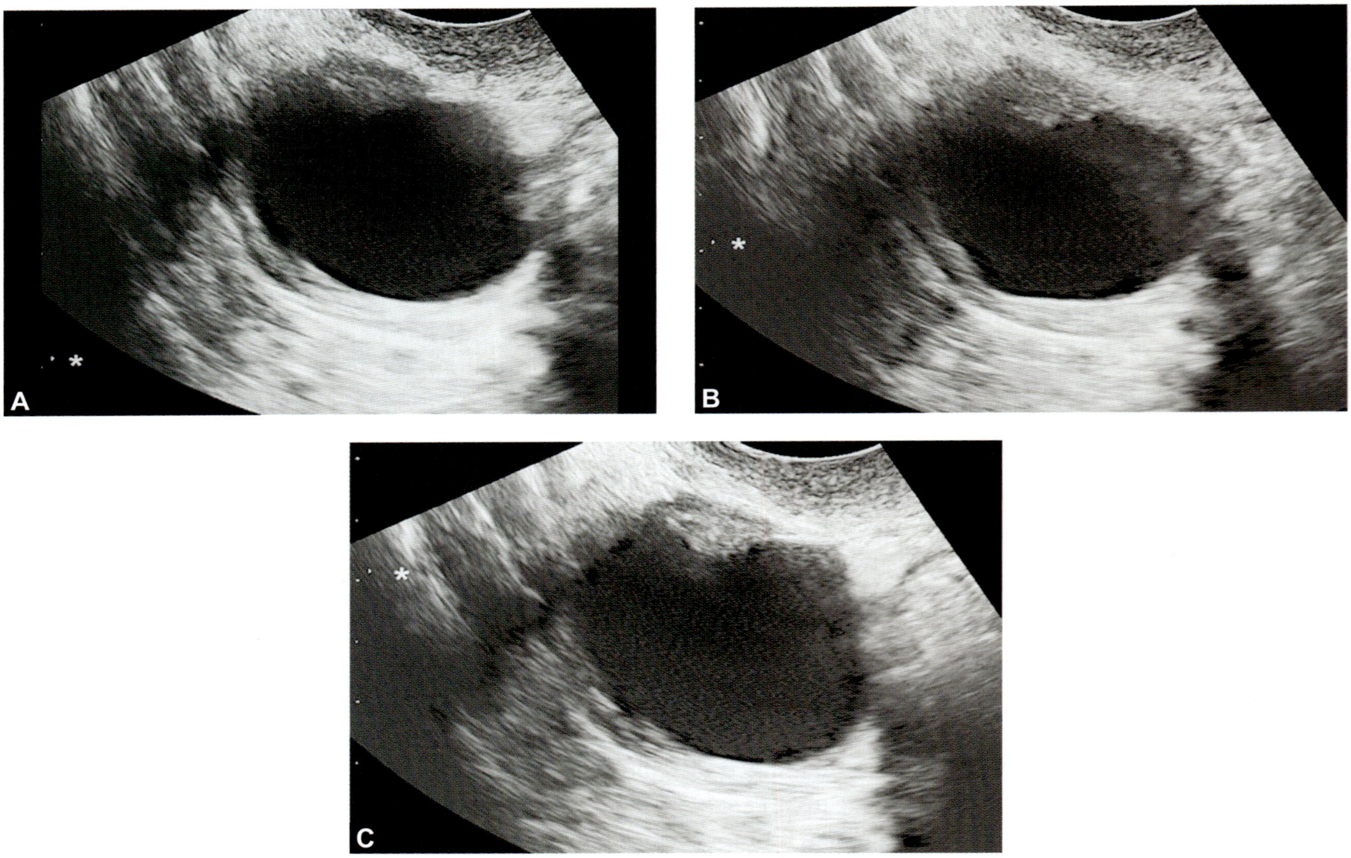

Figs. 2.2A to C: The resolution is maximum at the level, where the focus is placed. In images A to C, the level of the focus is indicated by an asterisk. (A) The focus is placed at a level outside the adnexal cyst in the lower part of the image; this is not a correct technique to evaluate the cyst, (B) the focus is placed at a level corresponding to the center of the cyst, and (C) the focus is placed at the level of the solid component in the cyst; this is where the focus should be placed to get the best view of the solid component. Please note how the image of the solid component (upper part of the image) changes when the location of the focus changes; the solid component is best seen in (C).

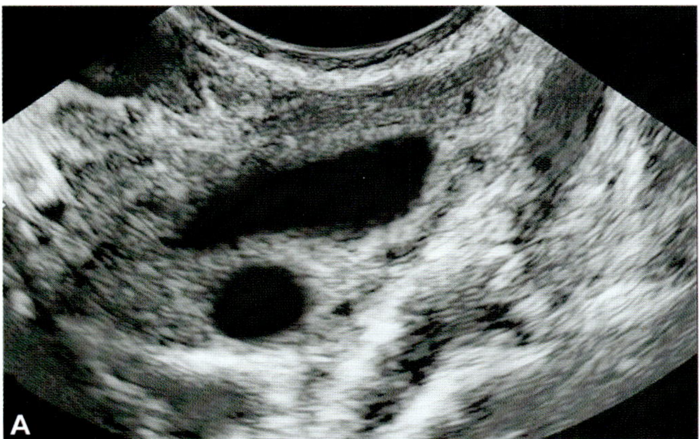

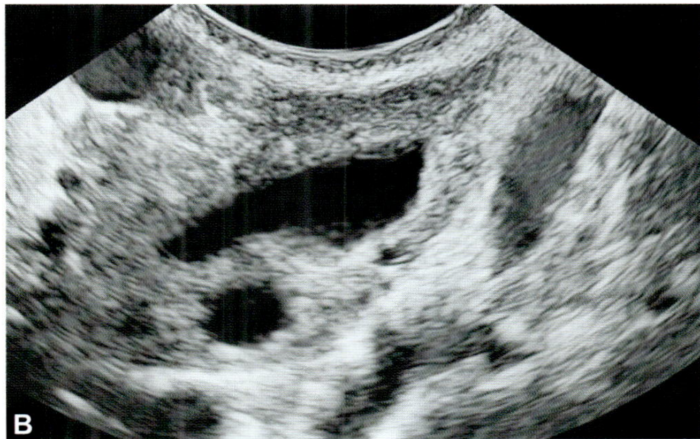

Figs. 2.3A and B: Adjust the gain to make the image (A) darker or (B) lighter. In (A) the gain is set at –7 (too dark) and in (B) the gain is set at +7.

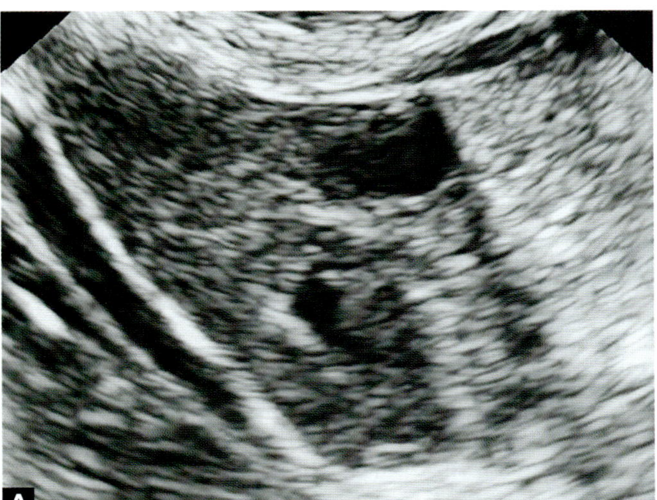

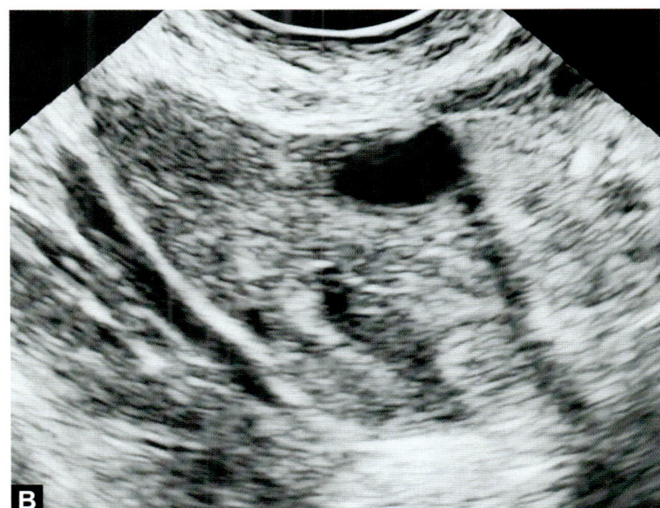

Figs. 2.4A and B: The same ultrasound image of an ovary with a corpus luteum obtained with (A) low and (B) high frequency. For maximum (axial) resolution, always choose the highest ultrasound frequency possible.

and persistence), but unlike those discussed earlier, they do not need to be adjusted in every patient.

In some cases, it is important to work with a high frame rate, e.g. if one wants to detect or study a moving structure such as an embryonic or fetal heart. To increase the frame rate, use high magnification (small depth and small scan angle, or "true" zoom function) and a single ultrasound focus. Moving structures are also seen more easily if persistence is decreased (the persistence function "averages" several images into one, so when persistence is decreased there is no "averaging").

Unfortunately, different companies use diverse terms to describe the same ultrasound function. Ask a representative of the ultrasound company to explain the functions of the system you are using!

Image Orientation

Irrespective of whether one performs a transabdominal, transvaginal, or transrectal scan there is a general agreement that the patient's right side should be shown on the left side of the ultrasound screen. When performing a transabdominal scan, cranial structures should be shown on the left side of the screen and caudal on the right side. Unfortunately, there is no consensus on image orientation for transvaginal scans. Some prefer to show the image with the transducer head ("footprint" and "apex of the pie") in the upper part of the image, others prefer to show it with the transducer head in the lower part of the image. For longitudinal sections through the pelvis, some show the bladder on the left side of the screen, others show it on the right side.

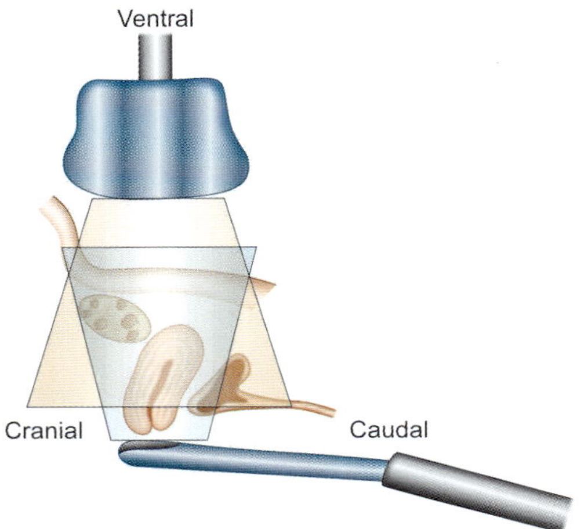

Fig. 2.5: Recommended image orientation for longitudinal scans through the pelvis. When scanning transabdominally, the transducer head ("footprint" and "apex of the pie") is shown on the top of the screen; when scanning transvaginally, it is shown at the bottom of the screen. In both cases, the cranial end of the patient is shown to the left on the screen and the caudal end (bladder) is shown to the right on the screen. For transabdominal imaging, this image orientation is internationally agreed, for transvaginal scanning it is recommended. On transverse scans—however they are obtained—the patient's right side is always shown on the left side of the screen and vice versa. (*Source:* Reproduced from Jurkovic D, Valentin L, Vyas S. Gynaecological Ultrasound in Clinical Practice: Ultrasound Imaging in the Management of Gynecological Conditions. London: RCOG Press; 2009, with the permission of the Royal College of Obstetricians and Gynecologists.)

To avoid confusion, it would be good if image orientation could be standardized also for transvaginal scans. In order to obtain transvaginal images that are similarly orientated to those of transabdominal images, the logical orientation would be one where the scan head is shown in the lower part of the image, and the bladder is shown on the right side of the ultrasound screen (Fig. 2.5). This orientation makes transvaginal images clearly distinguishable from transabdominal ones and it facilitates correlation between transvaginal and transabdominal images.

Why is a Systematic Scanning Technique Necessary?

There are two reasons to adopt a systematic scanning technique. First, it will ensure that a complete pelvic examination is performed. For example immediately after starting the scan, you notice a large ovarian cyst. You completely focus on the cyst, only to realize, once the patient has left, that you did not examine either her uterus or the contralateral adnexa. Second, if you always scan all the organs in the pelvis in a systematic manner as described in the following text, you will build up a reference of what is normal. This will increase your confidence in detecting pelvic pathology.

TRANSVAGINAL ULTRASOUND EXAMINATION

It is mandatory that transvaginal scans are performed with a completely empty bladder. Scanning a woman who has an incompletely empty bladder increases examination time and decreases image quality.

All probes should be cleaned after each patient examination. The probe should be covered with a protective sheath. Following each examination, the sheath should be disposed and the probe wiped clean and appropriately disinfected. The type of antimicrobial solution and method of disinfection depends on manufacturer and infectious disease recommendations. Contact your manufacturer and your department of hygiene to obtain information on how to clean your ultrasound probes! There must be a sufficient amount of coupling gel between the transducer head and the cover (so that there is no air between the transducer head and the cover), and the covered probe should be lubricated. The patient should be informed how the examination will be carried out, and she should be warned before the probe is inserted. Some patients may want to watch the screen during the examination—if technically feasible—others might prefer not to. Ask the patient about her preference.

When starting the examination, the ultrasound probe is placed in the introitus of the vagina so that a longitudinal view of the pelvic floor is obtained (Fig. 2.6).

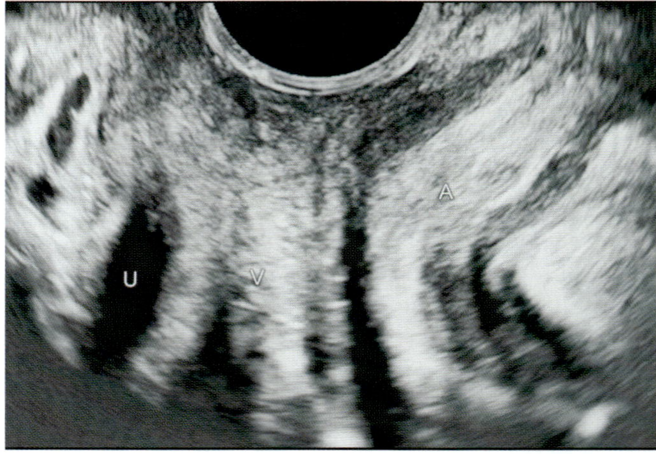

Fig. 2.6: Longitudinal ultrasound view of the pelvic floor. The ultrasound probe is placed in the introitus of the vagina. To the left is the urethra (U), in the middle—the vagina (V), and to the right—the anal canal (A).

Then the ultrasound probe is slowly introduced into the vagina while you watch the ultrasound screen to check if the bowel, urethra and bladder slide freely against the vaginal wall. In the top of the vagina, you will find the cervix. You might be able to see the vagina attach to the posterior aspect of the cervix (Figs. 2.7A and B). When the cervix has come into view, you start scanning the cervix and the corpus uteri.

Move the probe so that a longitudinal section through the cervical canal is shown on the screen (Figs. 2.7A and B). Follow the cervical canal upward toward the fundus uteri so that the cervical canal can be seen to adjoin the endometrium (Figs. 2.8A and B). Look through the corpus uteri from one side to the other until the whole uterine body has been scanned in a longitudinal section. Turn the transducer 90° so that a transverse section through the corpus uteri comes into view (Fig. 2.9). Now scan the uterus from the fundus to the portio of the cervix and back again.

To find the ovaries start from a transverse section through the uterine body. Identify the "corner" of the

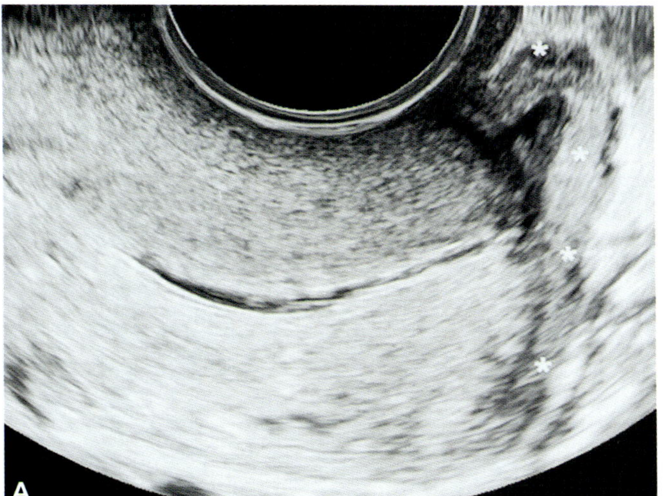

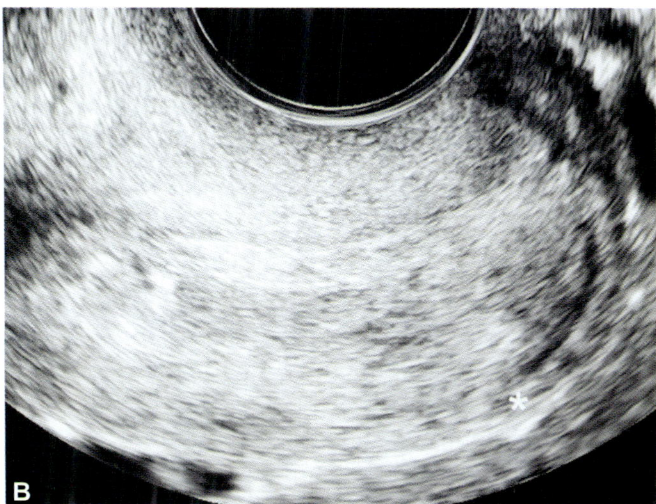

Figs. 2.7A and B: Longitudinal view of the cervix: (A) There is some fluid in the vagina which makes it easy to see the vaginal wall (asterisks). (B) The insertion of the vaginal wall at the back of the cervix is indicated by an asterisk.

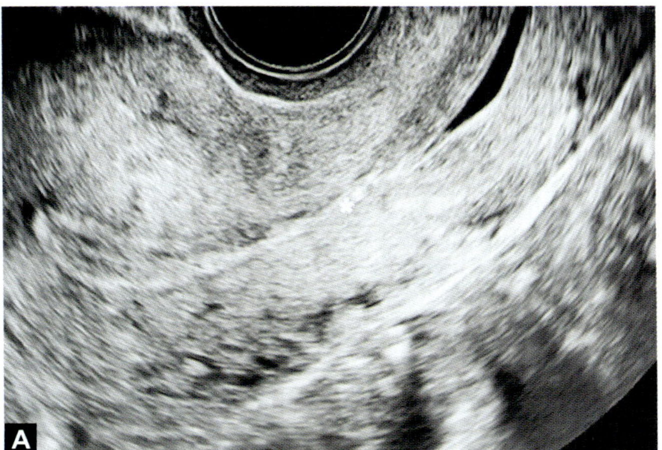

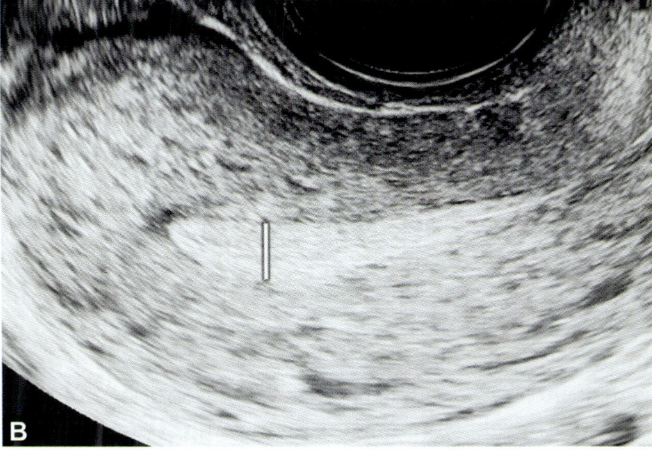

Figs. 2.8A and B: Longitudinal scan through the uterus: (A) The cervical canal can be seen to adjoin the endometrium (asterisk). Scan the uterine corpus from one side to the other, scrutinizing the myometrium and endometrium. (B) Endometrial thickness is measured on that longitudinal section through the uterus where it appears to be at its thickest. Use the "true" zoom function of the ultrasound system and measure from the endometrial-myometrial border on one side to that on the other (white line).[1]

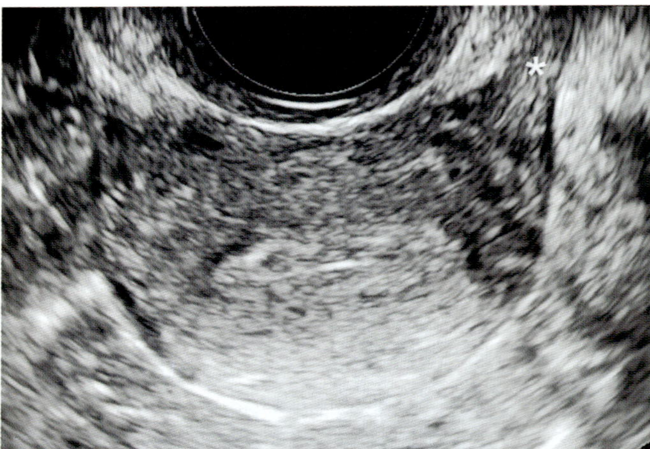

Fig. 2.9: Transvaginal scan showing a transverse section through the uterus. The width of the uterus is measured on a transverse section through the uterine body where it appears to be at its widest. The asterisk shows the "corner" of the uterus where the tube starts. If one is scanning transvaginally, this is the starting point when searching for the ovary.

uterus where the tube starts (Fig. 2.9) and follow the tube to the iliac vessels on the pelvic wall. A transverse view through the ovary will now come into view (Figs. 2.10A and B). Scan the ovary on a transverse section from "bottom" to "top" and then turn the transducer 90° so that a longitudinal section of the ovary is shown on the screen (Figs. 2.10A and B). Scan the ovary from one side to the other. Is the ovary tender? Is it mobile? Scan the area below and above the ovary on a transverse scan through the pelvis, and scan the area laterally and medially of the ovary on a sagittal scan through the pelvis. Are there any masses adjacent to the ovary? Go back to a transverse section of the uterus and perform exactly the same maneuver to find and examine the contralateral ovary.

Scan the pouch of Douglas. Is there any fluid? Peritoneal implants? Masses? (Figs. 2.11A and B). If there is fluid in the pouch of Douglas, you might be able to see a tube floating in the fluid (Figs. 2.11A and B). Scan the urinary bladder. Are the walls of the bladder normal? (Figs. 2.12A and B). Finally check for signs of adhesions and deep infiltrating endometriosis. Do the bladder and the urethra slide against the vaginal wall or are they fixed? Check the bowel (anal canal, rectum, and sigmoid) for presence of adhesions and deep infiltrating endometriosis. Start by a transverse scan through the anal canal by placing the ultrasound probe in the introitus of the vagina (the "fourchette") (Figs. 2.13A and B). Then turn the transducer 90° to obtain a longitudinal view of the anal canal and follow it upward to obtain longitudinal sections through the bowel (Figs. 2.13A and B). Follow the bowel cranially, looking for signs of endometriotic nodules and checking if the bowel slides freely against surrounding structures or if it is fixed against the uterus, ovaries, or other structures (Box 2.1).

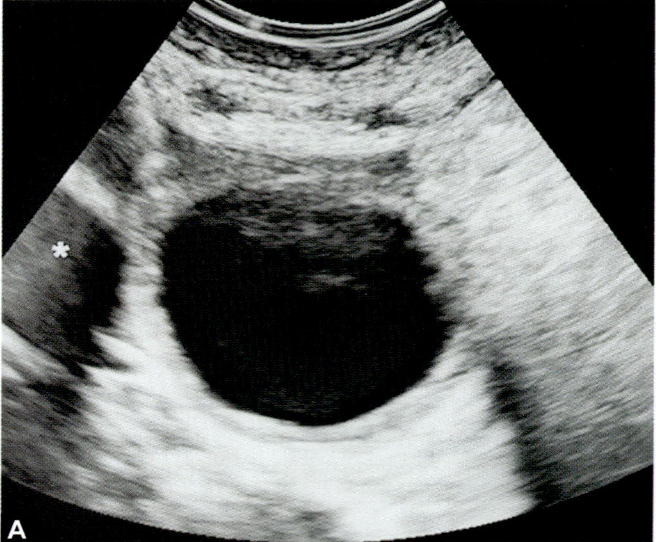

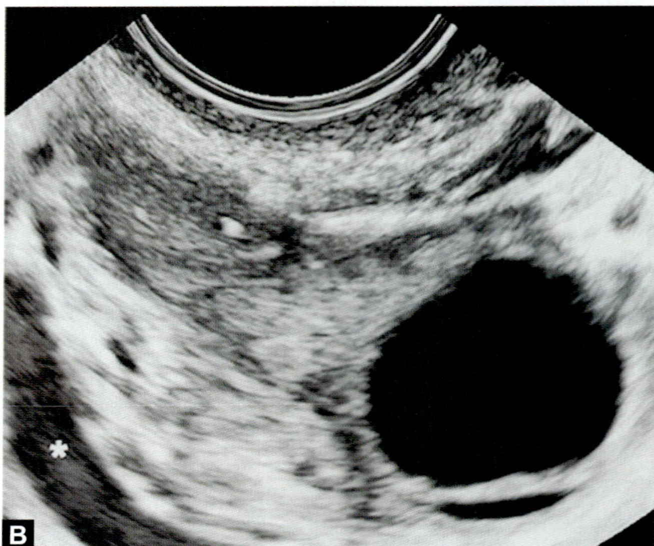

Figs. 2.10A and B: Transvaginal scan of the right ovary: (A) transverse section (B) longitudinal section obtained by rotating the ultrasound probe 90° from (A). The ovary lies close to the iliac vessels (asterisk). The ovary should be scanned on a transverse section from bottom to top and on a longitudinal section from one side to the other. The width of the ovary is measured on a transverse section through the ovary where it appears to be at its widest. The length and anterior-posterior diameter of the ovary are measured on a longitudinal scan through the ovary where it appears to be at its largest.

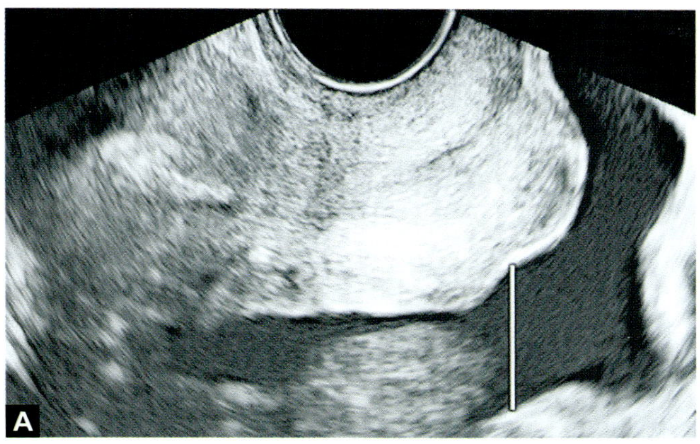

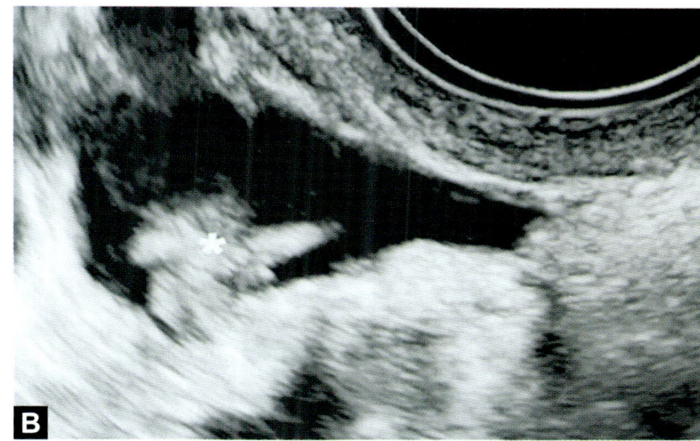

Figs. 2.11A and B: Fluid in the pouch of Douglas. More than a usual amount of fluid is seen here: (A) The amount of fluid is measured on a longitudinal section through the pelvis and the largest anterior-posterior measurement is reported (white line);[2] (B) a normal tube with fimbriae (asterisk) is seen floating in fluid in the pouch of Douglas.

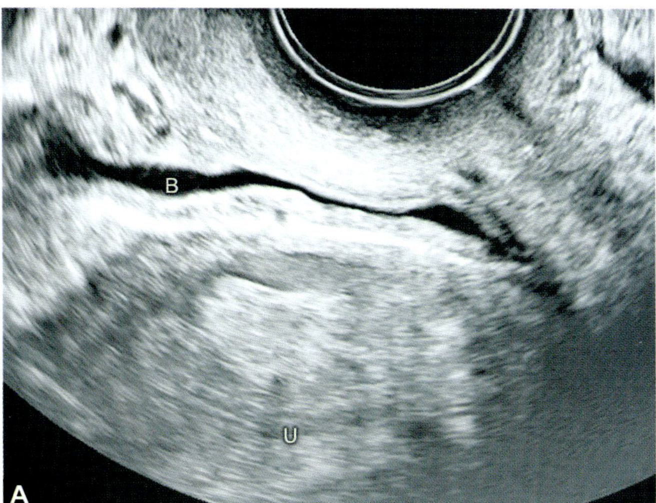

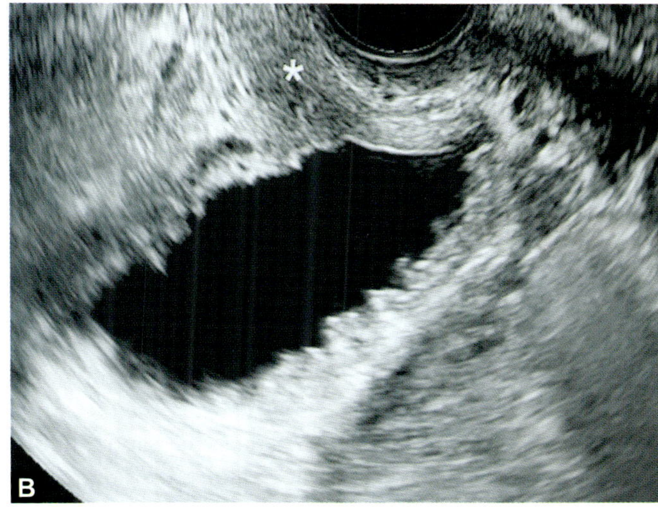

Figs. 2.12A and B: Transvaginal ultrasound image of a normal urinary bladder: (A) A small amount of urine is seen in this urinary bladder (B) there is too much urine in this bladder for the vaginal scan to be optimal, but to study the bladder wall in detail this amount of urine may be necessary (B, bladder; U, uterus; the asterisk in (B) denotes the urethra).

Box 2.1: Basic scanning technique

- Observe the urethra, bladder, anal canal, and rectum as probe slides in through the vaginal introitus and check the mobility of these organs
- See the uterus, the cervix, and endometrial cavity in a single section—longitudinal plane
- Scan across the uterus in long axis
- Rotate the probe 90° and scan across the whole uterus including cervix in transverse axis
- Direct the probe toward the lateral pelvic wall, scan across the ovary in both long and transverse axes
- Same procedure is to be done for the opposite ovary
- Check for any free fluid in pelvis

Measurements

Measuring endometrial thickness is an essential part of the examination in women with history of postmenopausal bleeding,[1] but the value of measuring endometrial thickness in women of fertile age is questionable, because endometrial thickness changes throughout the menstrual cycle. Measure endometrial thickness on a longitudinal scan through the uterus where the endometrium seems to be at its thickest. Measure from the endometrial-myometrial border on one side to that on the other[1] (Figs. 2.8A and B). Never measure endometrial thickness on a transverse scan

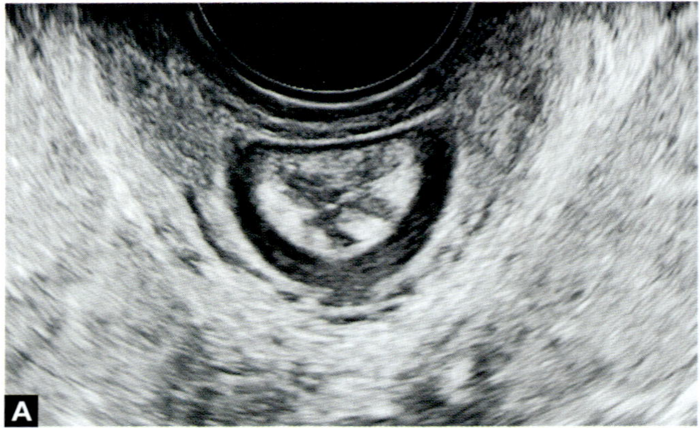

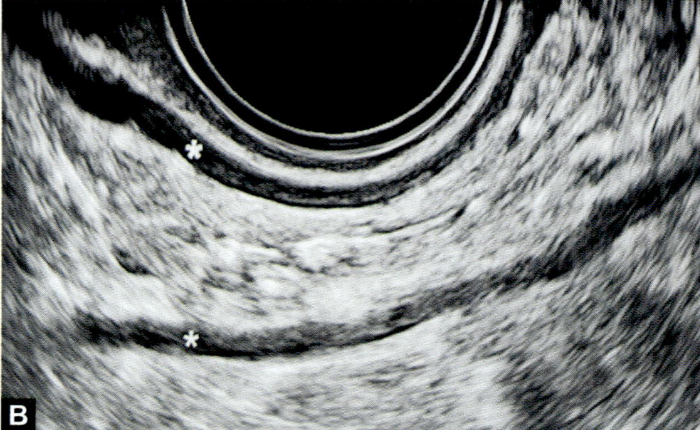

Figs. 2.13A and B: Transvaginal ultrasound images of normal bowel: (A) Transverse section through the anal canal, this image has been obtained with the ultrasound probe placed in the "fourchette"; (B) longitudinal section through the bowel, the muscular layer of the bowel (asterisks) is thin (normal). The two layers of the muscular layer of the bowel are separated by a very thin white line seen in the muscle layer closest to the transducer.

through the uterus, because the scanning plane might be oblique and this will result in a too large measurement value. The clinical usefulness of measuring the uterine and ovarian size is unclear. However, should you wish to assess the uterine size, the length should be measured by measuring the cervix and corpus uteri separately and adding the two measurements. Measure the anterior-posterior diameter of the uterus where it appears to be at its widest. The width of the uterus is measured on a transverse section through the uterine body where it appears to be at its widest. The width of the ovary is measured on a transverse section through the ovary where it appears to be at its widest. The length and anterior-posterior diameter of the ovary are measured where they appear to be at their largest on a longitudinal scan through the ovary. Reference values for uterine and ovarian size can be found in the literature.[3-6] The amount of fluid in the pouch of Douglas should be measured on a longitudinal scan through the pelvis and the largest anterior-posterior measurement should be used[2] (Figs. 2.11A and B).

TRANSRECTAL EXAMINATION

A transrectal scan can be suggested to the patient as an alternative to a transvaginal scan, if a transvaginal scan is impossible and a transabdominal scan yields insufficient information. The examination technique of a transrectal scan is the same as that of a transvaginal scan.

TRANSABDOMINAL GYNECOLOGICAL ULTRASOUND EXAMINATION

Transabdominal ultrasound examination is an alternative to transvaginal or transrectal scan in women in whom transvaginal or transrectal scans are contraindicated, impossible, or unacceptable. It is necessary to perform a transabdominal ultrasound examination in case of very large pelvic masses or masses located in the abdomen above the pelvis. To assess the spread of malignant pelvic tumors, it is also necessary to supplement the vaginal scan with an abdominal scan.

Transabdominal ultrasound examinations must be performed with a full urinary bladder. A full bladder will displace gas-filled bowel and allow the ultrasound beams to travel through fluid (i.e. urine) until they reach the uterus and ovaries. When a transabdominal scan is performed as a supplement to a vaginal scan, the full bladder technique is not always required.

One should start the abdominal ultrasound examination by obtaining a longitudinal view of the uterus. Try to see the cervical canal adjoining the endometrium. Scan the uterus from one side to the other and measure the endometrial thickness as previously described, i.e. on a longitudinal scan where the endometrium appears to be at its thickest. Turn the transducer 90° to obtain a transverse view of the uterus. Scan the uterus in the transverse plane from the fundus to the portio of the cervix and back again to the fundus (Figs. 2.14A to C).

To find the ovaries, start from a longitudinal section through the uterus (Fig. 2.14A). With a longitudinal view of the uterus on the screen, angle—do not slide—the transducer toward the iliac vessels on the pelvic wall where you will find the ovary (Figs. 2.15A and B). Scan through the whole ovary from one side to the other in the longitudinal scan plane. Then go back to the uterus, angle the transducer toward the contralateral pelvic wall until the

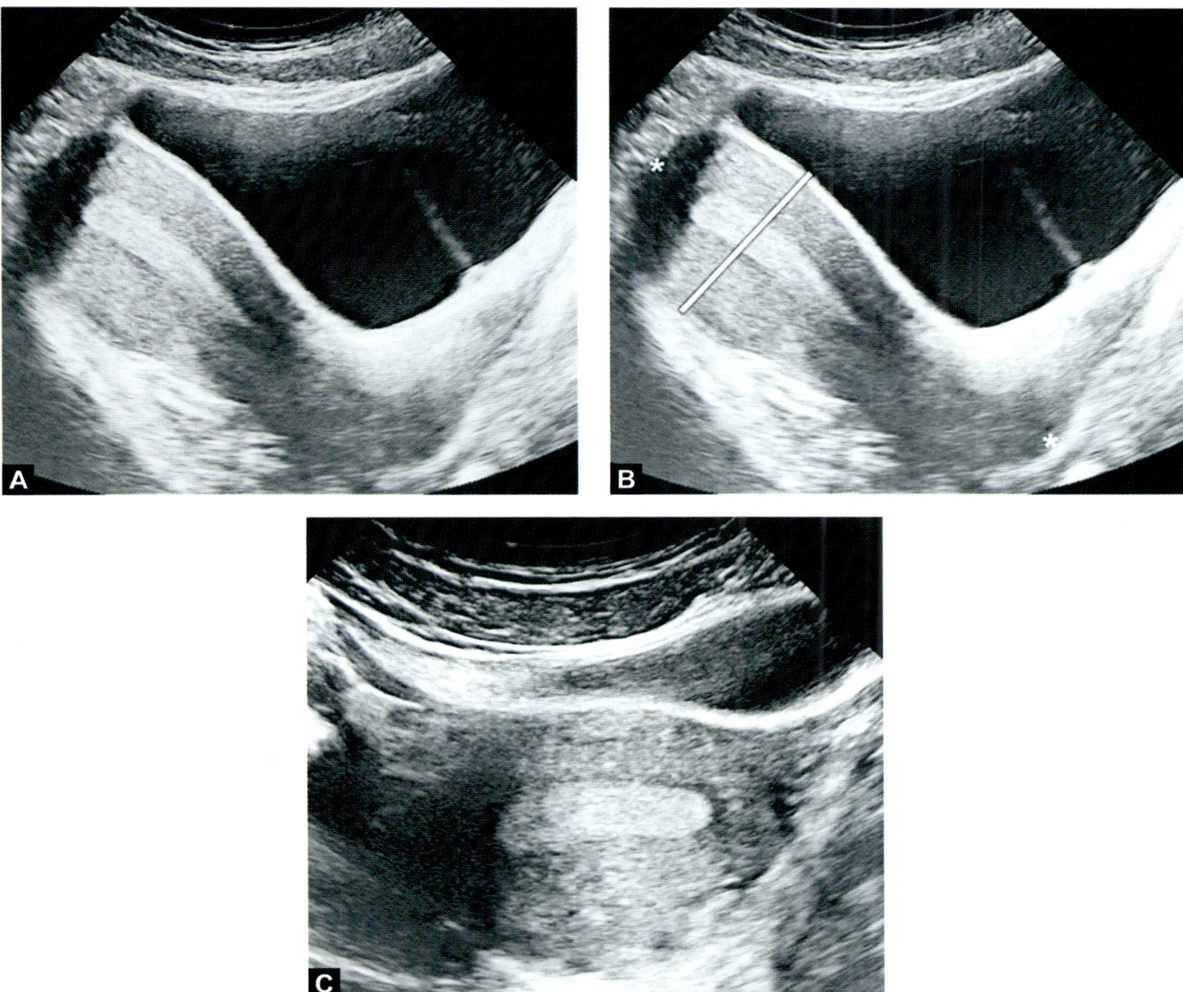

Figs. 2.14A to C: Abdominal ultrasound images of the uterus. (A) Longitudinal section through the uterus: the fundus uteri is shown to the left of the screen, the caudal end (cervix) is shown to the right of the screen, if the uterus is flexed, the lengths of the cervix and corpus uteri are measured separately and the two measurements are added. (B) The full length of the uterus is measured from the outer cervical os to the fundus (asterisks). The anterior-posterior diameter of the uterus is measured on a longitudinal sonogram where it appears to be at its widest (white line), and the endometrial thickness is measured on a longitudinal sonogram where it seems to be at its thickest in the same manner as when measuring it on a transvaginal ultrasound image. (C) Transverse view of the uterus: measure the width of the uterus where it appears to be at its widest on the transverse scan.

contralateral ovary comes into view, and scan the contralateral ovary in the same manner as described earlier.

Go back to a transverse section through the uterus, slide the transducer up and down—you might also need to angle it and rotate it—till you find a transverse section through one of the ovaries. Scan through the whole ovary in the transverse plane. Then do the same for the contralateral ovary (Figs. 2.15A and B).

The measurements of uterine and ovarian size are performed in the same manner as and when you perform a transvaginal scan (see subsection on the technique of transvaginal scan and figure legends).

NORMAL ULTRASOUND MORPHOLOGY OF THE UTERUS AND OVARIES IN WOMEN OF FERTILE AGE

Endometrial ultrasound morphology changes during the menstrual cycle (Figs. 2.16A to D).[7] In the beginning of the menstrual cycle, the endometrium is thin. During the follicular phase, the endometrium becomes thicker and manifests a "triple-layer" appearance. After ovulation, the "triple-layer" appearance of the endometrium disappears, and the endometrium becomes homogenously hyperechoic.

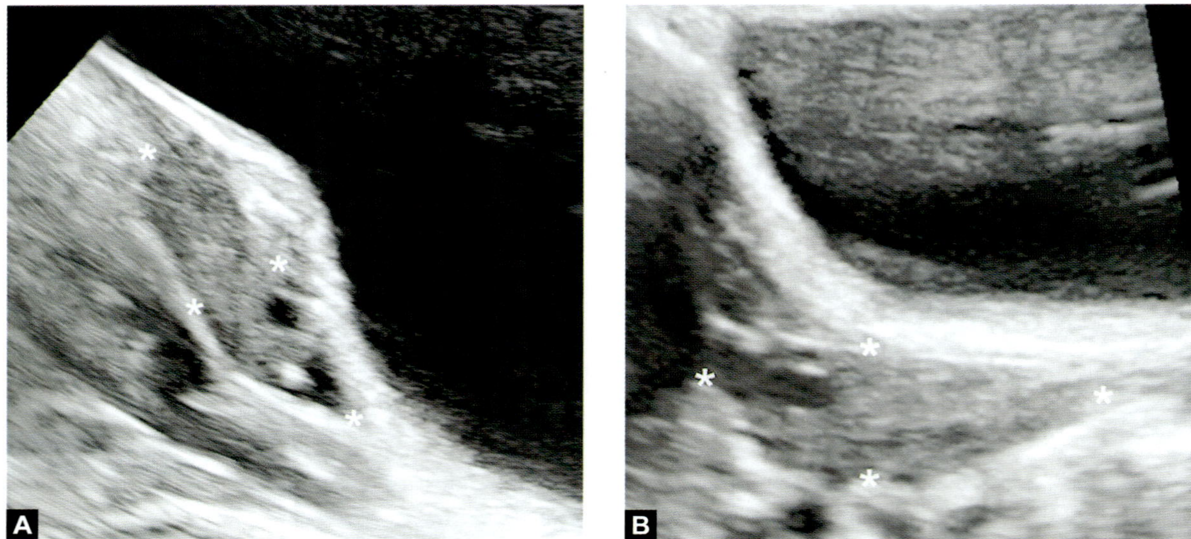

Figs. 2.15A and B: Abdominal ultrasound images of the right ovary. (A) Longitudinal section through the ovary and (B) transverse scan through the same ovary. The asterisks show the outlines of the ovary. Measurements of the ovary are taken in the same manner as when measuring on a transvaginal ultrasound image.

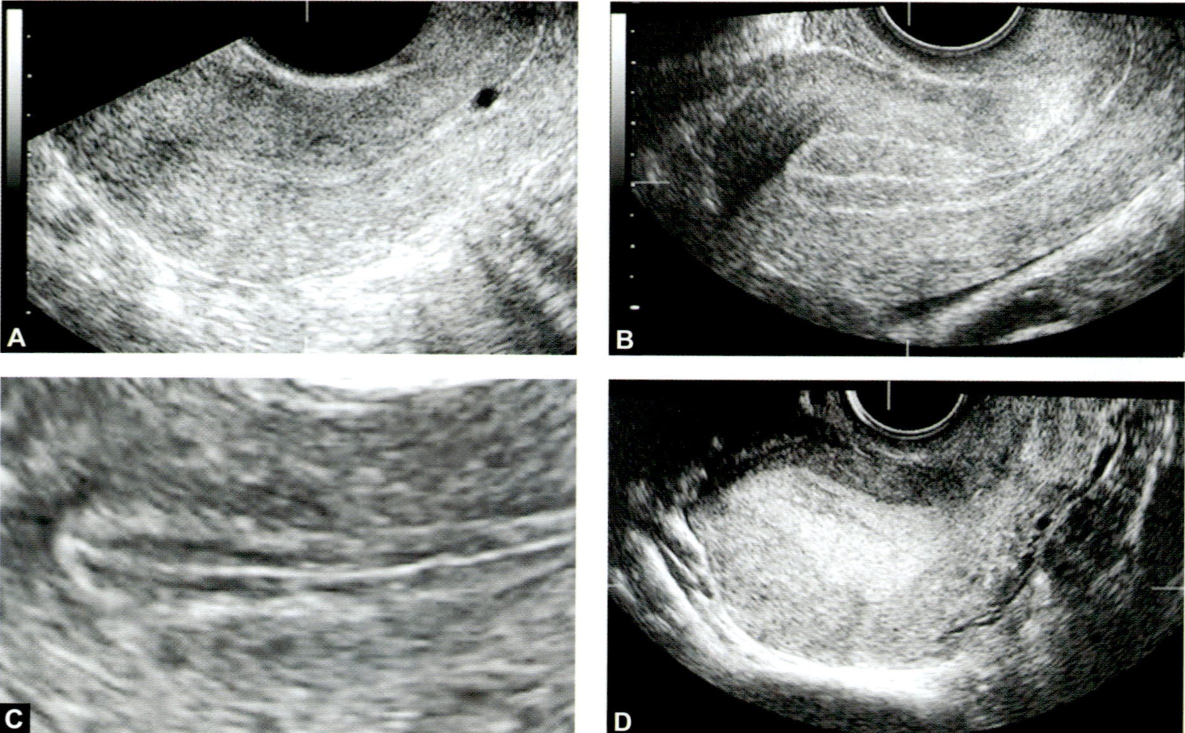

Figs. 2.16A to D: Transvaginal ultrasound images (longitudinal section through the uterus) of the endometrium in different phases of the menstrual cycle. (A) Shortly after menstruation, the endometrium appears as a thin white line; (B) in the mid and late proliferative phase of the menstrual cycle, the endometrium becomes thicker and manifests a "triple-layer" appearance; (C) on the day before ovulation, the endometrium still has a "triple-layer" appearance but there is a thick white line surrounding it; this probably reflects some progesterone production from the dominant follicle; and (D) in the luteal phase of the menstrual cycle, the endometrium is thick and homogenously hyperechoic (white).

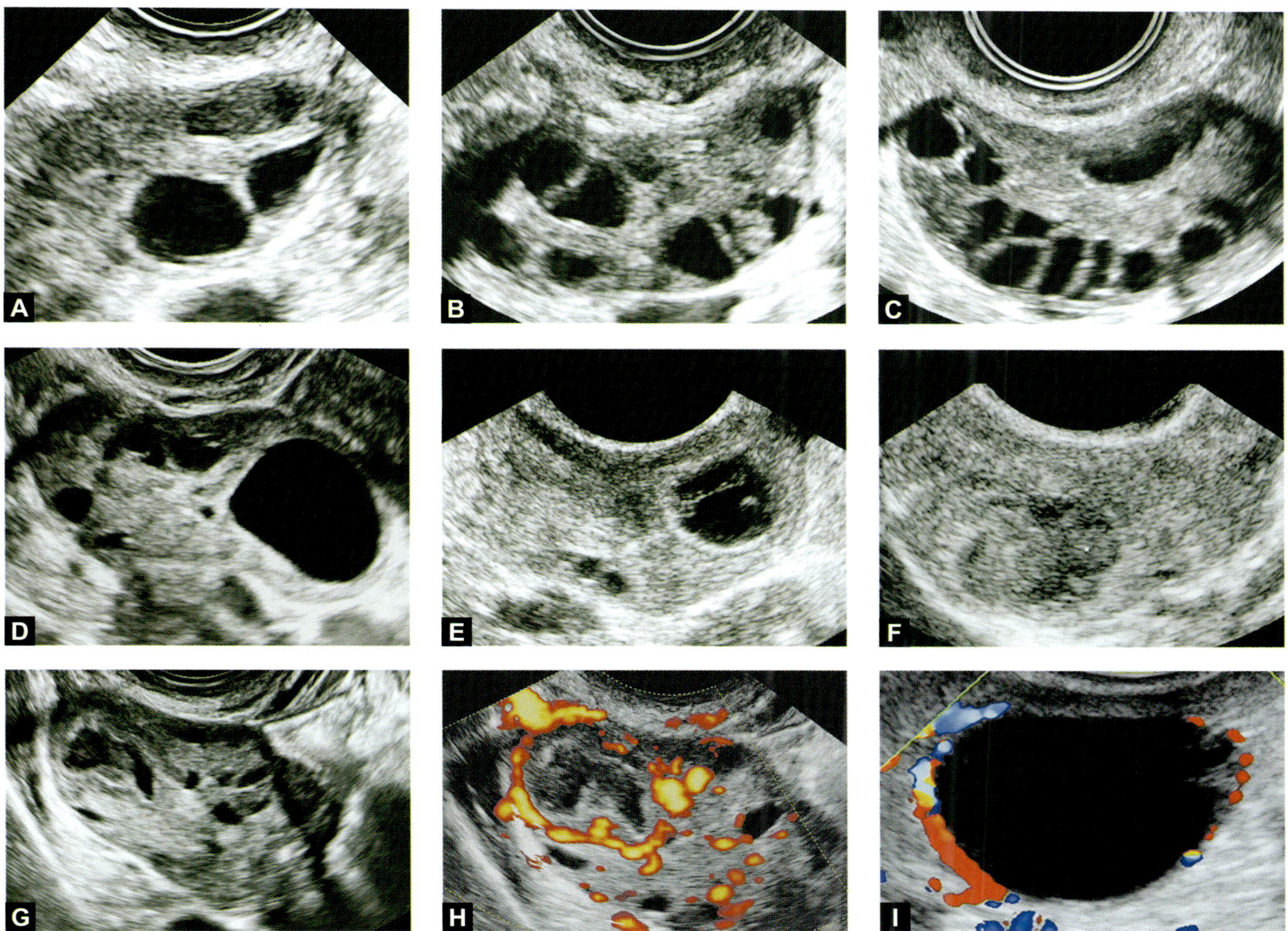

Figs. 2.17A to I: Transvaginal ultrasound images of ovaries in different phases of the menstrual cycle (A to C) show ovaries from different women in the early proliferative phase of the menstrual cycle. All three ovaries are normal but with a varying number of antral follicles; (D) dominant ovary in the mid proliferative phase of the menstrual cycle with one (dominant) follicle being larger than all the other ones and more than 10 mm in diameter; (E) ovary with cystic corpus luteum with echoes inside; (F) ovary with a corpus luteum that appears solid; (G) ovary with a corpus luteum with crenated wall; (H) power Doppler image of the corpus luteum depicted in (G); the thick color ring surrounding the corpus luteum reflects that the corpus luteum is richly vascularized; and (I) the color in the wall of a dominant follicle usually cannot be seen to surround the whole follicle, the color "ring" is thinner and the color hue is less intense.

Ovarian ultrasound morphology also changes during the menstrual cycle (Figs. 2.17A to I).[7,8] According to older literature, in the beginning of the menstrual cycle, there are usually 3–11 antral follicles (usually 6–7) less than or equal to 10 mm in diameter visible in each ovary on transvaginal ultrasound.[8] Recent publications suggest that the number of antral follicles seen on transvaginal ultrasound in the normal ovary is higher.[5,6,9] Moreover, the number of antral follicles seen at ultrasound examination decreases with age.[5,6]

The nondominant ovary does not change its appearance during the menstrual cycle.[8] In the early follicular phase, it is not possible to determine which ovary is going to become the dominant one, i.e. the one carrying the follicle destined to ovulate. The dominant ovary can usually be identified 6–9 days (mean 7 days) before the LH surge, i.e. between cycle days 5 and 12 (mean cycle day 8) as the ovary carrying a follicle larger than any of the other follicles and with a diameter of more than 10 mm.[8] The dominant follicle displays a linear growth rate of 1.4–2.2 mm (mean 1.7) per day.[8] At the time of the LH surge, the leading follicle has a diameter of 18–22 mm.[8] After ovulation, the follicle becomes a corpus luteum. The corpus luteum is usually smaller than the dominant follicle, its wall is thicker, and with high-resolution ultrasound systems, it may be possible to see the crenated appearance of its wall. Bleeding into the corpus luteum explains the presence of echoes in the corpus luteum at ultrasound examination.[7] The corpus luteum is well vascularized and its rich vascularization is detectable at color Doppler ultrasound examination.[10] Ultrasound images of corpora lutea are shown in Figures 2.17A to I.

NORMAL ULTRASOUND MORPHOLOGY OF UTERUS AND OVARIES IN POSTMENOPAUSAL WOMEN

While it is rare that we see postmenopausal women in a fertility clinic, occasionally we come across with women having premature ovarian dysfunction seeking treatment using donor eggs. The uterus and ovaries are smaller in postmenopausal women than in women of fertile age.[3] The endometrium has uniform ultrasound morphology because there are no cyclical hormonal changes. It is thin (usually no more than 5 mm thick) and hyperechoic.[3,4] The ovaries contain no follicles but one or more cystic structures with anechoic cyst contents up to 10 mm in diameter are often seen in healthy postmenopausal women and should be regarded as normal findings.[11] Ultrasound images of normal postmenopausal uteri and ovaries are shown in Figures 2.18A to D. It is often very difficult to get good ultrasound images of the uterus and the endometrium in postmenopausal women, because the uterus is often in an upright position. Moreover, the ovaries may be difficult to find, because they are small and devoid of antral follicles.

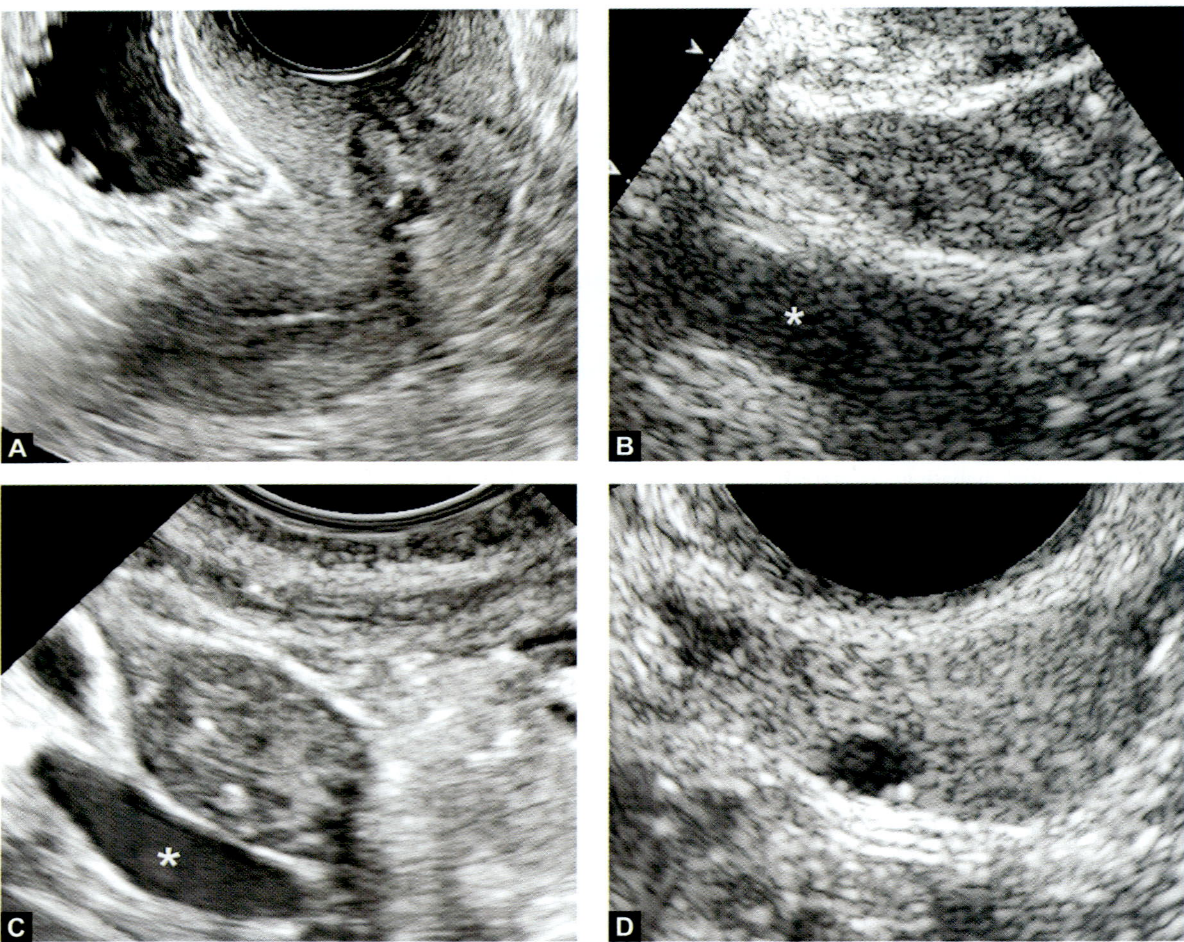

Figs. 2.18A to D: Transvaginal ultrasound images of normal postmenopausal uterus and ovaries: (A) Longitudinal section through the uterus. (B) The endometrium is thin and hyperechoic; (C) postmenopausal ovaries with no visible cystic structures (asterisk shows iliac vessel); and (D) postmenopausal ovary with a small anechoic cystic structure inside, presumably an inclusion cyst.[11]

URINARY BLADDER

The urinary bladder should be empty at transvaginal ultrasound examination. Nonetheless, it usually contains a small amount of urine, which makes it possible to examine the walls of the urinary bladder (Figs. 2.12A and B).

POUCH OF DOUGLAS

In women of fertile age, fluid is almost always seen in the pouch of Douglas, at least in the late follicular phase and in the secretory phase of the menstrual cycle[7] (Figs. 2.11A and B). In the early luteal phase, the pouch of Douglas normally contains 15–25 mL fluid.[7] It is not possible to give an exact cut-off in millimeter of what is a normal amount of pelvic fluid in a woman of fertile age, but fluid outside the pouch of Douglas, i.e. in the space between the uterus and the bladder is abnormal. An ultrasound finding of even a small amount of fluid in the pouch of Douglas in a postmenopausal woman is unusual, and a follow-up scan is advisable to exclude that the fluid is a first sign of ascites.

DOPPLER ULTRASOUND EXAMINATIONS OF NORMAL UTERUS AND OVARIES

There is no indication to perform a Doppler ultrasound examination of the uterus or ovaries if they appear normal at gray-scale ultrasound examination. However, color or power Doppler ultrasound can be used to confirm the presence of a corpus luteum. A corpus luteum is surrounded by a thick and bright ring of color reflecting the rich vascularization of the corpus luteum. A dominant follicle is less well vascularized and is surrounded by a thinner and less bright color ring (Figs. 2.17A to I).[10] Information on normal findings at transvaginal Doppler ultrasound examination of the uterus and ovaries in premenopausal and postmenopausal women are outside the remit of the book and can be found in the literature.[4,10,12-14] Application of Doppler ultrasound aid in the diagnosis of certain uterine and adnexal pathologies are detailed in the relevant chapters.

CONCLUSION

A successful performance of a gynecological ultrasound examination is possible only if the examiner knows how to optimize the image (magnification, gain, focus, and frequency), applies a systematic examination technique, and is familiar with the normal appearances of pelvic organs.

ACKNOWLEDGMENTS

The studies from my institution were supported by grants from the Malmo General Hospital Cancer Foundation, funds administered by the Malmo Health Care Administration, the Faculty of Medicine of Lund University, the Anna-Lisa och Sven-Erik Lundgren Foundation for Medical Research, the Ingabritt and Arne Lundberg Research Foundation, the Swedish Medical Research Council (grant nos. B96-17X-11605-01A, K98-17X-11605-03A, K2001-72X-11605-06A, K2002-72X-11605-07B, K2004-73X-11605-09A, and K2006-73X-11605-11-3), and two governmental grants (regionalt forskningsstod Skine, ALF-medel).

KEY POINTS

- Pelvic ultrasound examination can be performed transabdominally, transvaginally, or—in exceptional cases—transrectally
- Regardless of the route of examination, it is important to optimize the image and to perform the examination in a systematic manner
- Image depth, magnification, focus, gain, and frequency should be changed during every examination to optimize the image
- A systematic scanning technique is always adopted to ensure that a complete pelvic examination is performed and also to build up a reference of what is normal, which will increase our confidence in detecting pelvic pathology
- It is mandatory that transvaginal scans are performed with a completely empty bladder
- Transrectal scan is an alternative to a transvaginal scan, if a transvaginal scan is impossible and a transabdominal scan yields insufficient information
- It is necessary to perform a transabdominal ultrasound examination in case of very large pelvic masses or masses located in the abdomen above the pelvis
- There is no indication to perform a Doppler ultrasound examination of the uterus or ovaries if they appear normal at gray-scale ultrasound examination

REFERENCES

1. Epstein E, Valentin L. Managing women with postmenopausal bleeding. Best Pract Res Clin Obstet Gynecol. 2004;18:125-43.
2. Timmerman D, Valentin L, Bourne TH, et al. Terms, definitions and measurements to describe the sonographic

features of adnexal tumors: a consensus opinion from the International Ovarian Tumor Analysis (IOTA) Group. Ultrasound Obstet Gynecol. 2000;16:500-5.

3. Merz E, Miric-Tesanic D, Bahlman F, et al. Sonographic size of uterus and ovaries in pre- and postmenopausal women. Ultrasound Obstet Gynecol. 1996;7:38-42.
4. Sladkevicius P, Valentin L, Marsal K. Transvaginal greyscale and Doppler ultrasound examinations of the uterus and ovaries in healthy postmenopausal women. Ultrasound Obstet Gynecol. 1995;6:81-90.
5. Jokubkiene L, Sladkevicius P, Valentin L. Ovarian size and vascularization as assessed by three-dimensional grayscale and power Doppler ultrasound in asymptomatic women 20-39 years old using combined oral contraceptives. Contraception. 2012;86:257-67.
6. Jokubkiene L, Sladkevicius P, Valentin L. Number of antral follicles, ovarian volume, and vascular indices in asymptomatic women 20 to 39 years old as assessed by 3-dimensional sonography: a prospective cross-sectional study. J Ultrasound Med. 2012;31:1635-49.
7. Ritchie WG. Sonographic evaluation of normal and induced ovulation. Radiology. 1986;161:1-10.
8. Pache T, Hop WC, Wladimiroff JW, et al. Growth patterns of nondominant ovarian follicles during the normal menstrual cycle. Fertil Steril. 1990;54:638-42.
9. Dewailly D, Gronier H, Poncelet E, et al. Diagnosis of polycystic ovary syndrome (PCOS): revisiting the threshold values of follicle count on ultrasound and of the serum AMH level for the definition of polycystic ovaries. Hum Reprod. 2011;26:3123-9.
10. Sladkevicius P, Valentin L, Marsal K. Blood flow velocity in the uterine and ovarian arteries during the normal menstrual cycle. Ultrasound Obstet Gynecol. 1993;3:199-208.
11. Valentin L, Skoog L, Epstein E. The frequency and type of adnexal lesions in an autopsy material comprising postmenopausal women. An ultrasound study with histological correlation. Ultrasound Obstet Gynecol. 2003;22:284-9.
12. Sladkevicius P, Valentin L, Marsal K. Blood flow velocity in the uterine and ovarian arteries during menstruation. Ultrasound Obstet Gynecol. 1994;4(5):421-7.
13. Jokubkiene L, Sladkevicius P, Rovas L, et al. Assessment of changes in volume and vascularity of the ovaries during the normal menstrual cycle using three-dimensional power Doppler ultrasound. Hum Reprod. 2006;21:2661-8.
14. Jokubkiene L, Sladkevicius P, Rovas L, et al. Assessment of changes in endometrial and subendometrial volume and vascularity during the normal menstrual cycle using three-dimensional power Doppler ultrasound. Ultrasound Obstet Gynecol. 2006;27:672-9.

Chapter 3

Uterine Fibroids, Adenomyosis, and Congenital Uterine Anomalies

Janine Elson, Giuseppina Lamanna

Chapter Outline

ULTRASOUND OF THE UTERUS

Until recently, invasive procedures, such as diagnostic hysteroscopy and laparoscopy, have been the standard to look for uterine pathology at many fertility centers. Recent advances in gynecological ultrasonography have shown that ultrasound can replace routine invasive investigative procedures.

IMAGING METHODS

Transabdominal Sonography

Transabdominal imaging uses low frequency (3.75 MHz) and is useful to view large fibroids that are high in the pelvis. A full bladder provides a sonographic window for evaluation of the uterus and adnexa (Fig. 3.1). A full bladder has a teardrop-shaped appearance on the longitudinal view and is rectangular on the transverse view. The uterus (longitudinal orientation) is oval and more echogenic than the bladder and located posterior to the bladder, appearing to wrap under it, ending in the cervix and vaginal canal. The endometrial stripe is seen as an echogenic (bright) line in the central uterus. The vagina is a hypoechoic tubular structure posterior to the bladder and caudal to the uterus. A vaginal stripe can be identified. The cervix is seen between the uterus and vaginal canal.

Transvaginal Sonography

Endovaginal scanning uses a high-frequency transducer (6.5 MHz). Though multifrequency probes are now used for transvaginal scans also with frequencies ranging from 5 to 12 MHz. High-frequency probes provide high-quality images of the myometrium and endometrium and therefore, transvaginal scanning is commonly performed for detailed evaluation of uterus. The uterus usually is identified easily posterior to the bladder, which is preferred to be emptied prior to transvaginal scanning. In the longitudinal or sagittal view, with the orientation arranged as shown in Figure 3.2, and if the uterus is anteverted, the fundus is located on the left side of the imaging screen, with the cervix on the right. With this orientation, if the uterus is retroverted the fundus is seen on the right side of the screen and the cervix on the left (Fig. 3.3). The entire uterus may not be seen at one time or on one particular endovaginal view. The uterus is pear-shaped on the longitudinal view and round on the transverse view. The endometrial stripe is located within the central uterus and is connected to the endocervical canal; its thickness and pattern varies with the phase of menstrual cycle (Fig. 3.4).

Transvaginal color flow Doppler ultrasonography is helpful in localizing vessels within uterine lesions and may be useful in differentiating various uterine pathologies. It has also been reported useful in evaluation of functional

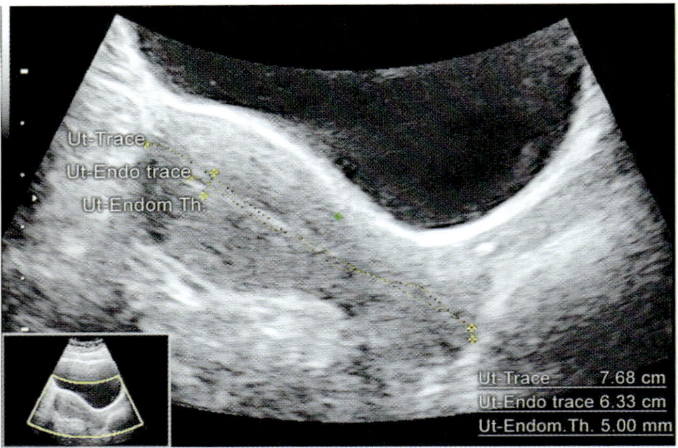

Fig. 3.1: Transabdominal scan: Longitudinal view of the uterus and cervix.

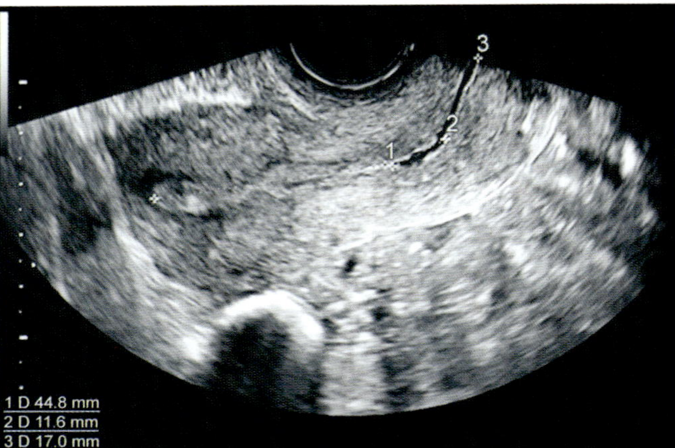

Fig. 3.2: Transvaginal scan: Longitudinal view of an anteverted uterus.

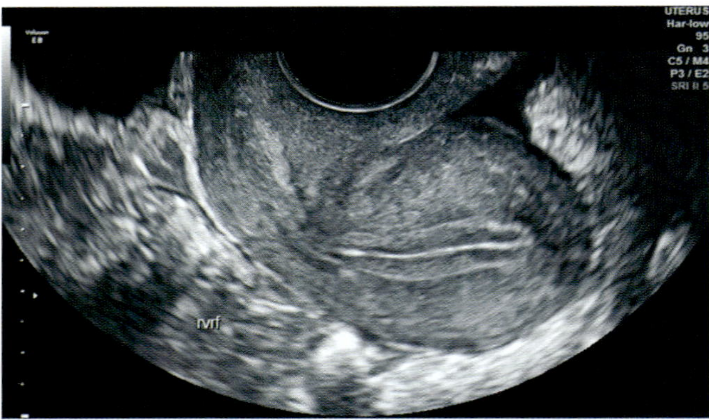

Fig. 3.3: Retroverted uterus with proliferative endometrium.

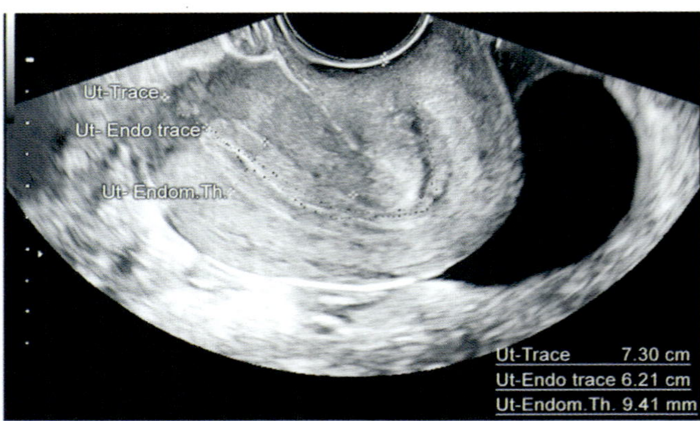

Fig. 3.4: Trilaminar endometirum as seen in proliferative phase.

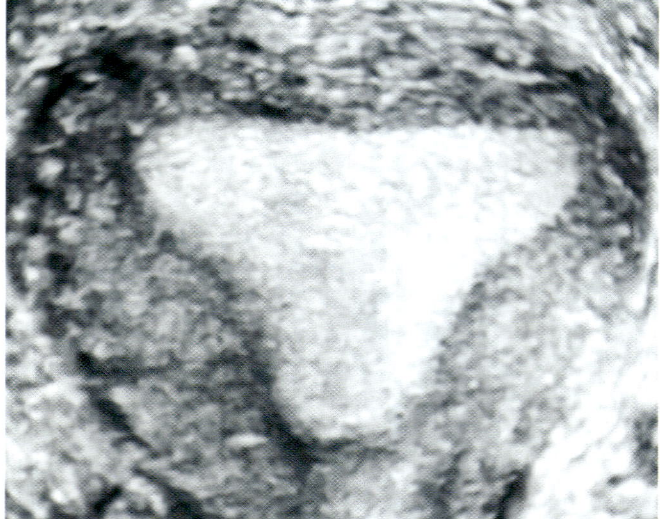

Fig. 3.5: Three-dimensional (3D) image of uterus allows viewing coronal plane of the normal uterine cavity.

component of endometrium with endometrial and subendometrial blood flow has been implicated in predicting conception following various fertility treatments in subfertile women.

Transvaginal three-dimensional (3D) imaging is as reliable as two-dimensional (2D) imaging in evaluating the uterus. It offers the advantage of providing coronal plane (Fig. 3.5), which is unique to 3D scanning. Three-dimensional ultrasound is considered as gold standard tool in diagnosing congenital uterine anomalies, while it has an increasing role in preoperative mapping of fibroids and adenomyosis. Other key advantage of 3D ultrasound is that it may allow the storage of volumes for later analysis by the sonographer or offline review by other operators, or teaching, although real-time analysis remains the most accurate diagnostic tool.[1]

Saline Infusion Sonography

The uterine cavity can be explored by saline infusion sonohysteroscopy [aquascan, saline infusion sonography (SIS)]. A bivalve speculum is placed in the vagina and the cervix cleaned. A thin catheter, preferably with an inflatable balloon tip, is placed through the cervix to the level of internal os and the speculum then withdrawn. The transvaginal probe is then inserted and the uterus viewed in the longitudinal plane and the catheter position checked. Between 5 and 10 mL of sterile saline is then introduced into the uterine cavity allowing its integrity to be checked. This technique has the advantage over hysteroscopy in that it allows both the endometrial cavity and myometrium to be assessed simultaneously. If 3D imaging is required then a 3D volume can be acquired to allow simultaneous multiplanar display to obtain coronal plane, which is not viewed by 2D SIS alone.

UTERINE FIBROIDS OR MYOMAS

Uterine fibroids are the commonest benign uterine tumors and are seen in 20–40% of women of child-bearing age.[2] When assessing fibroids by ultrasound, the number, site, and size as well as their relation to the endometrial cavity are noted. Fibroids are seen as distinct, well circumscribed usually heterogeneous lesions arising from the myometrium. They may be hypoechoic, hyperechoic, or show signs of calcification. Occasionally, they will be undergoing cystic degeneration and this is seen as hypoechoic areas within a hyperechoic lesion. It is important to assess fibroids in both the longitudinal and transverse planes and to note their position in relation to the anterior and posterior walls of the uterus and to carry out measurements in three perpendicular planes. Fibroids should then be categorized as intramural, those confined within the myometrium (Fig. 3.6); subserous, when greater than 50% protrudes through the serosal surface; and submucosal, when they distort the endometrial cavity (Figs. 3.7A and B).

Submucosal fibroids can further be subcategorized to grade 0, grade 1, and grade 2 depending on its relation to endometrial cavity.[3] Grade 0 indicates that the fibroid is present 100% within the endometrial cavity; grade 1 indicates greater than 50% of the fibroid present within the endometrial cavity, and grade 2 indicates less than 50% of the fibroid present within the endometrial cavity (Figs. 3.8 and 3.9).

Saline infusion sonography offers the advantage of delineating the endometrial cavity and helps in diagnosing

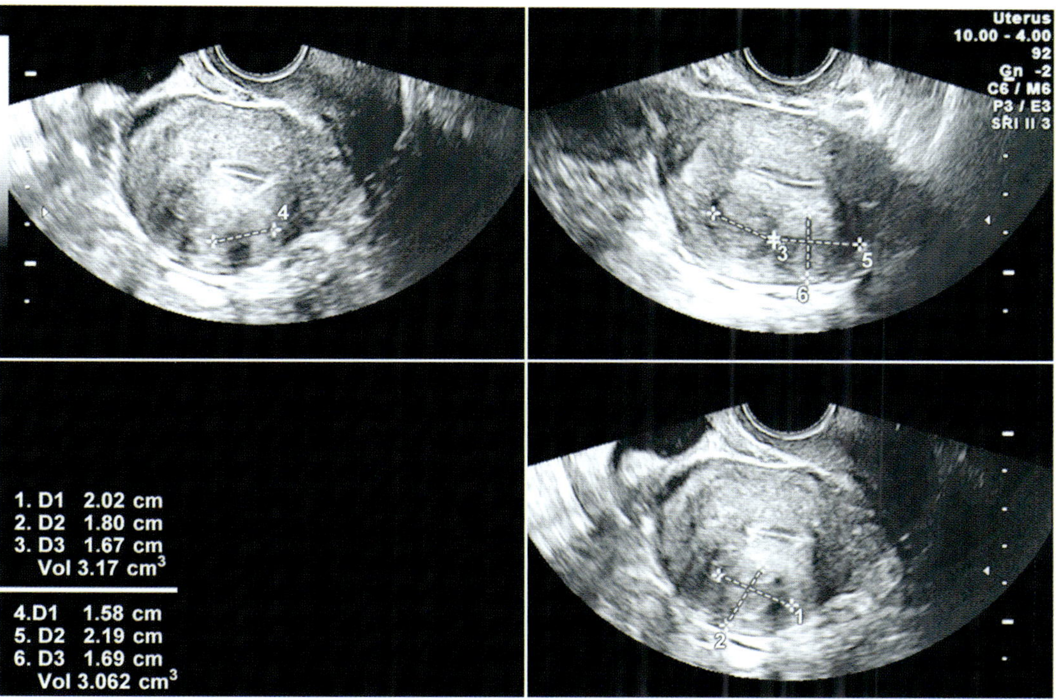

Fig. 3.6: Intramural fibroids.

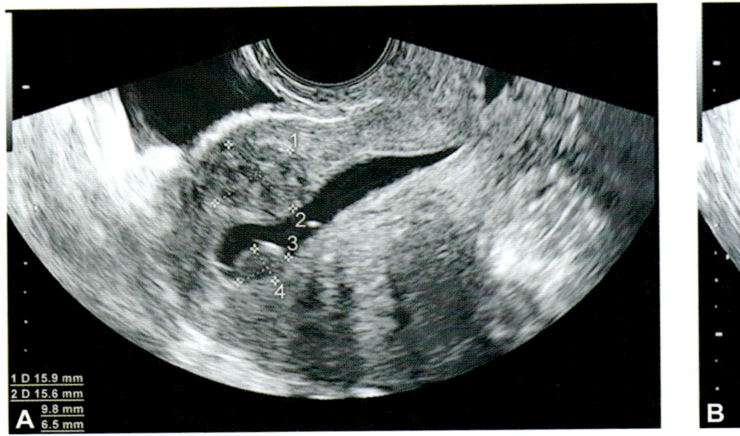

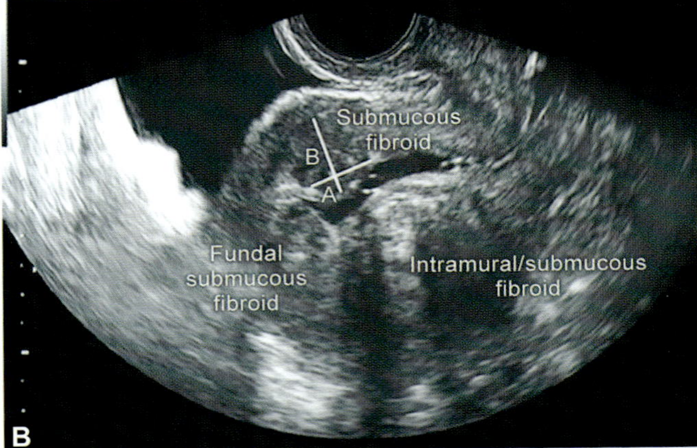

Figs. 3.7A and B: Images showing fibroid mapping of multiple fibroids.

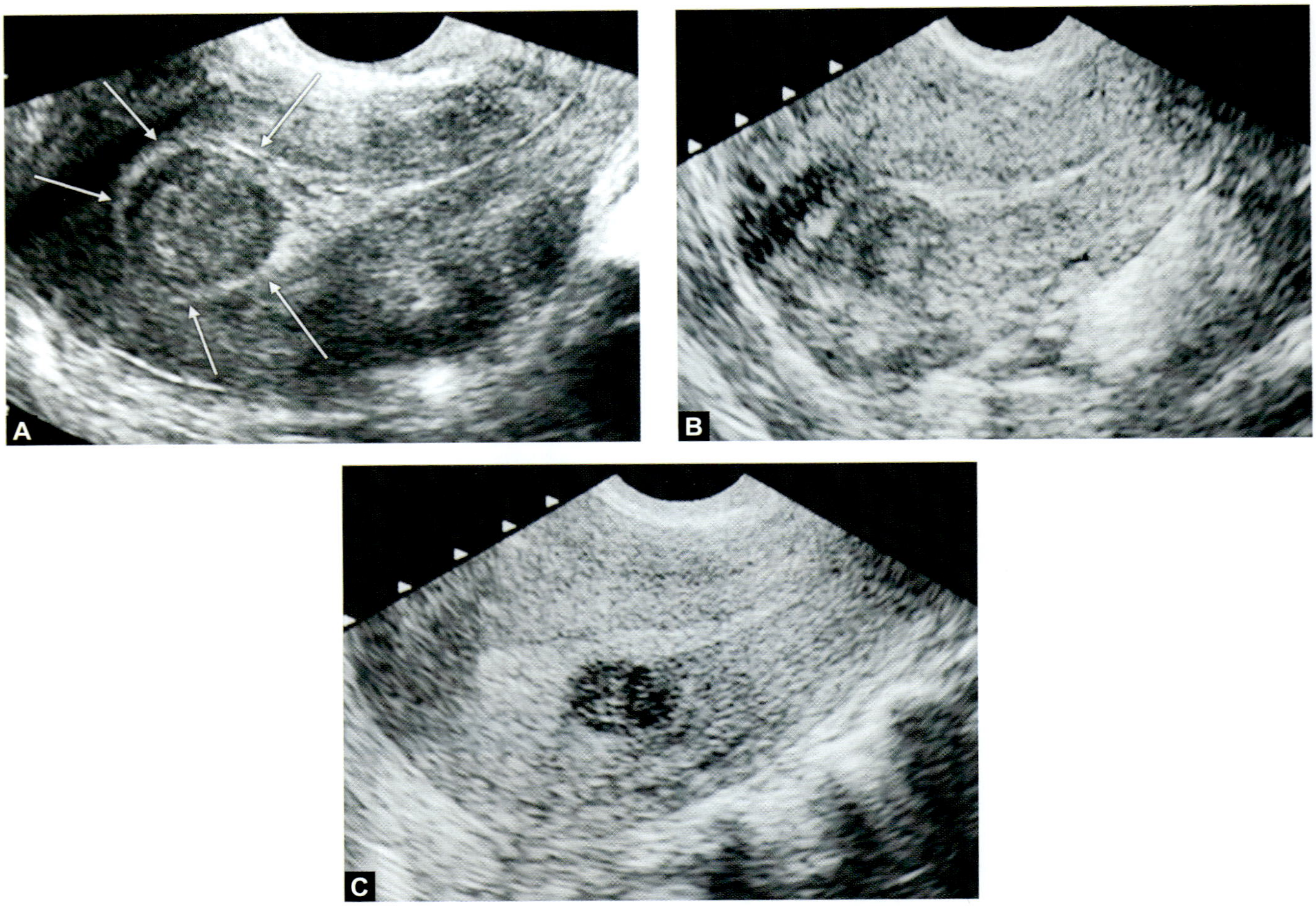

Figs. 3.8A to C: Submucous fibroids of (A) grade 0, (B) grade 1, and (C) grade 2 on two-dimensional (2D) ultrasound.

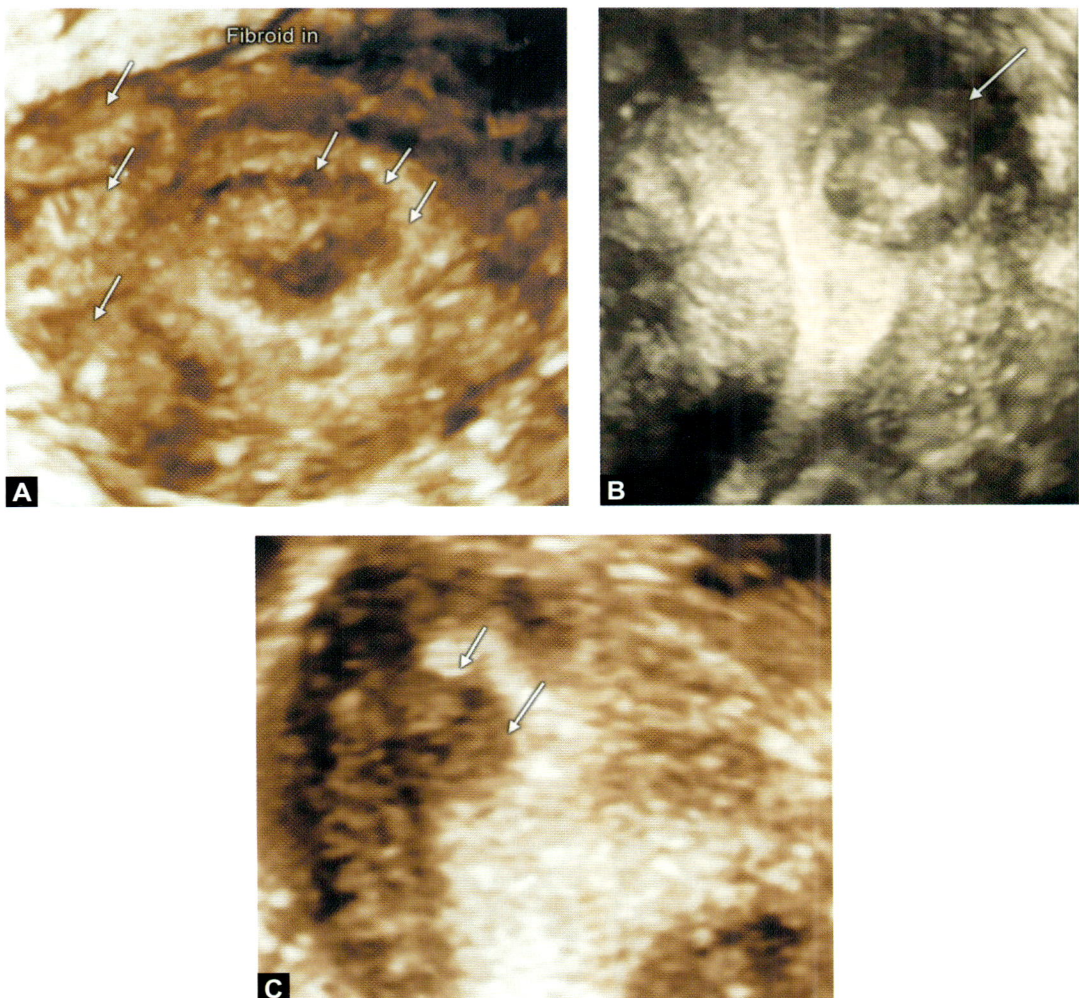

Figs. 3.9A to C: Submucous fibroids of (A) grade 0, (B) grade 1, and (C) grade 2 on three-dimensional (3D) ultrasound (coronal plane).

submucous fibroids. It is comparable to hysteroscopy in detecting the presence of submucous fibroids, and enables measurements to be taken. However, its value in determining the extent of protrusion into the endometrial cavity is limited. Using 3D, SIS allows for a more accurate assessment of the cavity from the visualization of coronal plane (Fig. 3.10). The degree of protrusion into the cavity can be calculated by measuring both the section of the fibroid protruding into the cavity (A) and the part confined to the myometrium (B) and calculating the protrusion ratio as $A/(A + B) \times 100$ (Fig. 3.7B). These measurements have been shown to have good reproducibility amongst operators and can be used to predict the likelihood of successful hysteroscopic surgery.[4] Fibroids greater than 38 mm and with 43% or less protrusion have been shown to be more likely to need a two-stage resection.[5]

Color flow or Doppler can be used to look for vascularization and is usually seen as capsular flow with a vascular rim around the fibroid (Figs. 3.11A to D), though degenerated fibroids may show internal vascularity. The use of 3D ultrasound is largely in improving mapping of fibroid localization prior to surgery.

Leiomyosarcoma

Leiomyosarcomas are rare and seen in around 2 per 1,000 surgically removed fibroids. They are usually solitary, greater than 10 cm in size and their distinguishing sonographic feature is central vascularization.[6] Though vascularity is also seen in degenerated fibroids, it is difficult to ascertain the malignant nature of the lesion, unless the capsule is broken (Figs. 3.12A and B).

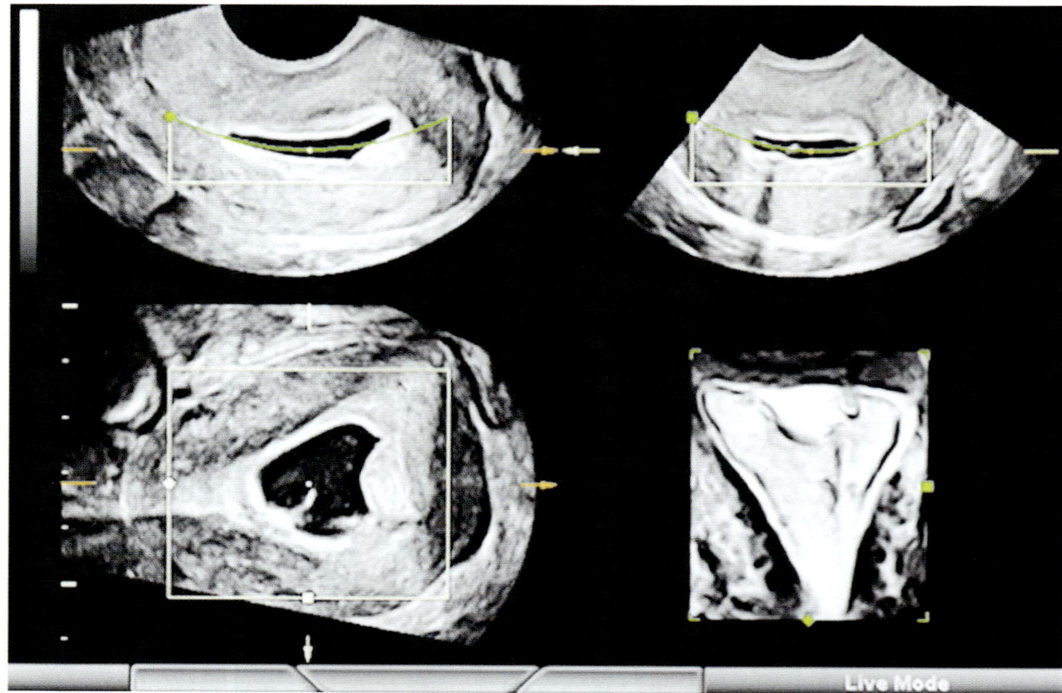

Fig. 3.10: Three-dimensional (3D) SIS showing submucosal fibroid.

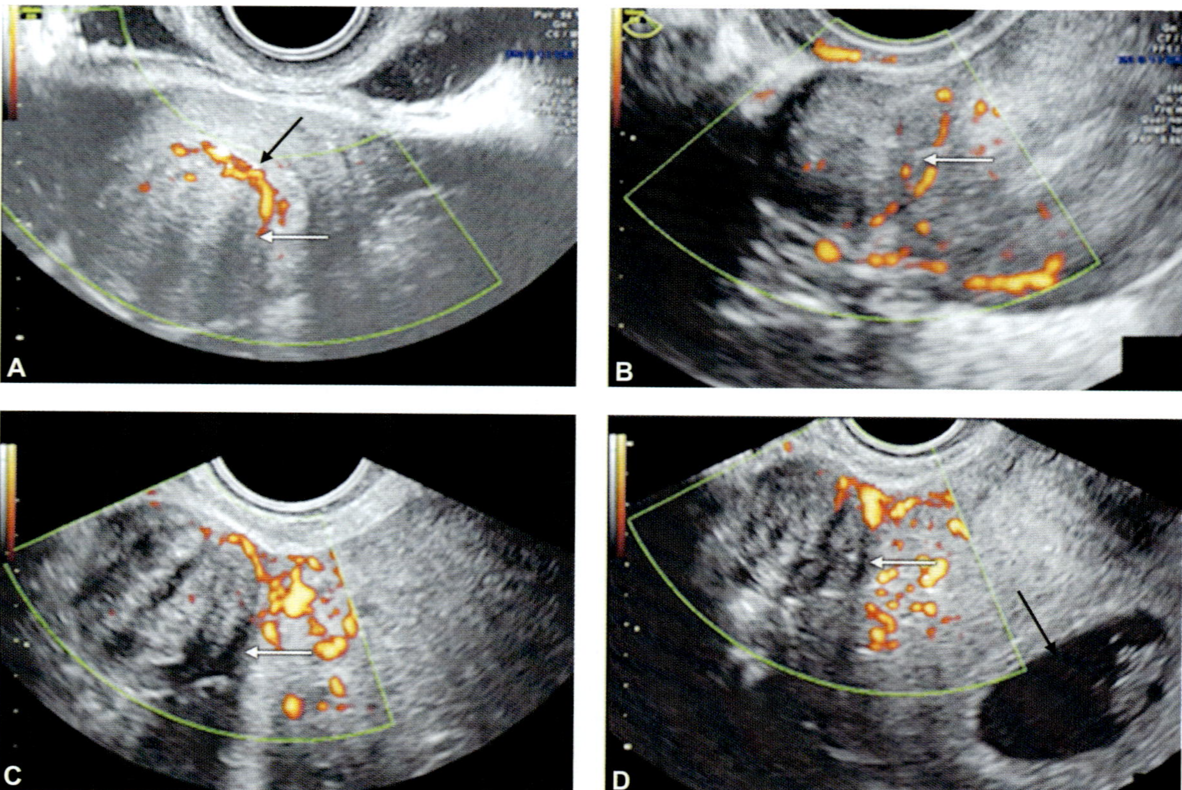

Figs. 3.11A to D: Doppler of fibroid uterus. Image (A) demonstrates a submucosal fibroid (white arrow) indenting the endometrial cavity. A typical "rim-like" pattern of blood vessels is noted (black arrow). Images (B to D) demonstrate a subserosal fibroid (white arrow). On image (D), a gestation sac is noted (black arrow).

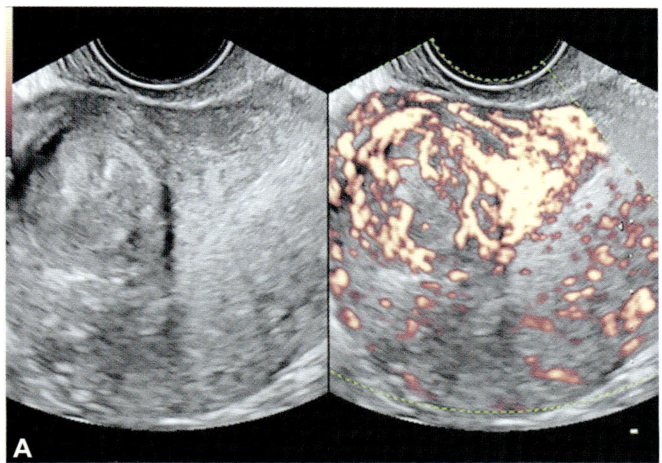

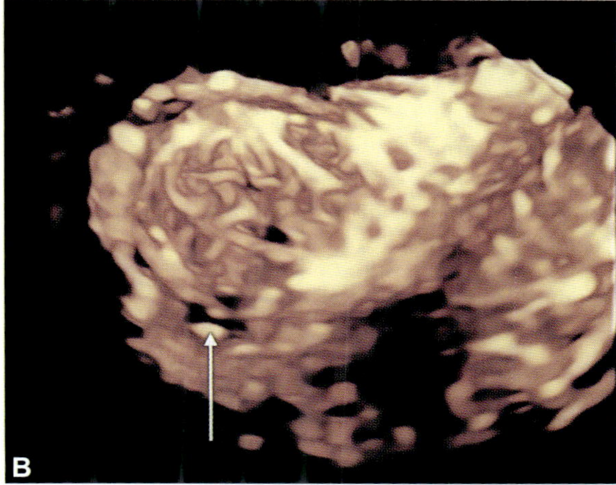

Figs. 3.12 A and B: Internal vascularity is seen in the fibroid suggesting a possibility of malignant change.

Management of Fibroids in the Subfertile Patient

Myomectomy is recommended for any fibroid that is within or distorting the endometrial cavity. Several preoperative assessment tools for submucous fibroids exist. The ESGE scoring system using grades 0–2 as previously described looks at the degree of intramural extension (Type 0: Completely intracavitary, Type 1: Less than 50% intramural extension and Type 2: More than 50% intramural extension). Surgery can usually be performed hysteroscopically for submucous fibroids grade 0 or 1, and via open surgery or laparoscopically for grade 2 submucous fibroids. The STEPW classification described by Lasmar et al. looks at size, topography, extension, penetration, and wall and it is used to underline the complexity of hysteroscopic myomectomy.[7] There is good evidence from randomized controlled trials that removal of submucous fibroids increases spontaneous pregnancy rates in the subfertile population.[8] There is also evidence that resection of submucous fibroids in the population undergoing in vitro fertilization (IVF) restores their success rates to those of women with normal cavities.[9] There is no evidence that the use of gonadotropin-releasing hormone (GnRH) analogs prior to surgery improves outcome, although it may have a role in anemic patients and those with large fibroids.[10] While there is evidence that noncavity distorting intramural fibroids compromise the chance of pregnancy following IVF treatment,[11] the role for myomectomy for such fibroids on improving pregnancy rates is more controversial. However, some research has shown an improvement in IVF success rates with removal of intramural fibroids more than 4 cm,[12] others have not found that the presence of fibroids affects pregnancy rates.[13] There is no evidence that removal of subserous fibroids improves either the chance of spontaneous conception or the success with fertility treatment.[13,14] There is evidence, however, that removal of intramural or subserosal fibroids may improve pregnancy outcome by a reduction in miscarriage rates.[15] Myomectomy for intramural and subserosal fibroids can be removed either via open or laparoscopic surgery although there is no evidence that either method has superior outcome with regards to fertility than the other.[16] There is some evidence that laparoscopic myomectomy may be associated with reduced morbidity, a shorter hospital stay, less blood loss,[17] and perhaps a lower rate of uterine rupture in subsequent pregnancy. The safety of alternatives to surgery, such as myolysis or uterine artery embolization (UAE), has yet to be established. Pregnancies have been reported with following UAE, but it is associated with a higher risk of miscarriage[18] and higher follicle-stimulating hormone (FSH) levels following the procedure. Around 1–2% of women undergoing UAE may suffer premature ovarian failure. It may have a role with proper counseling of the patient, in those women not suitable for surgical myomectomy.

ADENOMYOSIS

Adenomyosis presents with the clinical symptoms for dyspareunia, dysmenorrhea, and menometrorrhagia. Pathologically, it is defined as the presence of endometrial

Box 3.1: Sonographic features of adenomyosis

- Uterine enlargement not explained by presence of myomas
- Asymmetrical thickening of anterior or posterior wall
- Lack of contour abnormality or mass effect
- Anechoic lacunae (myometrial cysts)
- Heterogeneous poorly circumscribed areas within the myometrium
- Increased echotexture of the endometrium and subendometrial echogenic linear striations

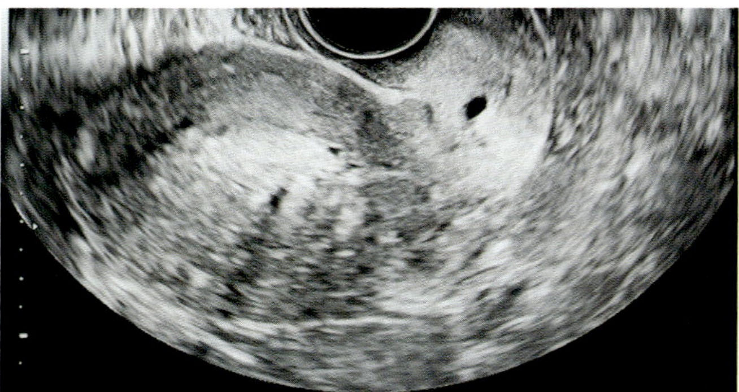

Fig. 3.13: Adenomyosis showing heterogeneous tissue in the posterior wall.

glands and stroma found within the myometrium with associated hypertrophy and hyperplasia of the surrounding myometrium. Clinical diagnosis is difficult. While there is a lack of epidemiological data linking adenomyosis to subfertility, the high prevalence of adenomyosis in women having endometriosis and other available indirect data indicate that adenomyosis may be linked to subfertility, possibly due to structural and functional changes of the endomyometrial junctional zone (JZ) leading to impaired embryo implantation.

A number of diagnostic features on transvaginal ultrasound have been described in Box 3.1.

A regularly enlarged uterus with a globular appearance, the presence of subendometrial echogenic linear striations, and myometrial cysts have the most accurate correlation with histopathology. The finding of a heterogeneous myometrium, however, is highly sensitive but not very specific when it comes to diagnosing adenomyosis[19] (Fig. 3.13).

In order to try and improve the accuracy of diagnosing adenomyosis via ultrasound, 3D techniques have been employed. Adenomyosis leads to diffuse or focal thickening of the endomyometrial JZ, which can be seen on ultrasound as the subendometrial halo- or hypoechoic

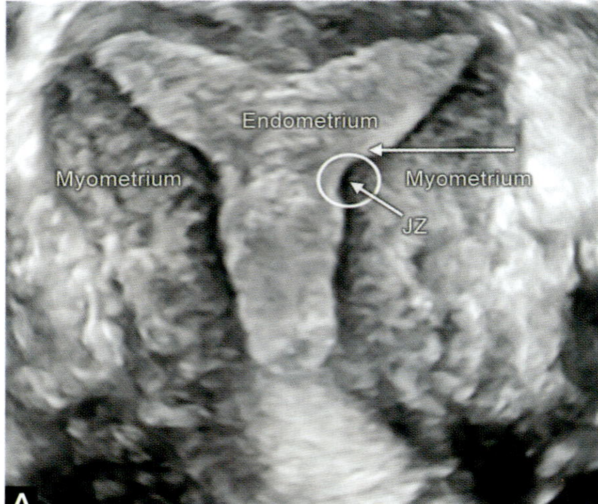

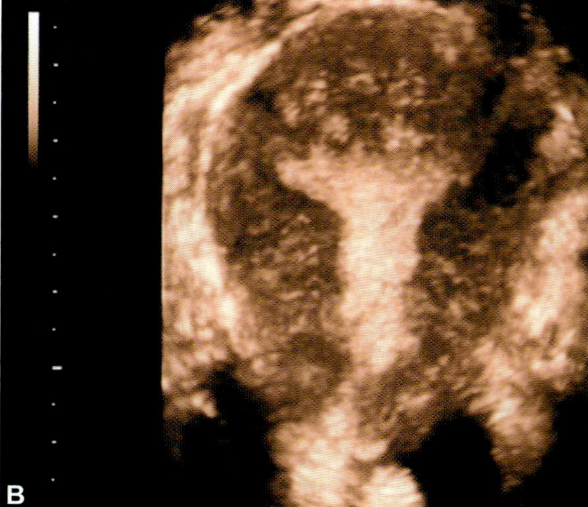

Figs. 3.14A and B: Coronal view of uterus: (A) Demonstrates hypoechoic junctional zone; (B) demonstrates irregular endometrial-myometrial junction and protrusions of endometrium into the inner myometrium, which are early features of adenomyosis.

area seen below the endometrial basal layer. Using 3D ultrasound to acquire the uterine volume and hence the coronal plane of the uterus, and then carrying out volume contrast imaging and volume rendering on the images, the JZ can be seen as hypoechoic area around the endometrium (Figs. 3.14A and B). Measurements of the JZ can then be taken to objectively assess the presence of adenomyosis. The JZ maximum (JZmax) is defined as the largest JZ thickness measured on coronal or longitudinal section at any level of the uterus; the JZ minimum (JZmin) is defined as the smallest JZ thickness measured on coronal or longitudinal section at any level of the uterus, and

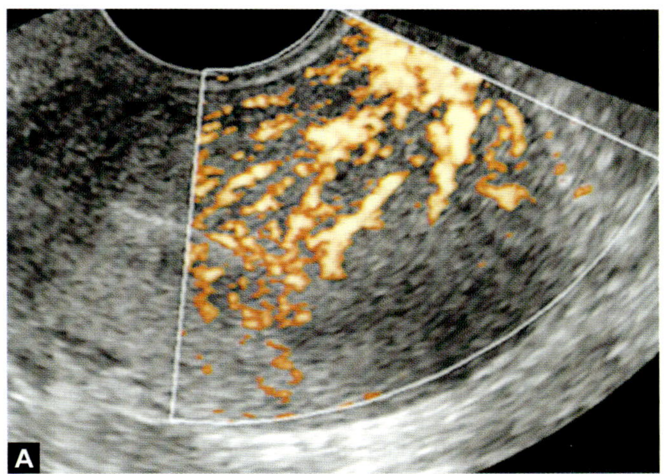

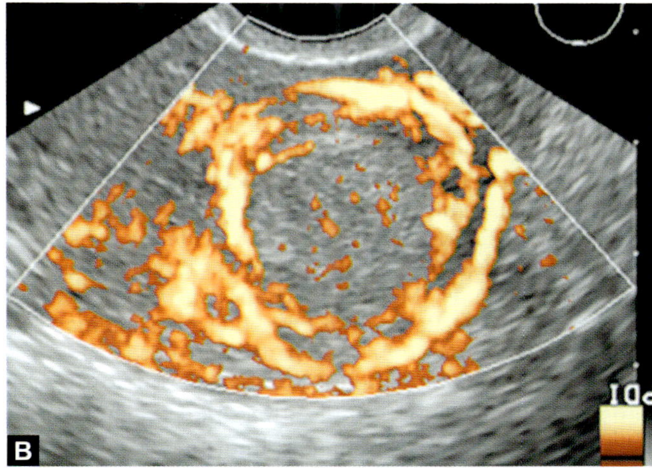

Figs. 3.15A and B: Doppler imaging of (A) an adenomyomatous uterus and (B) a fibroid uterus. While vessels are seen traversing through areas of adenomyosis (A), peripheral rim of vasculature is seen in fibroids (B).

the difference between them (JZdif) is the JZdif = JZmax – JZmin. Junctional zone alteration is defined as distortion and infiltration of the hypoechoic inner myometrium by hyperechoic endometrial tissue or ill-defined JZ. The 3D ultrasound findings with the most sensitivity for adenomyosis are a JZmax of greater than or equal to 8 mm, and JZdif greater than or equal to 4 mm and JZ alteration.[20] However, although 3D ultrasound has a greater sensitivity, it is not more specific than 2D ultrasound in the diagnosis of adenomyosis. Doppler ultrasound adds the diagnostic ability with finding of vessels traversing straight through areas of adenomyosis in contrast to peripheral rim of vasculature as seen in fibroids (Figs. 3.15A and B).

Management of Adenomyosis

Management of adenomyosis for those wishing to retain their fertility is challenging and requires particular expertise.

While the role of surgery for improving fertility in women having adenomyosis is controversial, surgery is not generally recommended for the sole purpose of improving the chances of conception. Cytoreductive laparoscopic or open surgery is the main option, although patients have an increased risk of uterine rupture in any subsequent pregnancy, especially if a significant amount of myometrium needs to be excised. Localized disease or adenomyomas is the easiest to excise laparoscopically as this tissue resembles fibroids. Fujishita et al.[21] described an open procedure known as transverse H technique, which consists one vertical and two crossing horizontal incisions to allow the removal of extensive adenomyosis, and reported spontaneous pregnancies following this method of excision. Diffuse adenomyosis is the most difficult to manage. Radical resection of the endometrium with triple flap reconstruction of the uterus has been described. This involves bisecting the uterus, excising the adenomyomatous layer, and then stripping the serosal surface of the lower uterine flaps to reconstruct the myometrium. Sixty-one percent of patients are reported as having conceived following surgery, and 88% of them having a cesarean section.[22]

CONGENITAL UTERINE ANOMALIES

Congenital uterine anomalies occur because of failure of Müllerian duct formation, fusion, or resorption in the fetus. Their exact prevalence is difficult to assess due to the lack of standard diagnostic criteria but is thought to be around 5% in general population, 6–8% in infertile women, 13–16% in women who have had one or more miscarriages, and 25–32% in women who have experienced to have both subfertility and recurrent miscarriage.[23] The anomalies may be divided into those associated with canalization defects—arcuate, subseptate, and septate and those associated with unification defects—bicornuate and unicornuate with or without rudimentary horn. Traditionally, these are classified according to the American Fertility Society (AFS) guidelines, although these are dependent on individual clinician interpretation. Some reproductive outcome studies have shown that septate and subseptate uteri are more commonly associated with infertility,[24] and arcuate uteri are associated with second trimester miscarriage.

Salim et al. in 2003[25] found that it was not the finding of an anomaly that was more common in women with recurrent miscarriage but those women with recurrent pregnancy loss had a greater degree of distortion of the uterine cavity. Unification defect anomalies are not associated with infertility, but with obstetric complications such as miscarriage and premature labor. All anomalies appear to be associated with fetal malpresentation.[26]

The double endometrial echo complex seen on a transverse plane with conventional 2D ultrasound is indicative of a uterine anomaly (Fig. 3.18) but this is observed with arcuate, septate, and bicornuate uteri. A transverse slice through the fundus of an arcuate uterus can give the view of a double endometrial echo complex, although this mildest form of uterine anomaly, with a shallow internal fundal indentation of 1 cm or less, is of doubtful clinical importance. This is undoubtedly the area where 3D ultrasound has contributed the most and has become the current gold standard for diagnosis of these anomalies. The main benefit of 3D ultrasound for diagnosing uterine anomaly is that it allows us to image both internal and external (serosal surface) contour of the uterine fundus simultaneously in the coronal plane, which is frequently impossible to obtain using 2D ultrasound. This view allows the user to identify easily an abnormal uterus and then classify the abnormality (Figs. 3.16 to 3.20). Three-dimensional ultrasound enables the clinician ability to diagnose the anomaly without resorting to the invasive surgery or more invasive diagnostic options such as saline infusion sonohysterography.

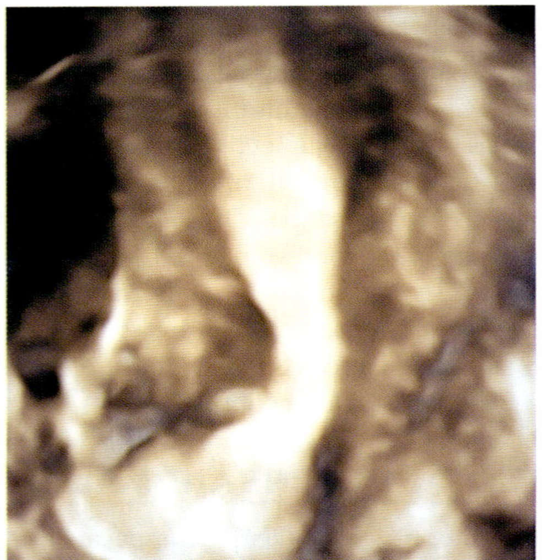

Fig. 3.16: Unicornuate uterus (3D coronal view).

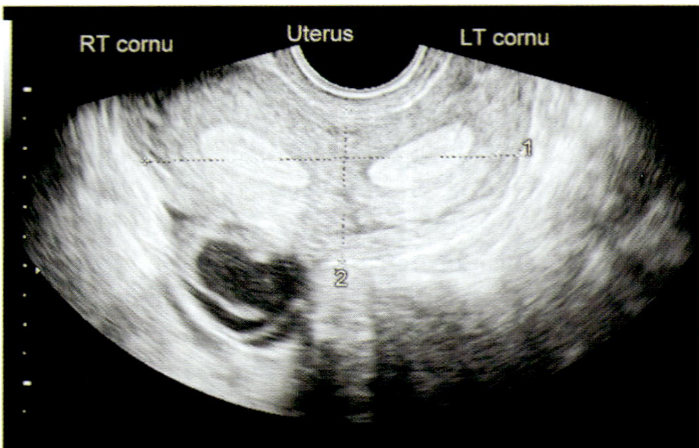

Fig. 3.18: Two-dimensional (2D) image of two endometrial complexes on a transverse plane of a uterus indicates that there is an anomaly.

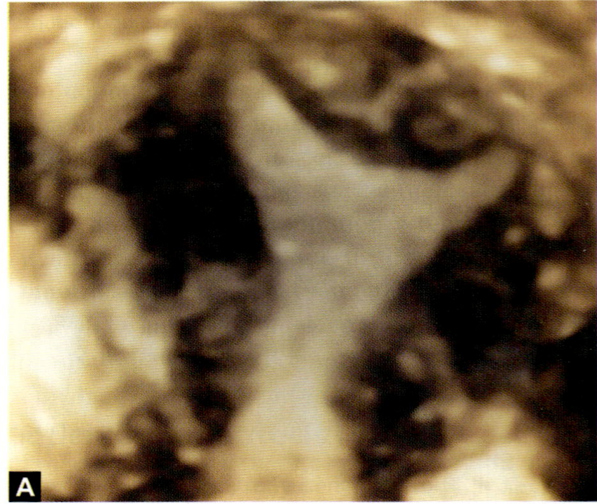

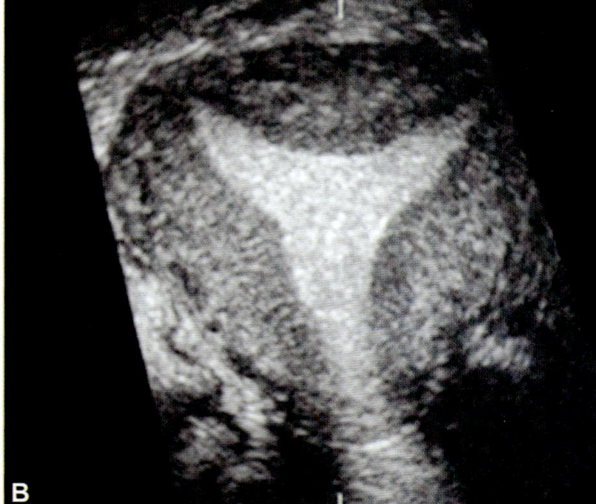

Figs. 3.17A and B: Arcuate uteri (3D coronal view).

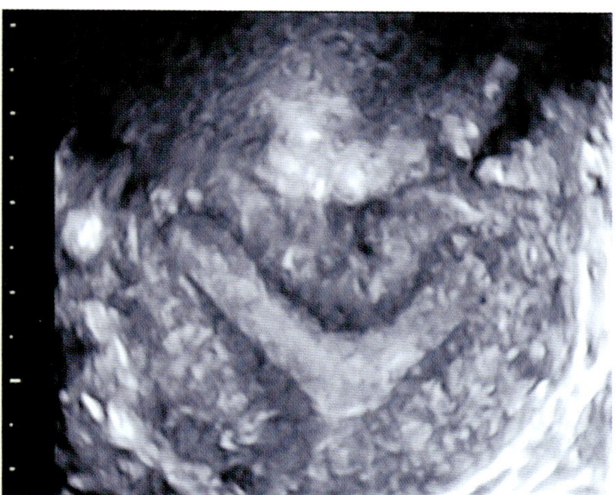

Fig. 3.19: Three-dimensional (3D) coronal plane of a bicornuate uterus.

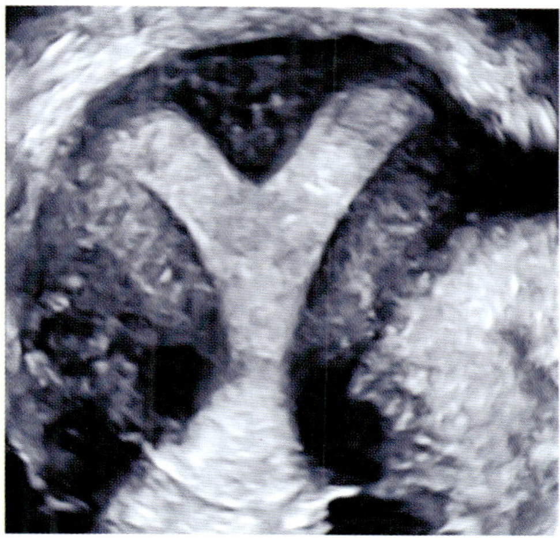

Fig. 3.20: Three-dimensional (3D) image of a subseptate uterus.

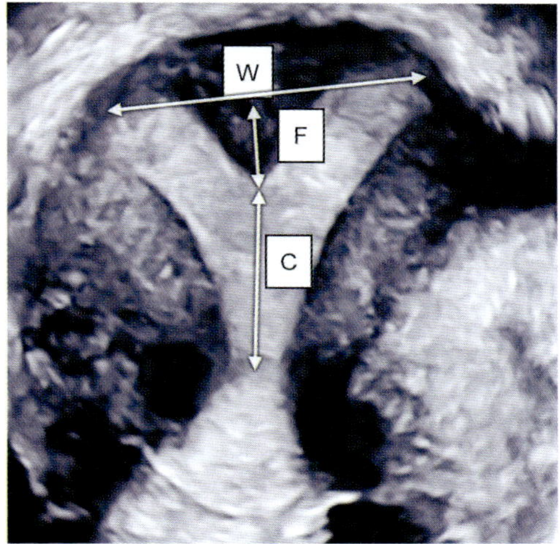

Fig. 3.21: Measurement methods to assess the degree of distortion of uterine cavity in a subseptate uterus.

Although the method for diagnosis is agreed, set international ultrasound criteria have yet to be agreed upon. However, criteria for the classification of 3D uterine anomalies have been well described in the literature.[25] The morphology of the uterus is best examined in the coronal plane, using the interstitial portions of the Fallopian tubes as reference points. Three measurements should be taken: (1) "*W*," the width of the uterine cavity which is measured as the distance between the internal tubal ostia, (2) "*F*," the septum length or fundal indentation which is measured as the distance from the midpoint of a line joining the tubal ostia and the tip of the fundal indentation or septum, and (3) "*C*," the length of the unaffected cavity from the tip of the septum or fundal indentation to the internal os, and then the diagnosis made with the diagnostic criteria as shown in Table 3.1. The degree of distortion of the cavity can be calculated by $F/(F + C)$ (Fig. 3.21).[25] Good interobserver and intraobserver reproducibilities for these measurements have been shown. Saline infusion sonography has been suggested as a method for diagnosing rudimentary horns as saline can be clearly seen in the unicornuate uterus, with no passage into the rudimentary horn.[27]

The European Society for Human Reproduction and Embryology (ESHRE) and the European Society for Gynecological Endoscopy (ESGE), through a structured Delphi procedure jointly published the ESHRE/ESGE classification, which is currently considered to be the most updated classification in the literature.[28] It also provides a pictorial guide—similar to the AFS classification—to aid diagnosis based on the imaging results. Furthermore, it includes quantitative definitions to guide the diagnosis and differentiation between anomalies. For example, an internal indentation at the fundal midline exceeding 50% of the uterine wall thickness has been used to diagnose the septate uterus, while an external indentation at the fundal midline exceeding 50% of the uterine wall thickness has been used to diagnose the bicorporeal uterus. However, although this classification attempted to address all the shortcomings of the past, it has not been received without criticism, as some authors have observed an increase in the diagnosis of the septate uterus compared with former classifications, which they feel may cause confusion in terms of clinical management.[29]

Table 3.1: Modified criteria for classification of congenital uterine anomalies based on three-dimensional (3D) ultrasound[24]

Uterine morphology	*Fundal contour*	*External contour*
Normal	Straight or convex	Uniformly convex or with indentation <10 mm
Arcuate	Concave fundal indentation with central point of indentation at obtuse angle (>90°)	Uniformly convex or with indentation <10 mm
Subseptate	Presence of septum does not extend to cervix, with central point of septum at an acute angle (<90°)	Uniformly convex or with indentation <10 mm
Septate	Presence of uterine septum that completely divides cavity from fundus to cervix	Uniformly convex or with indentation <10 mm
Bicornuate	Two well-formed uterine cornua, with a convex fundal contour in each	Fundal indentation >10 mm dividing the two cornua
Unicornuate with or without rudimentary horn	Single well-formed uterine cavity with a single interstitial portion of Fallopian tube and concave fundal contour	Fundal indentation >10 mm dividing the two cornua if rudimentary horn present

Management of Congenital Uterine Anomalies

One of the difficulties with the lack of set ultrasound criteria for the diagnosis of congenital uterine anomalies is that the data regarding prevalence and relevance of these anomalies in the subfertile patient and those with pregnancy complications are therefore very varied. Some studies have found that the rate of first trimester miscarriage is associated with subseptate uteri, and second trimester miscarriage with an arcuate uterus.[30] Hypothetically, restoration of normal morphology of the uterus is thought to improve reproductive outcomes. However, to date, there has been no randomized controlled trial of metroplasty versus expectant management in septate or subseptate uteri. Although observational studies have found a benefit in removing the septum in subfertile women,[8,31] a Cochrane review of the evidence for hysteroscopic metroplasty in women with recurrent miscarriage and a septate uterus in 2011 found no evidence to recommend it as routine practice. Rudimentary horns can be excised laparoscopically to prevent the risk of hematometra or pregnancy occurring in the horn, although the presence of associated renal tract anomalies needs to be ruled out prior to any surgery.[32]

CLINICAL CASES

Case 1

A 41-year-old woman presented to the clinic having being trying to conceive for the last year. An anti-Müllerian hormone (AMH) was within the low-fertility range. A 2D ultrasound scan showed the suspicion of submucosal type 0 fibroids which was confirmed on 3D SIS (Fig. 3.22). The woman underwent a hysteroscopy which confirmed the presence of submucosal fibroids, which were resected during the same procedure.

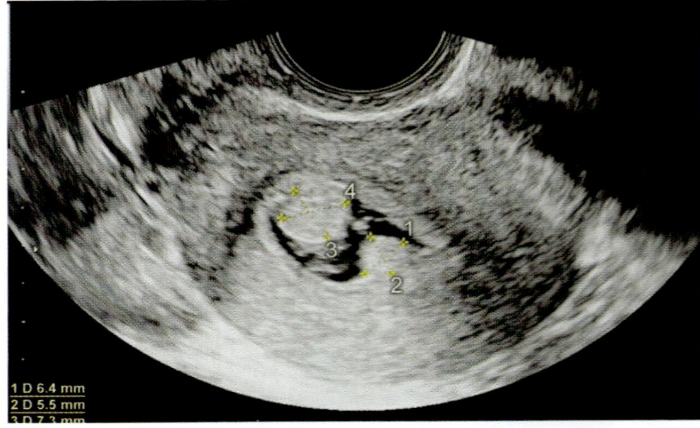

Fig. 3.22: Two-dimensional (2D) ultrasound scan showing the suspicion of submucosal type 0 fibroids which was confirmed on saline infusion sonography (SIS).

Case 2

A 37-year-old lady presented with a history of a septal metroplasty 6 years earlier for a subseptate uterus, three unsuccessful intrauterine insemination treatments and three unsuccessful IVF cycles. She had low ovarian reserve. A 3D ultrasound of the uterus showed a residual uterine septum (Fig. 3.23). She underwent a second hysteroscopic procedure to resect the residual septum. The

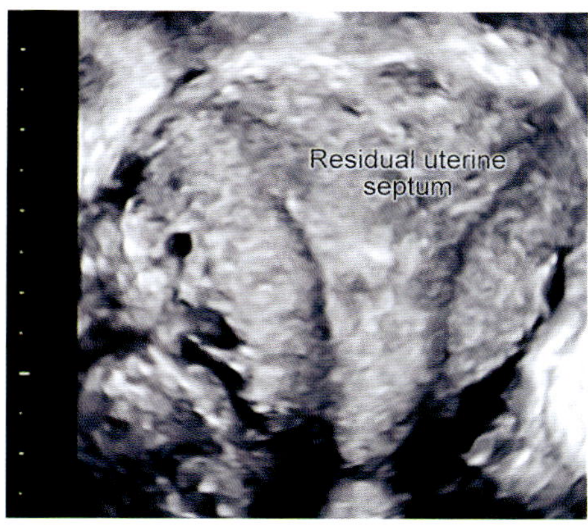

Fig. 3.23: Three-dimensional (3D) ultrasound of the uterus showing a residual uterine septum.

couple then underwent treatment with ovulation induction and timed sexual intercourse, which resulted in a successful pregnancy.

CONCLUSION

Uterine fibroids, particularly submucosal and intermural, adenomyosis and congenital uterine anomalies, can all be associated with subfertility. Transvaginal ultrasound is the main tool used for diagnoses of these conditions. Two-dimensional ultrasound can be used to diagnose intramural and subserosal fibroids and adenomyosis, and may raise the suspicion of submucous fibroids or congenital uterine anomalies. Three-dimensional ultrasound is the gold standard for diagnosis of congenital uterine anomalies and improves the detection of adenomyosis. Two-dimensional or 3D SIS increases the diagnostic accuracy for determining pathologies that affect the endometrial cavity such as submucous fibroids.

Submucosal fibroids should be removed hysteroscopically if type 0 or 1, and as a combined procedure if type 2 to improve fertility outcomes. Consideration should be given to the removal of intramural fibroids particularly over 4 cm, and if there has been pregnancy loss or failed fertility treatment before. Laparoscopic myomectomy may be the better technique if there is sufficient expertise, but the evidence is not strong enough to recommend it over open myomectomy completely. In those women, not suitable for myomectomy, UAE may have a role to play.

Surgical management of adenomyosis is complex and associated with increased risk of uterine rupture in subsequent pregnancies. It should only be offered where there is sufficient expertise and with consideration of the risks, in those women with previously unsuccessful fertility treatment.

Careful consideration of previous history and the risk of surgery also need to be taken into account for those women with congenital uterine anomalies, as there is insufficient evidence to recommend metroplasty routinely, although it may be of benefit to some women.

KEY POINTS

- Transvaginal ultrasound is the method of choice for imaging the uterus
- Three-dimensional ultrasound is the gold standard for diagnosing congenital uterine anomalies
- Saline infusion sonography should be used for evaluating the uterine cavity in particular assessing submucosal fibroids prior to surgery
- Type 0 and type 1 submucosal fibroids should be removed hysteroscopically in a subfertility patient
- Three-dimensional ultrasound may improve the sonographic diagnosis of adenomyosis
- Septate and subseptate uteri are associated with subfertility
- Removal of the septum may improve pregnancy rates in subfertile women

REFERENCES

1. Van den Bosch T, Valentin L, Van Schoubroeck D, et al. Detection of intracavitary uterine pathology using offline analysis of three-dimensional ultrasound volumes: interobserver agreement and diagnostic accuracy. Ultrasound Obstet Gynecol. 2012;40:459-63.
2. Ryan GL, Syrop CH, Van Voorhis BJ. Role, epidemiology, and natural history of benign uterine mass lesions. Clin Obstet Gynecol. 2005;48:312-24.
3. Lee C, Salim R, Ofili-Yebovi D, et al. Reproducibility of the measurement of submucous fibroid protrusion into the uterine cavity using three-dimensional saline contrast sonohysterography. Ultrasound Obstet Gynecol. 2006;28:837-41.
4. Wamsteker K, De Blok S, Gallinat A, et al. Fibroids. In: Lewis BV, Magos AL (Eds). Endometrial Ablation. Edinburgh: Churchill Livingstone; 1993. pp. 161-81.
5. Mavrelos D, Naftalin J, Hoo W, et al. Preoperative assessment of submucous fibroids by three-dimensional saline contrast sonohysterography. Ultrasound Obstet Gynecol. 2011;38:350-4.
6. Exacoustos C, Romanini ME, Amadio A, et al. Can grayscale and color Doppler sonography differentiate between uterine leiomyosarcoma and leiomyoma? J Clin Ultrasound. 2007;35:449-57.

7. Lasmar RB, Lasmar BP, Celeste RK, et al. A new system to classify submucous myomas: a Brazilian multicenter study. J Minim Invasive Gynecol. 2012:19(5):575-80.
8. Shokeir T, Abdelshaheed M, El-Shafie M, et al. Determinants of fertility and reproductive success after hysteroscopic septoplasty for women with unexplained primary infertility: a prospective analysis of 88 cases. Eur J Obstet Gynecol Reprod Biol. 2011;155:54-7.
9. Surrey ES, Minjarez DA, Stevens JM, et al. Effect of myomectomy on the outcome of assisted reproductive technologies. Fertil Steril. 2005;83:1473-9.
10. Mavrelos D, Ben-Nagi J, Davies A, et al. The value of preoperative treatment with GnRH analogues in women with submucous fibroids: a double-blind placebo-controlled randomized trial. Hum Reprod. 2010;25(9):2264-9.
11. Sunkara SK, Khairy M, El-Toukhy T, et al. The effect of intramural fibroids without uterine cavity involvement on the outcome of IVF treatment: a systematic review and meta-analysis. Hum Reprod. 2010;25:418-29.
12. Hart R, Khalaf Y, Yeong CT, et al. A prospective controlled study of the effect of intramural uterine fibroids on the outcome of assisted conception. Hum Reprod. 2001;16:2411-7.
13. Oliveira FG, Abdelmassih VG, Diamond MP, et al. Impact of subserosal and intramural uterine fibroids that do not distort the endometrial cavity on the outcome of in vitro fertilization-intracytoplasmic sperm injection. Fertil Steril. 2004;81:582-7.
14. Casini ML, Rossi F, Agostini R, et al. Effects of the position of fibroids on fertility. Gynecol Endocrinol. 2006;22:106-9.
15. Campo S, Campo V, Benagiano G. Adenomyosis and infertility. Reprod Biomed Online. 2012;24:35-46.
16. Metwally M, Cheong YC, Horne AW. Surgical treatment of fibroids for subfertility. Cochrane Database Syst Rev. 2012;11:CD003857.
17. Jin C, Hu Y, Chen XC, et al. Laparoscopic versus open myomectomy—a meta-analysis of randomized controlled trials. Eur J Obstet Gynecol Reprod Biol. 2009;145(1):14-21.
18. Homer H, Saridogan E. Uterine artery embolization for fibroids is associated with an increased risk of miscarriage. Fertil Steril. 2010;94:324-30.
19. Kepkep K, Tuncay YA, Göynümer G, et al. Transvaginal sonography in the diagnosis of adenomyosis: which findings are most accurate? Ultrasound Obstet Gynecol. 2007;30:341-5.
20. Exacoustos C, Brienza L, Di Giovanni A, et al. Adenomyosis: three-dimensional sonographic findings of the junctional zone and correlation with histology. Ultrasound Obstet Gynecol. 2011;37:471-9.
21. Fujishita A, Masuzaki H, Khan KN, et al. Modified reduction surgery for adenomyosis. A preliminary report of the transverse H incision technique. Gynecol Obstet Invest. 2004;57(3):132-8.
22. Osada H, Silber S, Kakinuma T, et al. Surgical procedure to conserve the uterus for future pregnancy in patients suffering from massive adenomyosis. Reprod Biomed Online. 2011;22(1):94-9.
23. Chan YY, Jayaprakasan K, Zamora J, et al. The prevalence of congenital uterine anomalies in unselected and high-risk populations: a systematic review. Hum Reprod Update. 2011;17:761-71.
24. Saravelos SH, Cocksedge KA, Li TC. Prevalence and diagnosis of congenital uterine anomalies in women with reproductive failure: a critical appraisal. Hum Reprod Update. 2008;14:415-29.
25. Salim R, Regan L, Woelfer B, et al. A comparative study of the morphology of congenital uterine anomalies in women with and without a history of recurrent first trimester miscarriage. Hum Reprod. 2003;18(1):162-6.
26. Chan YY, Jayaprakasan K, Tan A, et al. Reproductive outcomes in women with congenital uterine anomalies: a systematic review. Ultrasound Obstet Gynecol. 2011;38: 371-82.
27. Ercan CM, Coksuer H, Pehlivan H, et al. Saline infusion sonography in the accurate diagnosis of a rudimentary horn pregnancy. J Obstet Gynaecol. 2012;32:311-2.
28. Woelfer B, Salim R, Banerjee S, et al. Reproductive outcomes in women with congenital uterine anomalies detected by three-dimensional ultrasound screening. Obstet Gynecol. 2001;98(6):1099-103.
29. Grimbizis GF, Gordts S, Di Spiezio Sardo A, et al. The ESHRE/ESGE consensus on the classification of female genital tract congenital anomalies. Hum Reprod. 2013;28:2032-44.
30. Ludwin A, Ludwin I. Comparison of the ESHRE-ESGE and ASRM classifications of Müllerian duct anomalies in everyday practice. Hum Reprod. 2015;30(3):569-80.
31. Tomaževič T, Ban-Frangež H, Virant-Klun I, et al. Septate, subseptate and arcuate uterus decrease pregnancy and live birth rates in IVF/ICSI. Reprod Biomed Online. 2010;21(5):700-5.
32. Kadan Y, Romano S. Rudimentary horn pregnancy diagnosed by ultrasound and treated by laparoscopy—a case report and review of the literature. J Minim Invasive Gynecol. 2008;15:527-30.

Chapter

4

Assessment of Uterine Cavity

Jane Stewart

Chapter Outline

- Introduction
- Endometrial Cavity on Ultrasound Scan
- Abnormalities of the Endometrium
- Structural Abnormalities of the Uterus
- Reporting Endometrial Findings on Ultrasound Scanning of the Uterus
- Other Ultrasound Modalities
- Conclusion
- Key Points

INTRODUCTION

The normal endometrium is a dynamic tissue, which changes on a daily basis in response to the hormone changes of the hypothalamo-pituitary-ovarian (HPO) axis. The sole function of the endometrium is to provide a suitable milieu and surface to allow implantation of the developing embryo when it arrives in the uterine cavity in order to establish a pregnancy. Thus, the changes occurring in the endometrium are exquisitely timed and tuned to ovulation, allowing a narrow window of opportunity for implantation to occur. These changes are far from fully understood, and diagnostic tests to establish implantation problems are lacking in the armamentarium of infertility tests. While ultrasound scanning can be used to observe the structural and textural changes of the endometrium, these observations provide a poor surrogate for the subtleties of endometrial biochemical function. That is not to say that ultrasound does not have a place in the detection of endometrial abnormalities but its limitations must be acknowledged.

This chapter describes the ultrasound monitoring of the endometrium in its normal physiological cycle and where abnormalities of this may be of importance. Moreover, the pathologies relevant to fertility, which can be diagnosed or assessed by the use of ultrasound in its various modalities, are highlighted. Pregnancy-related endometrial changes are described in relation to findings before the appearance of the gestational sac or in the case of ectopic gestation. Ultrasonically detectable pregnancy is described in full elsewhere. This chapter concentrates on "standard" two-dimensional (2D) ultrasound readily available to ultrasonographers working in the field. Three-dimensional (3D), Doppler and contrast modalities have, however, also been discussed.

ENDOMETRIAL CAVITY ON ULTRASOUND SCAN

Most fertility-related pelvic ultrasound examinations are undertaken transvaginally. The general process of setting up for and undertaking a vaginal scan are described in Chapters 1 and 2; however, to attain appropriate insight into the endometrium, it is essential that a scan is properly set up and the sonographer appropriately trained.

General assessment of the endometrium is undertaken with examination of the uterus; however, it is worth more than a cursory look and indeed more than a simple assessment of endometrial thickness (ET). Moreover, it is essential to have appropriate background information—menstrual history, current use of any hormonal preparations, and date of the last menstrual period (LMP)—in order to interpret endometrial scan findings (Box 4.1).

Ultrasound of the uterus is undertaken in both the longitudinal and transverse planes. A second look concentrating on the endometrial cavity may be very revealing. The

Box 4.1: Information required to interpret findings on ultrasound examination of the endometrium

- Premenopausal or postmenopausal
- Date of last menstrual period
- Length or regularity of menstrual cycle
- Use of hormonal preparations
- Any relevant symptoms

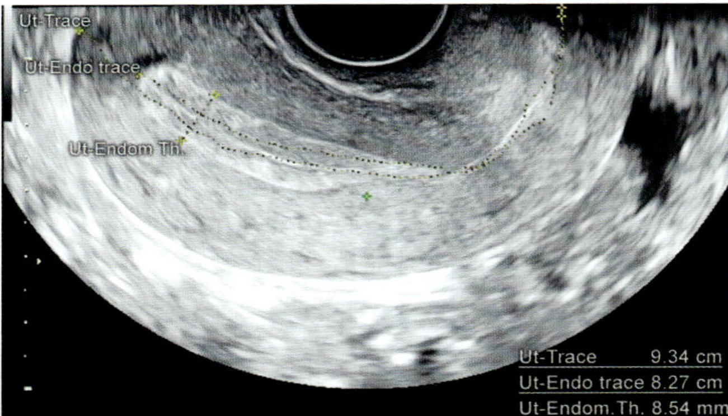

Fig. 4.1: Longitudinal view of uterus with linear echo.

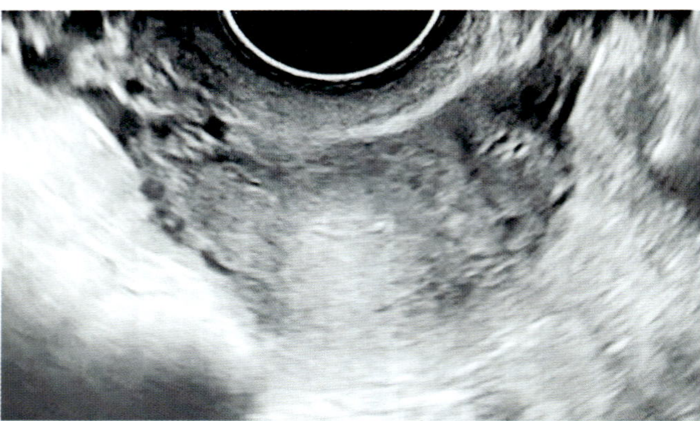

Fig. 4.3: Transverse section of uterus: At uterocervical junction.

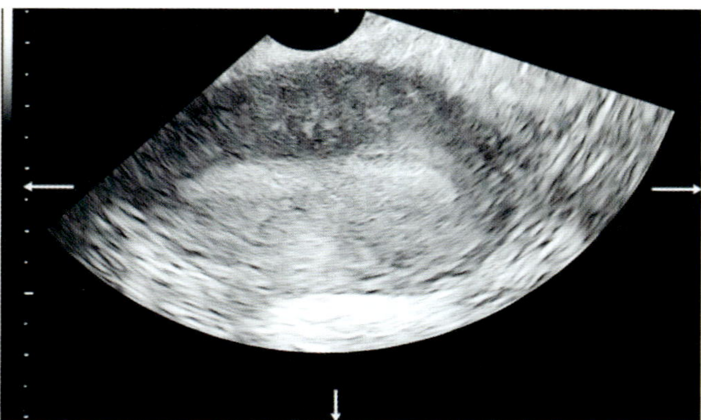

Fig. 4.5: Transverse section of uterus: At fundus.

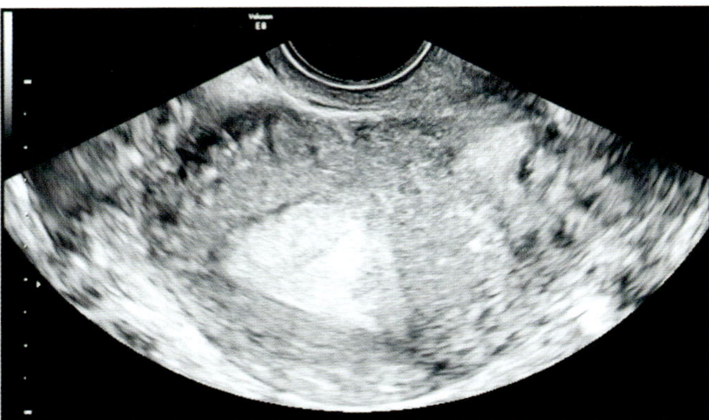

Fig. 4.2: Oblique view of the uterus demonstrating triangular shape of endometrial cavity.

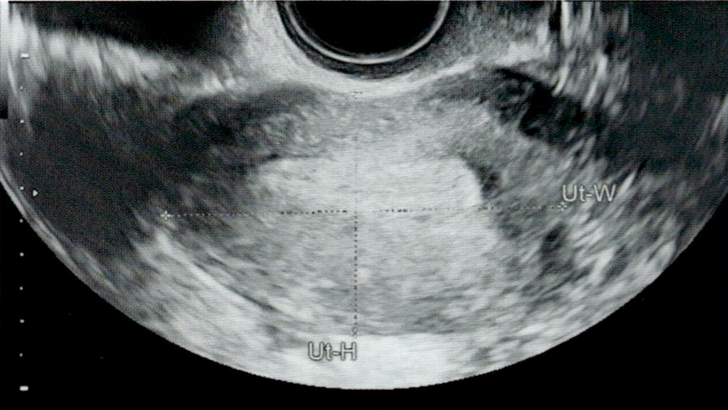

Fig. 4.4: Transverse section of uterus: Mid cavity.

endometrium lines the uterine cavity and appears as two layers of tissue meeting at an interface, which can generally be seen as a bright midline reflective echo (Fig. 4.1). The endometrium itself is a flattened triangular shape, filling the cavity from the endocervix caudally to the fundus (Fig. 4.2), extending outward toward the tubal ostia at either cornu. The transverse view demonstrates the ovoid anteroposterior shape of the endometrium and can be followed from its narrowest point at the uterocervical junction to the fundus where its extensions into the cornua give way to the intramural portions of the Fallopian tubes (Figs. 4.3 to 4.5). It follows the contours of the myometrium and careful examination may demonstrate a variation in its shape in keeping with uterine structural abnormalities.

The Endometrial (Menstrual) Cycle

While the first day of the period is generally known as day 1 of the menstrual cycle, menses is shedding of the endometrium as a result of loss of hormonal support following ovulation that does not result in pregnancy. Shedding of the so-called functional layer of the endometrium occurs at menstruation leaving the lower basal layer adjacent to the myometrium from which regeneration of the endometrial tissue occurs. Following menstruation, the endometrium is thin and appears as a single linear bright echo in both longitudinal and transverse planes on ultrasound scan (Figs. 4.6 and 4.7). There may be a fluid or mixed echogenic area within the endometrial cavity, which separates the thin endometrial surfaces and represents blood, clot, and debris within the cavity (Fig. 4.8). This clears as menses progresses.

As the ovary enters the follicular phase, the developing follicles increasingly produce estrogen, which stimulates regeneration of the endometrium and it proliferates over the following days. The proliferative endometrium is characterized by a relative sonolucency and appears as a so-called triple echo (Fig. 4.9). Complimenting this finding there is likely to be a demonstrable dominant follicle in one of the ovaries (Fig. 4.10). The central echo is that of the endometrial surface interface, with a less echogenic thickening layer adjacent and a defining bright echo at the junction with myometrium. Following ovulation in response to progesterone production by the corpus luteum, the endometrium becomes denser, sometimes consolidating and appearing slightly thinner but with the development of echogenicity from the peripheries inward (Figs. 4.11 and 4.12). This finding corresponds with and typifies the secretory phase of the menstrual cycle and a corpus luteum will be present in the ovary (Fig. 4.13).

Endometrial Thickness

In the postmenopausal woman, an acceptable "unstimulated" endometrial echo is considered to be less than or

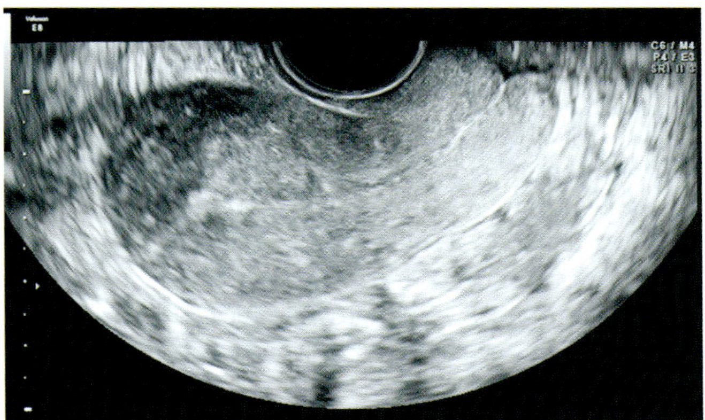

Fig. 4.6: Longitudinal view of postmenstrual uterus with thinned endometrium.

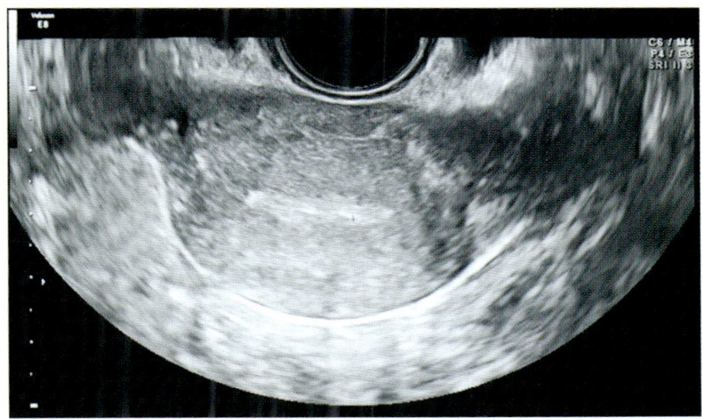

Fig. 4.7: Transverse view of postmenstrual uterus with thinned endometrium.

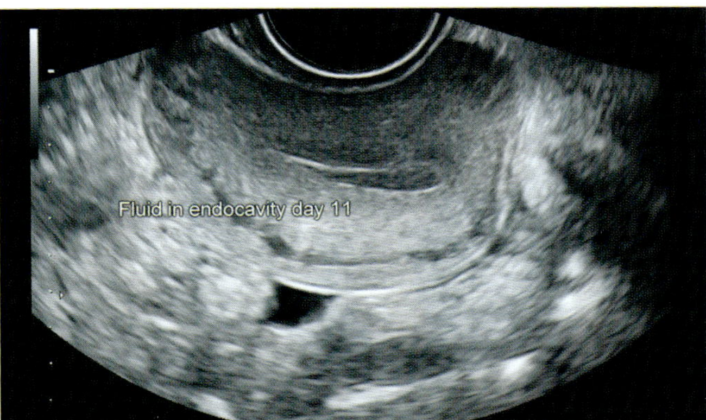

Fig. 4.8: Longitudinal view of uterus with fluid in cavity and thin endometrium.

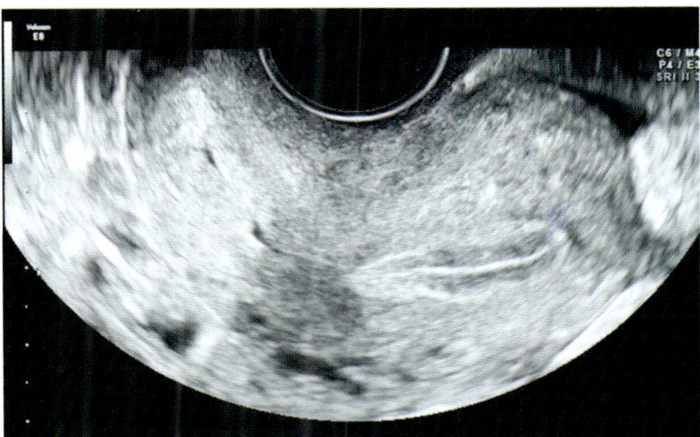

Fig. 4.9: Longitudinal view of proliferative endometrium.

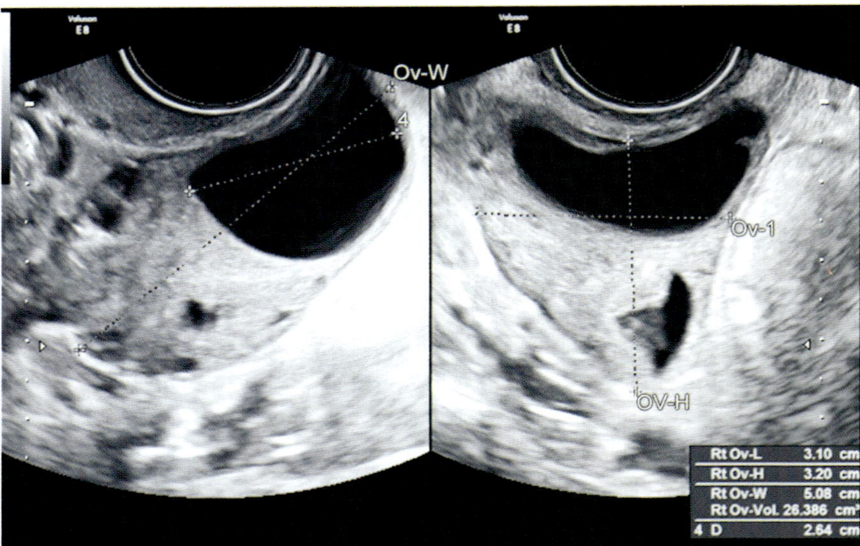

Fig. 4.10: Mature follicle in normal ovary.

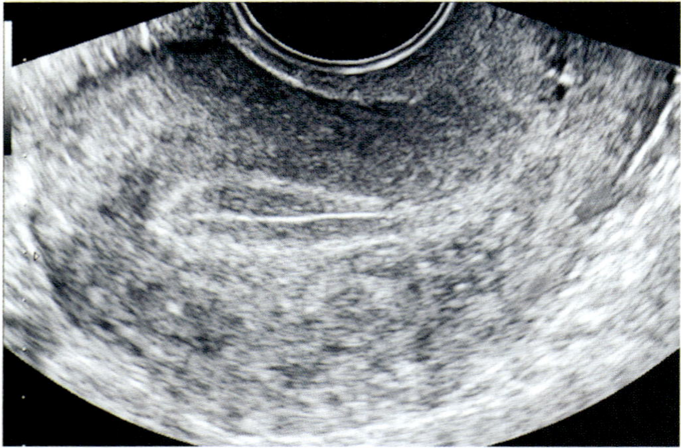

Fig. 4.11: Longitudinal view of early luteal endometrium with peripheral echogenicity.

equal to 4 mm.[1] A postmenstrual endometrial echo may approximate to this and a thin endometrium after menses is considered to exclude significant hyperplasia as well as being used to confirm downregulation in many fertility treatments (Fig. 4.14). During the proliferative phase, the endometrium develops its functional layer gradually becoming thicker with a typical ET of 10–15 mm at midcycle. Following ovulation, the ET changes little although there is occasionally an apparent consolidation or alternatively a possible further increase in thickness until the endometrium is again shed at menses.

The measurement of ET is often used as a surrogate of function. An endometrium, which responds to hormonal changes by appropriate expansion, may be presumed to function normally, although clearly this may be far from the case. Through assisted reproductive technologies (ARTs), it has been considered that an endometrium which does not reach "sufficient" thickness is less likely to allow implantation of a good-quality embryo.[2,3] The identification of a lower threshold, below which pregnancy will not occur, remains elusive as pregnancies have been reported in women with relatively thin endometria sometimes with high rates.[4,5] It has been suggested in addition that an ET of over 14 mm may also not function normally reducing the chance of successful ART pregnancy,[6] although others disagree.[7,8] A recent meta-analysis of ET and ART pregnancy concluded that there is no clinical significance to the finding of a mean ET 1 mm greater in pregnancy versus nonpregnancy cycles;[9] however, this does not preclude the possibility that there is a lower (or upper) threshold beyond which a woman may be considered to have an implantation problem. Others suggest that it is the rate of expansion of ET that is important rather than the final measurement.[10] While this has been observed in ART cycles, less is known about the implications of a thin endometrium in natural conception and the nature of any pathology inferred is unknown.[11] The range of ET seen in midcycle is large, and a cyclical maximum appropriate for implantation is undefined, with 7–15 mm easily within the norm.

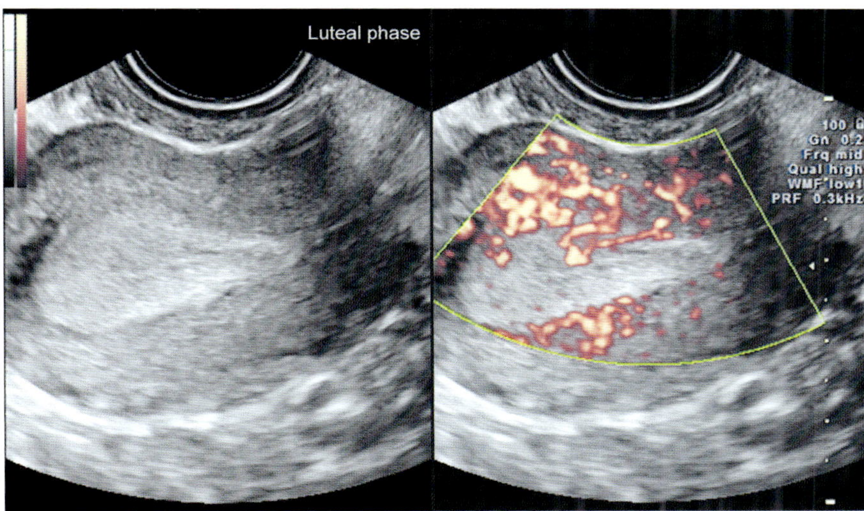

Fig. 4.12: Late luteal phase longitudinal view.

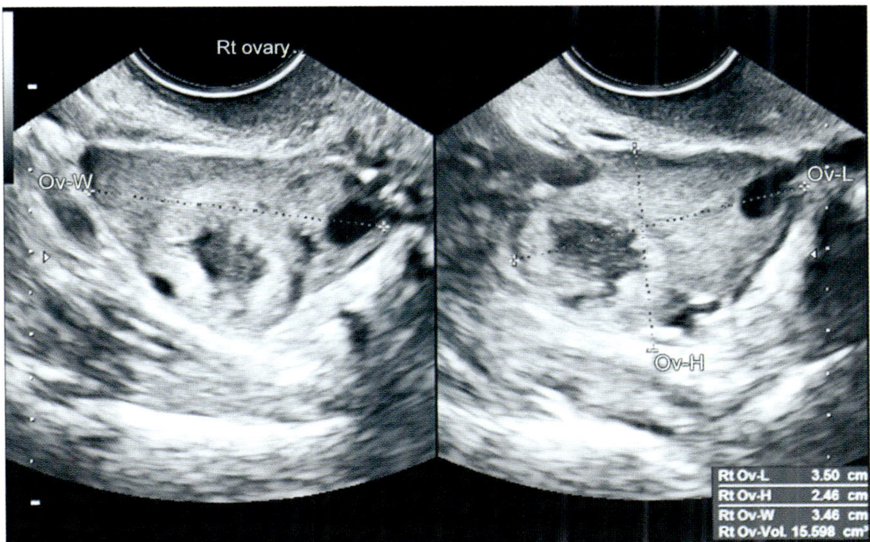

Fig. 4.13: Typical corpus luteum.

Measuring Endometrial Thickness

Since the endometrium lines the complete uterine cavity, measuring its thickness is open to significant variation resulting in error of interpretation, an oblique view, for instance will overestimate the measurement. In order to ensure both intraoperative and interoperative reproducibility, a standard approach is necessary. Thus, to maintain consistency and ensure the best value from the measurement, ET should be measured in the longitudinal (sagittal) view, midway along the cavity taking an anteroposterior measurement perpendicular to the midline echo. The measurement should reach both echo margins (Figs. 4.15 and 4.16).

Early Pregnancy Changes

Human chorionic gonadotropin (hCG) production by an early conceptus is responsible for the maintenance of the corpus luteum. The consequent continued production of estrogen and progesterone maintains the secretory endometrial integrity past the time where menses would otherwise have taken place and results in so-called decidualization. Ultrasonography of decidualized endometrium reveals

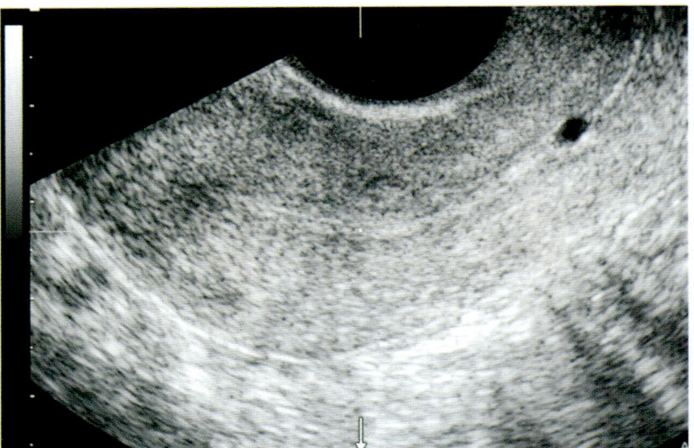

Fig. 4.14: Longitudinal view of postmenses thin endometrium.

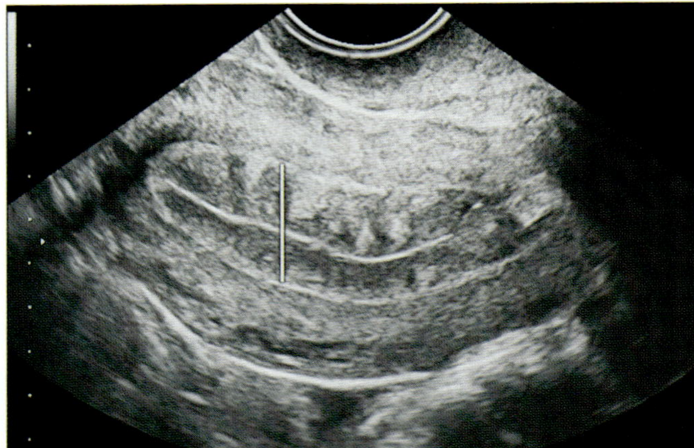

Fig. 4.15: Incorrect measurement.

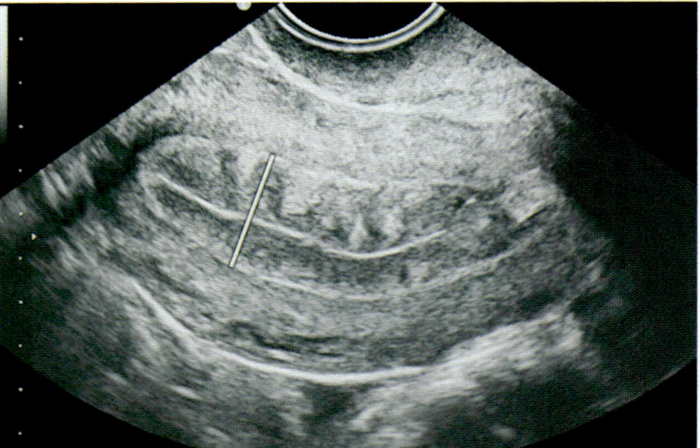

Fig. 4.16: Correct measurement.

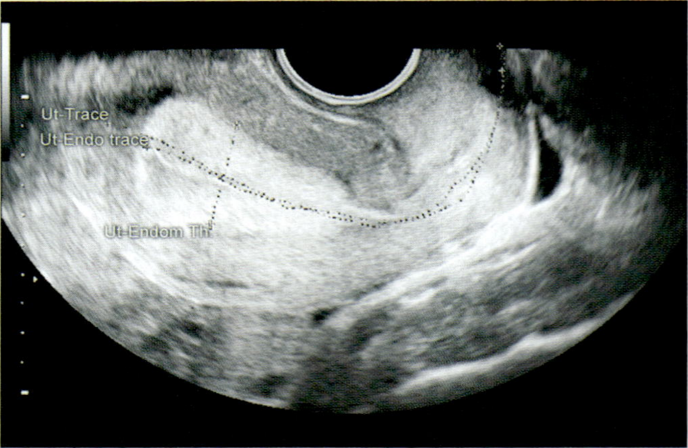

Fig. 4.17: Longitudinal view of thick decidualized endometrium.

a dense, thickened structure similar to that seen in the luteal phase but may be much thicker (20–30 mm) (Fig. 4.17).[12]

After about a week from the expected missed period (fifth week of gestation), a gestational sac may be seen within the uterus (Figs. 4.18A and B). Prior to this appearance, however, the decidualized endometrium with an intrauterine gestation is indistinguishable from that occurring, when the pregnancy is extrauterine or ectopic. Hence, there are no definitive endometrial features to confirm the site of the gestation at this stage.

ABNORMALITIES OF THE ENDOMETRIUM

Since the endometrium is a sensitive tissue responding to hormonal stimulation, any abnormalities of the HPO axis will have a downstream effect on the endometrium. Hence postmenopausal women, including young women exhibiting premature ovarian failure without hormone replacement, would be expected to have a thin, unstimulated endometrium comparable to a postmenstrual appearance. Stimulation by exogenous hormones or aberrant endogenous secretion will result in the corresponding "physiological" appearance. Persistent noncyclical hormonal stimulation can ultimately result in pathological change within the endometrium itself. A prime example of this would be endometrial hyperplasia resulting from unopposed tonic estrogen secretion by the ovaries of an anovulatory woman with polycystic ovarian syndrome. The hyperplastic endometrium can become grossly thickened resulting in breakthrough "dysfunctional" bleeding, mitotic change can occur and subsequently, malignant change. Endometrial appearances in this situation will not fit with the hormonal milieu and hence a mismatched ultrasound appearance is a cause for concern. Moreover,

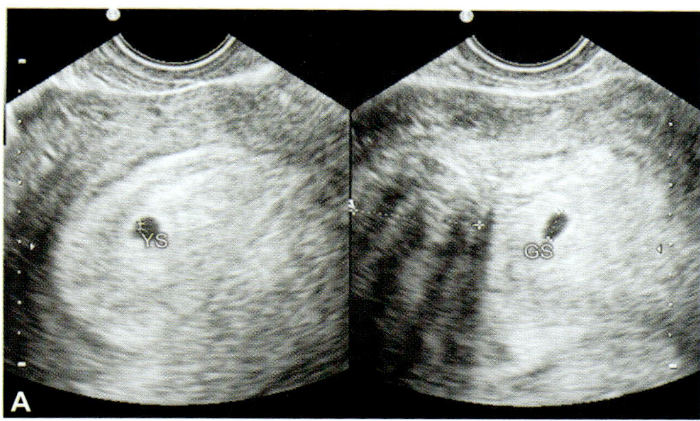

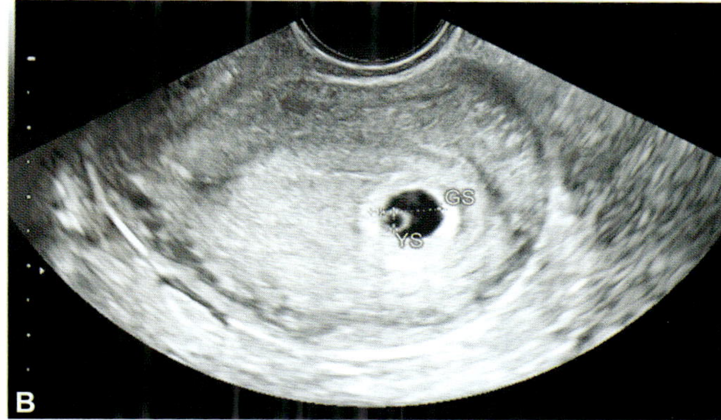

Figs. 4.18A and B: Longitudinal view of endometrium with gestational sac.

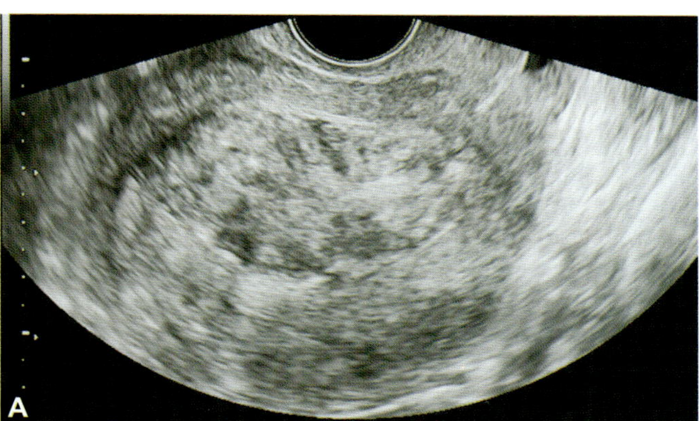

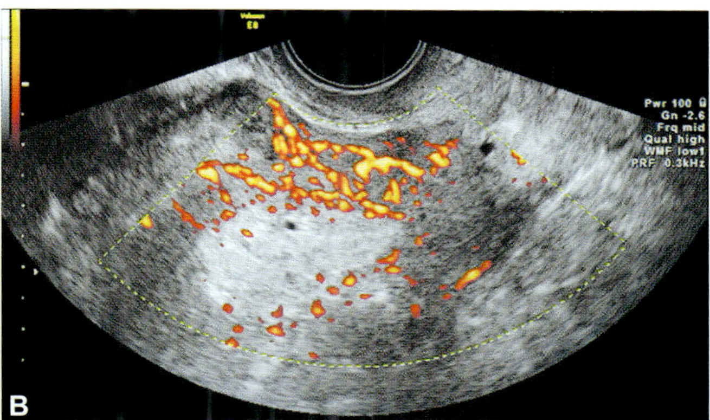

Figs. 4.19A and B: Longitudinal view of endometrial hyperplasia.

primary abnormalities of the endometrium and endometrial cavity may be observed at ultrasound scan which may then require further elucidation and management.

Endometrial Thickness and Texture

In a woman who does not exhibit a regular ovulatory cycle, a thick endometrium may be the result of hyperplasia and on occasion endometrial carcinoma. This is a particular concern in women with oligo- or amenorrhea or dysfunctional uterine bleeding in association with polycystic ovarian syndrome. The tonic production of estrogen in these women without regular progesterone withdrawal may result in endometrial overgrowth, hyperplasia, and malignant change. It is therefore worth noting and managing in this setting. The hyperplastic endometrium appears thickened often over 15 mm with a patchy appearance of mixed echogenicity so that the triple echo is not seen and the endometrial interface may not be well defined (Figs. 4.19A and B). Such an endometrium will not be fully shed even after a bleed induced by exogenous progesterone treatment and should be further investigated and managed to exclude the presence of or development of carcinoma in situ. A frank carcinoma may also be detected in this situation by extension of the "fluffy" endometrium beyond the myometrial margin denoting invasion into the muscle layer (Figs. 4.20A and B).

Adenomyosis may also be apparent on ultrasound of the uterus, marking the benign presence of endometrial-type tissue within the myometrium. The appearance is not always easy to define but may be seen as pools of glandular-like tissue, sometimes blurring the endometrial-myometrial interface making the ET appear greater than it is or on occasion being mistaken for an atypical fibroid (Fig. 4.21).

An endometrial cavity which appears heterogeneous in thickness and texture may occur when there are endometrial adhesions and synechiae as may be found in

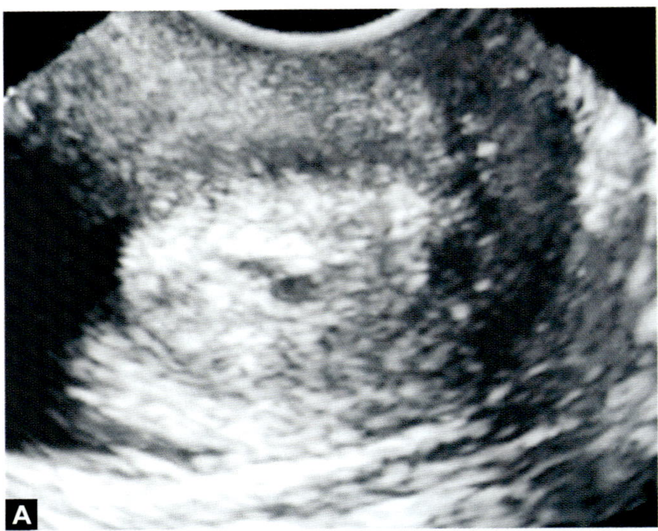

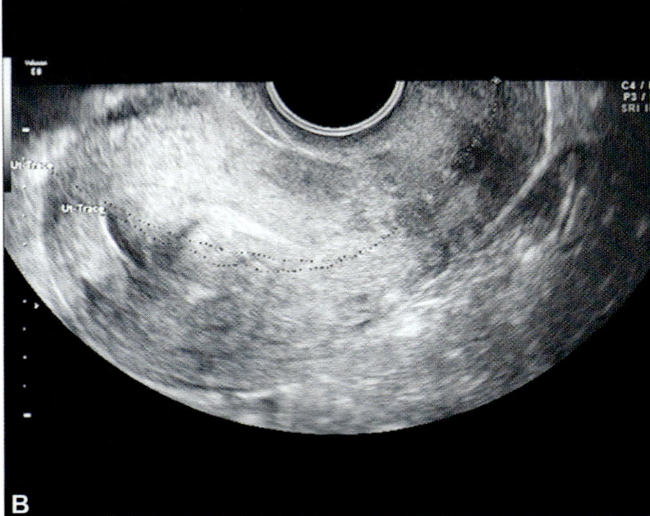

Figs. 4.20A and B: Longitudinal view of endometrial malignancy with loss of endomyometrial junction.

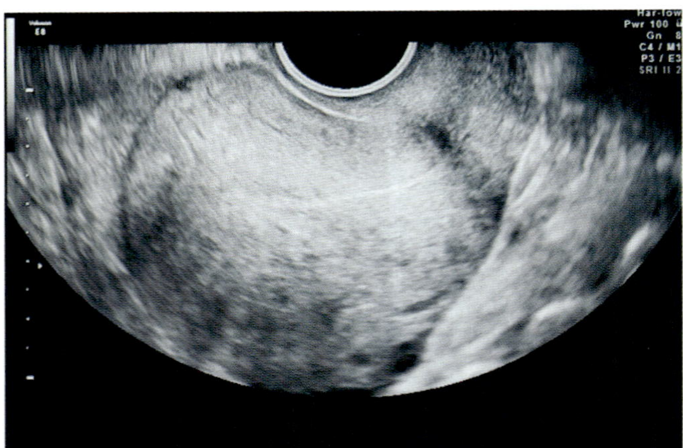

Fig. 4.21: Adenomyosis uterus. Note asymmetrical wall thickness.

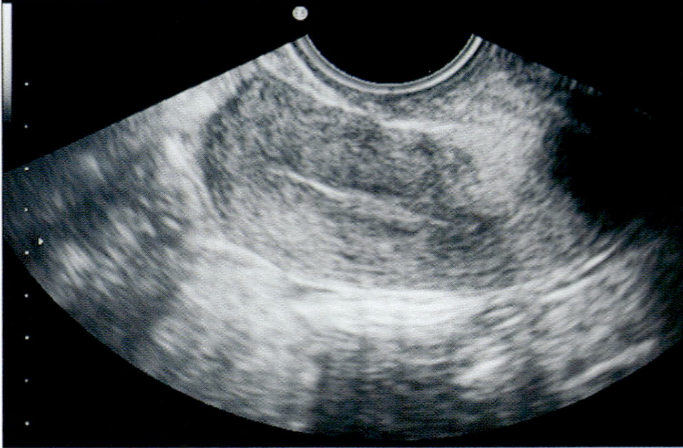

Fig. 4.22: Asherman's syndrome. Note heterogenous thin endometrium with bright linear echo.

Asherman's syndrome and warrants further assessment in the infertile woman (Fig. 4.22).

Endometrial Assessment in Infertility Treatment

The assessment of ET as a marker of function is a tool most commonly used in fertility treatment (discussed previously). In this setting, it may be used to determine the duration of treatment, for example, duration of estrogen stimulation in an egg donation or frozen embryo cycle where exogenous estrogen is administered to replace ovarian hormones causing endometrial proliferation. Only when sufficient thickness (usually at least 6 mm) is achieved, would embryo transfer be planned and progesterone prescribed to convert the endometrium to a secretory and receptive state, embryo transfer being timed accordingly.

Endometrial thickness and texture are also assessed through the stimulation phase of an in vitro fertilization (IVF) cycle and the loss of the triple echo may denote a lower chance of pregnancy.[13] It is unlikely that this is revealing an abnormality of the endometrium; however, as much as a normal response to premature progesterone secretion from stimulated ovaries associated with lower pregnancy rates.[14] Whether or not such a change is evident enough to abandon embryo transfer will remain a dilemma for fertility practitioners as long as the outcome for frozen embryo transfer remains lower than that of fresh. With progress in freezing techniques and improved quality of frozen-thawed embryos, this may become a more important point of assessment[15] and a combination of thin endometrium with a dense echo may be prognostic enough to make that recommendation,[16] although previous attempts to "score" the endometrium for implantation on these parameters have not been helpful.[17] Occasionally, despite high levels of endogenous (or exogenous) hormones, the endometrium fails to achieve the desired thickness. Not only there is a presumption that the function of the endometrium is compromised (lower-pregnancy rates) but also there is a "fault" in the endometrium itself causing this perceived deficiency. While it is possible that this is the case in some women perhaps as a result of receptor abnormalities or cellular response capabilities; there is no good physiological, molecular, or even histological data to corroborate such assumptions. It is not appropriate therefore to extrapolate a thin endometrial measurement to mean a fundamental abnormality of endometrial function and more importantly that any therapeutic measure that increases ET will hence improve that function. This simplistic view has nevertheless been examined with studies assessing the use of aspirin and sildenafil citrate (Viagra) amongst others in attempts to achieve increased ET by affecting, for example, vascular change in the endometrial basal vessels. While a single study on Viagra suggests some benefit in women with thin endometria,[18] aspirin has not met with a successful increase in pregnancy rates,[19] serving to confirm the disassociation between ET and function. Thus, while it is pertinent to examine and record ET and texture for prognostic reasons, care should be taken not to overinterpret the significance of the result.

STRUCTURAL ABNORMALITIES OF THE UTERUS

While 3D ultrasound and other imaging such as magnetic resonance imaging (MRI) can provide explicit structural information, a fastidious 2D scan of the endometrium may provide the first clues to a uterine structural abnormality. While the management of these abnormalities is generally conservative and the pros and cons of surgical resolution are beyond the scope of this chapter, it remains important to be aware of such findings in the fertility clinic not least for the management of subsequent pregnancy. While structural abnormalities, like congenital anomalies, uterine fibroids and adenomyosis, are detailed in Chapter 3, this chapter briefly discusses these pathologies, but focuses mainly on endometrial polyps, intrauterine adhesions, and methods to evaluate uterine cavity.

Congenital Abnormalities of the Uterus

In the longitudinal view, spanning across the body of the uterus may reveal the presence of a midline abnormality as the fundal portion appears to dip down from one cornu at the midline and reappear rising to the contralateral. This may represent a frank bicornuate uterus if the myometrial fundal profile follows suit (Figs. 4.23 and 4.24) or depending on the breadth and depth of the apparent defect a heart-shaped cavity (broad) or midline septum, the latter possibly evident through the entire length of the cavity and moreover, if carefully imaged, two fully separate cavities leading to separate cervical canals may be seen.

When a transverse image is viewed (Fig. 4.25), the shape of the endometrium can be further elucidated. As discussed earlier, at the fundus, two separate endometrial

Fig. 4.23: Bicornuate uterus: Change in fundal length on spanning.

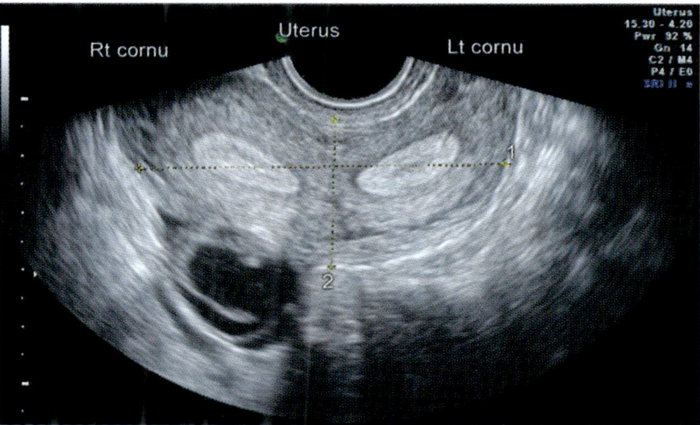

Fig. 4.24: Oblique view: Bicornuate uterus.

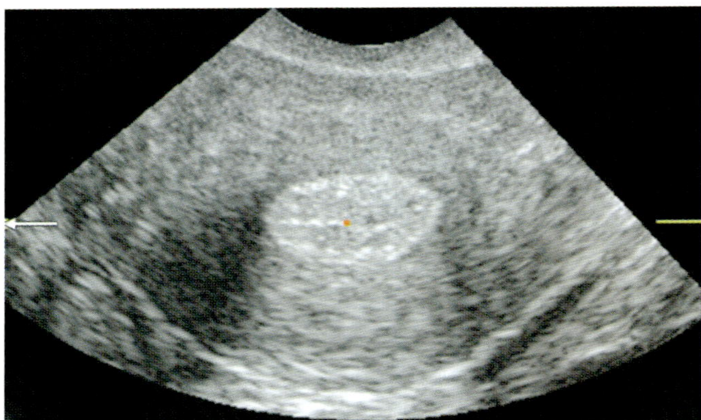

Fig. 4.25: Transverse section: Normal cavity.

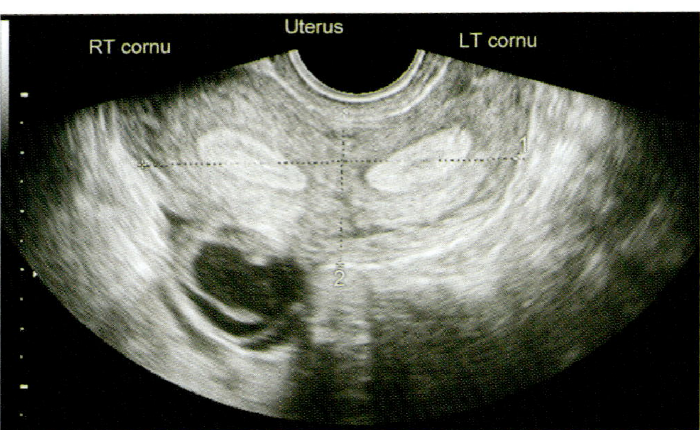

Fig. 4.26: Transverse section of uterus showing two endometrial complexes suggesting a duplication abnormality.

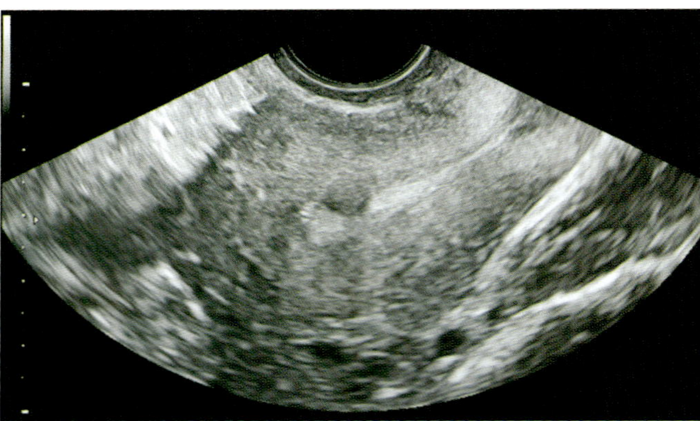

Fig. 4.27: Submucous fibroid.

echoes may be seen denoting incomplete fusion of the cavity (Fig. 4.26). This may run the full length of the endometrium down to separate cervical canals or merge at some point. Again the myometrial echo viewed in tandem will give further information. On rare occasions, noncommunicating horns of hemiuterus may be identified sometimes exhibiting hematometrium, and then associated with cyclical pain or indeed hematometrium in the otherwise normal uterus of a young woman with an obstructive abnormality, e.g. imperforate hymen. However, clear the findings, it remains pertinent to consider further assessment; examination, imaging, and laparoscopy to fully understand the extent of the abnormality and related features (vaginal septum, renal tract anomalies, etc.).

Fibroids

While fibroids are, strictly speaking, myometrial in origin they may have an impact on the endometrial cavity. Submucosal fibroids by definition lie just below the endometrial basal layer pushing into the endometrial cavity (Fig. 4.27), similarly pedunculated intracavitary fibroids protrude into the uterine cavity lying between the endometrial surfaces (Figs. 4.28A and B). Both submucosal and intracavitary fibroids may thus distort the uterine cavity (as may large endometrial intramural fibroids) and may consequently have an effect on function. Although evidence for altered endometrial physiology in the presence of fibroids is lacking, the structural deformation of the uterine cavity may hinder implantation or pregnancy development and warrant further consideration. Previous systematic reviews indicated that submucosal fibroids and intramural fibroids regardless of whether they distort the endometrial cavity or not have a detrimental effect on fertility.[20,21] While removal of submucous fibroids confers benefits, the effect of surgical treatment to intramural fibroids is unclear.[20]

Endometrial Polyps

Endometrial polyps are the most common structural abnormalities of endometrium with its prevalence ranging from 10% in asymptomatic women to 26% in women with unexplained subfertility.[22] Endometrial polyps are generally benign tags of tissue forming within the endometrial cavity (Fig. 4.29). These may be single or multiple and can be detected at only a few millimeters in size but can grow to several centimeters. Importantly, their appearance may be transient, either disappearing after menses or only being evident at particular times of the menstrual cycle. This transience is particularly the case with small polyps less than 10 mm in size and which are

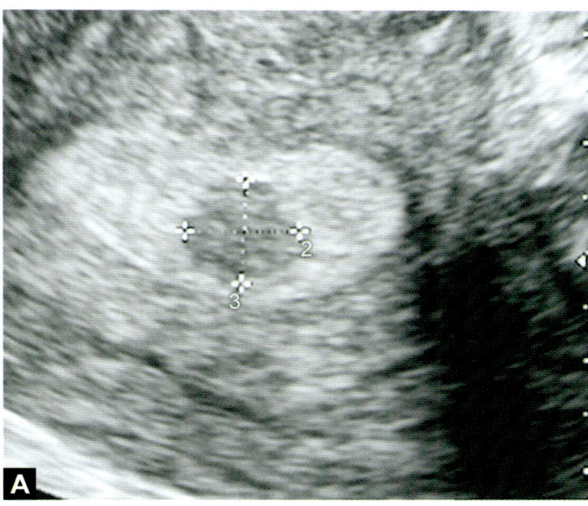

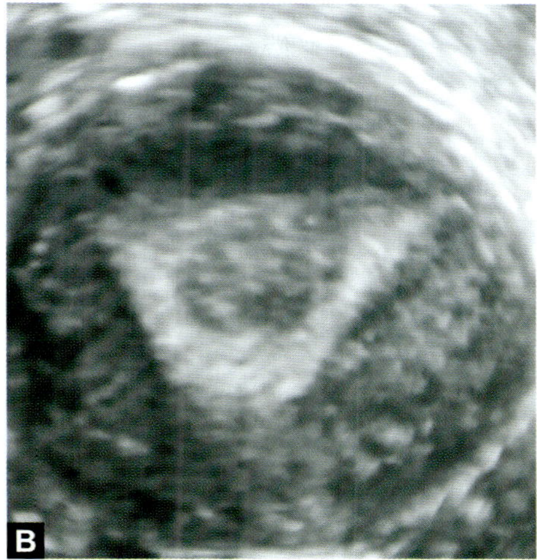

Figs. 4.28A and B: Intracavitary fibroid.

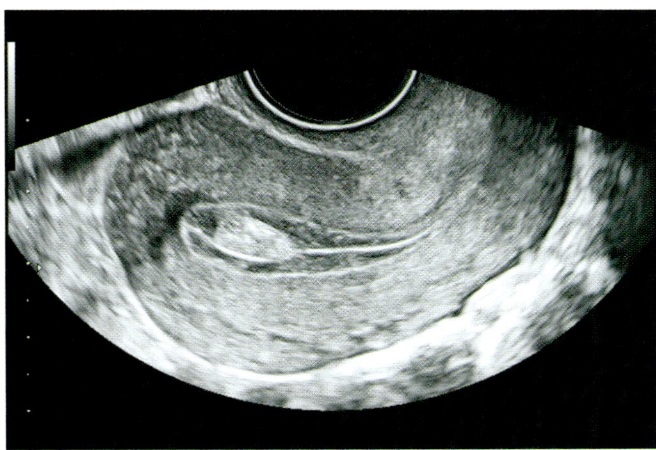

Fig. 4.29: Endometrial polyp.

notorious for "disappearing" when definitive diagnosis or treatment is attempted. This also raises the question of their importance in infertility with opinions varying from the need to seek and treat any apparent uterine anomaly to an acceptance that they are a physiological variant of proliferation which can be safely ignored. Pragmatically, it is appropriate to consider removal of larger (>1 cm) persistent polyps since, as for intracavitary fibroids, their physical presence may interfere with implantation as an intrauterine foreign body.[23] As polyps are relatively frequent in subfertile women, most clinicians recommend removal prior to commencement of any fertility treatment. While there is no robust evidence to support this, the only randomized controlled study of polypectomy versus polyp biopsy through hysteroscopy in an intrauterine insemination (IUI) population of 215 subfertile women reported a significant improvement in the pregnancy rate in the polypectomy group.[24] To this end, it is worthwhile detecting such structures at ultrasound assessment of the pelvis for fertility with consideration of further intervention. Small polyps may be best seen distorting a thin postmenstrual endometrium. Review at this time may also confirm their persistence since a transient polyp may be shed with the endometrium at menstruation and not reform.

On ultrasound, polyps are seen as small, well-defined masses within the endometrial cavity. They typically assume a slightly higher echogenicity than the endometrium itself. Small polyps may be best seen distorting a thin postmenstrual endometrium, or deshaping the smooth curve of the central line of the endometrium in proliferative phase. Review at this time may also confirm their persistence since a transient polyp may be shed with the endometrium at menstruation and not reform. Doppler ultrasound can be used to visualize feeding vessels to the polyp (the "pedicle sign") (Fig. 4.30) and improve the detection rate to a level comparable with hysteroscopy, studies suggest a sensitivity and specificity for color Doppler ultrasound of 95% and 80%, respectively. Saline infusion sonohysterography may also be used to improve the detection rate and reduce the number of false-positive results. It often helps to define the position and size of the polyp, which can allow surgeons to modify their approach and resect the larger, more broad-based polyps rather than list them for simple polypectomy.

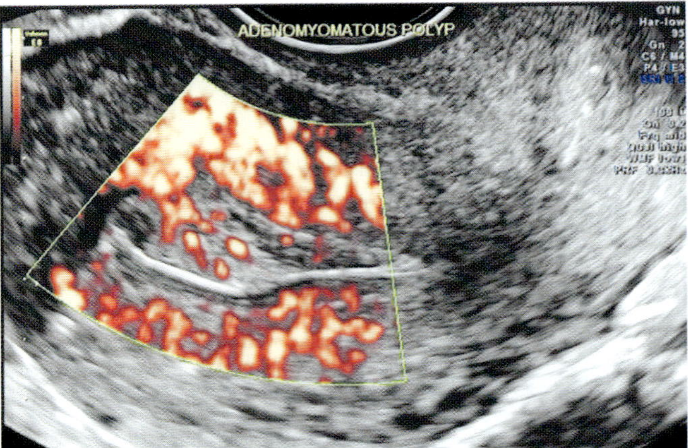

Fig. 4.30: Endometrial polyp with pedicle sign.

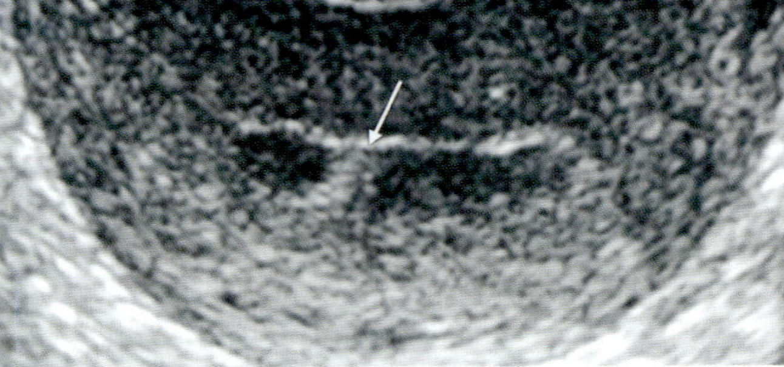

Fig. 4.31: Intrauterine adhesions (arrow).

Intrauterine Adhesions

Any inflammatory process can cause scarring and on occasion inflammation within the uterine cavity can cause adhesions. Previously, intrauterine adhesions were most commonly associated with vigorous curettage at so-called therapeutic dilatation and curettage (D&C) for menstrual problems or following surgical evacuation of pregnancy tissue. Dilatation and curettage is rarely undertaken in this way now and with gentler suction curettes the problem of adhesions is much less common. They can still occur after a formal endometrial ablation procedure and also following pregnancy-related infection, or uterine tuberculosis. The pathological appearance is of fibrous bands traversing the endometrial cavity with the formation of synechiae. In the menstruating woman, these may retain shed endometrial tissue and blood. Transvaginal ultrasound may not always reveal adhesions but a markedly damaged cavity; so-called Asherman's syndrome may demonstrate a mixed echogenic appearance with dense, thinner areas interspersed with thicker hypoechoic areas (Fig. 4.31), in keeping with the disordered appearance within the cavity seen at hysteroscopy. Saline infusion sonography (SIS) may be helpful in confirming the diagnosis with the ultrasound (Figs. 4.32A and B).

Other Intrauterine Findings

On occasion while examining the endometrium at ultrasound scan, other unexpected findings occur, e.g. intrauterine devices (IUDs) or portions of IUDs thought to have been removed, fragments of fetal bone, remnants from previous late miscarriages or terminations of pregnancy which can become embedded in the endometrium (Fig. 4.33), and of course on occasion and more happily an intrauterine pregnancy.

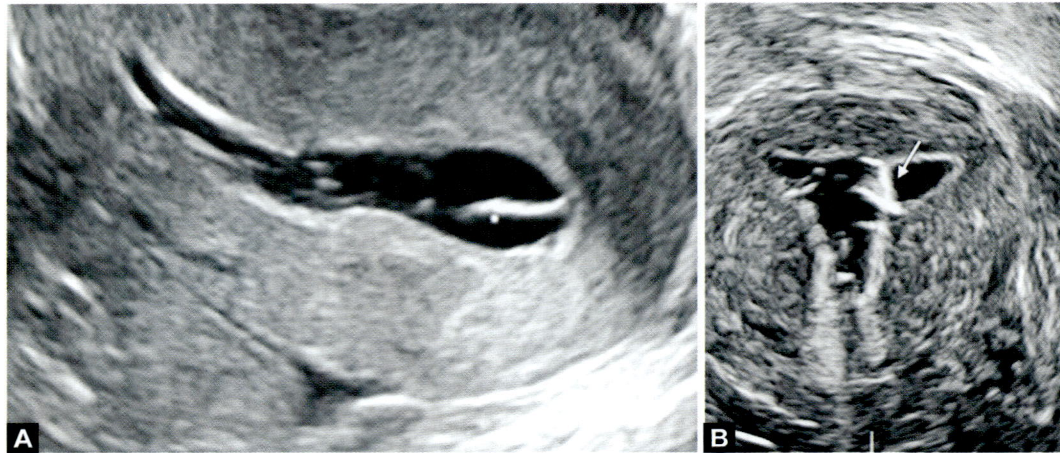

Figs. 4.32A and B: Intrauterine adhesions: Saline infusion sonography (SIS).

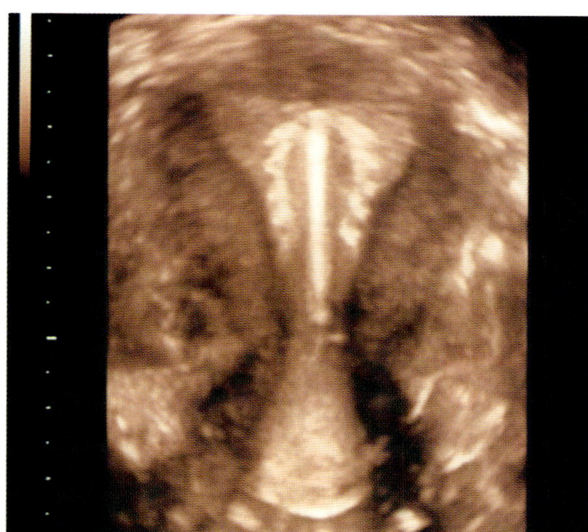

Fig. 4.33: Intrauterine device (IUD) in situ.

REPORTING ENDOMETRIAL FINDINGS ON ULTRASOUND SCANNING OF THE UTERUS

An individual undertaking pelvic assessment by ultrasound may be a trainee ultrasonographer undertaking the scan as a technical reporting exercise or a trained clinician who will make treatment decisions directly based on the scan as it is undertaken. In either case, information on the scan result should be appropriately recorded such that it need not be repeated by another practitioner in order to make appropriate ongoing clinical decisions.[23] Reporting methods may vary depending on the facilities available and may include pertinent images, still or video; however, the basic recorded information regarding endometrium should include both contextual information (Box 4.1) and findings (Box 4.2). Presenting complaint, menstrual status (including LMP), use of hormonal preparations as well as findings, ET, endometrial texture, and regularity of outline including any abnormal structural findings (including contour, polyps, and fibroids) are reported on endometrial ultrasound.

Box 4.2: Reporting on endometrial ultrasound

Contextual information (*see* Box 4.1)

Findings:

- Endometrial texture (triple echo, density, and uniformity)
- Outline (regular and clear)
- Structural abnormalities (contour, polyps, and fibroids—give measurements)
- Endometrial thickness

OTHER ULTRASOUND MODALITIES

Three-Dimensional Ultrasound of the Endometrium

Three-dimensional ultrasound is a tool useful in assessment of uterine structure in particular. While a good impression of a uterine structural abnormality can be obtained with 2D ultrasound, further refinement in diagnosis may be indicated. Three-dimensional ultrasound allows simultaneous display of three perpendicular (longitudinal, transverse, and coronal) planes. Due to its unique ability to demonstrate coronal plane, 3D ultrasound provides a clear structural view of the uterine shape and of course the uterine cavity defined by the endometrial tissue within it. The combined information can give an extremely good rendition of the abnormality[25] (Fig. 4.34). Three-dimensional ultrasound is similarly valuable in mapping the positions of fibroids including their impact on the endometrial cavity and in the diagnosis and assessment of endometrial polyps (Figs. 4.35 and 4.36).

With regard specifically to endometrial examination, 3D ultrasound confers the ability to estimate endometrial volume. Using the virtual organ computer-aided analysis (VOCAL) (GE Medical Systems, Zipf, Austria), a dedicated program for volume measurements, a 3D model of the endometrium can be generated by manually tracing the myometrial-endometrial contour as the dataset is rotated about its central axis through 180°. It may be considered that this may be a more valuable assessment of endometrial function than a simple ET measurement and probably, since it is a semiautomated calculation based on a

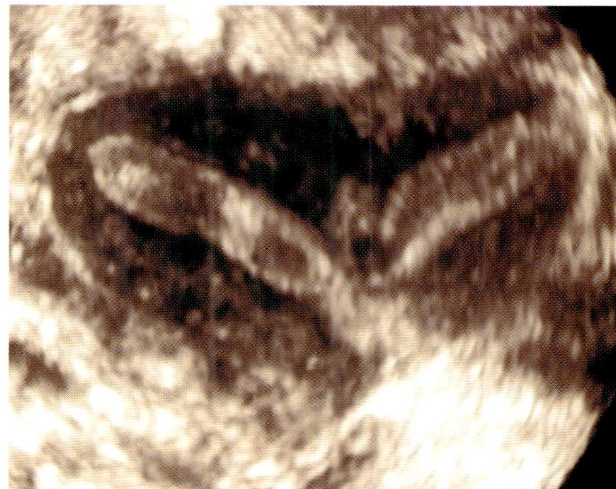

Fig. 4.34: Three-dimensional (3D) ultrasound (US) of bicornuate uterus.

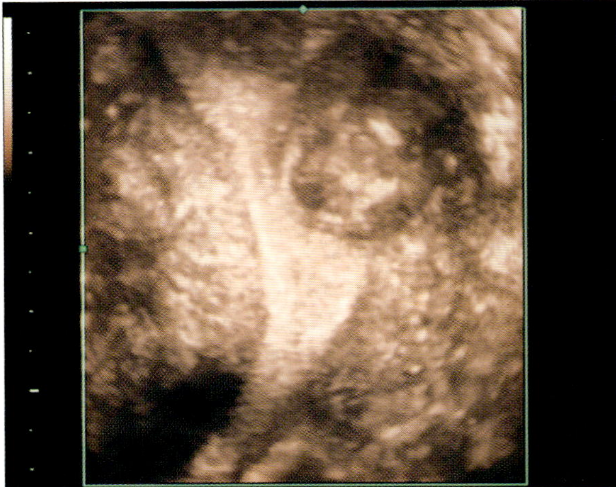

Fig. 4.35: Three-dimensional (3D) ultrasound (US) of fibroid uterus.

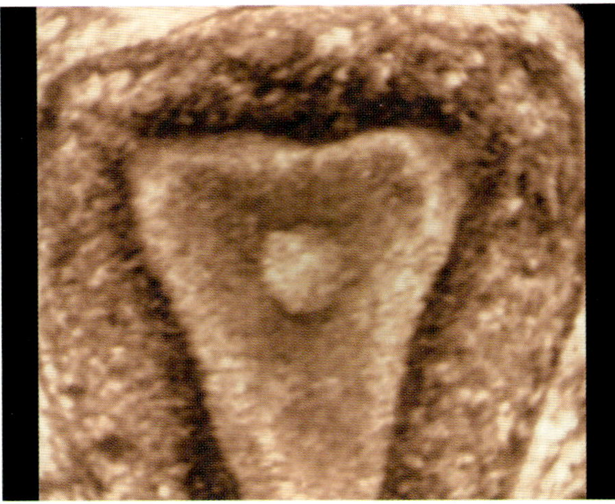

Fig. 4.36: Three-dimensional (3D) ultrasound (US) of endometrial polyp.

sweep image of the whole uterus, is more reproducible.[25,26] There is contradictory evidence for the correlation of endometrial volume with pregnancy in IVF cycles,[25,26] but if the limitations of the physical measurement of the endometrium in assessing function are acknowledged there is little that the volume alone can contribute further. While the first-ever study, and most of the subsequent studies suggest endometrial volume measurements, on the day of hCG, oocyte retrieval or embryo transfer, do not correlate with pregnancy following IVF treatment,[26-28] a proportion report a significantly lower-pregnancy rate if the endometrial volume is below 2.0–2.5 cm^3 with pregnancy highly unlikely to occur in association with an endometrial volume below 1 cm^3.[29,30] Although an endometrial volume of more than 2 cm^3 is reported to be a prerequisite for good endometrial receptivity, the specificity is so low that it appears to lack any clinical value.[31]

Three-dimensional ultrasound is not universally available. It is valuable in the structural appreciation of the uterine cavity and endometrium, but is not a prerequisite to good diagnostic ultrasound scanning.

Contrast Hysterography and Saline Infusion Sonography

Hystero-contrast-sonography (HyCoSy) is a contrast ultrasound technique whereby bubble-generating particles or foam are introduced into the uterine cavity, via a catheter inserted through the cervix, during ultrasound monitoring. The air-containing bubbles produce a high-contrast fluid which flows through the uterine cavity and into the Fallopian tubes and into peritoneal cavity. This is undertaken under direct ultrasound monitoring providing a valuable dynamic view of the structures. This technique is primarily used to define the Fallopian tubes and confirm tubal patency as part of the work-up of a subfertile couple.[32] The advantage of HyCoSy over other imaging techniques is that it is a dynamic examination, may be undertaken outside of the X-ray department and incorporates a baseline ultrasound study of the pelvis avoiding a second or prior procedure. In addition, there is no radiation dose. Since the process also outlines the uterine cavity, additional information on the endometrium may also be obtained; filling masses such as fibroids and polyps; however, these may be better outlined by the infusion of a small amount of saline into the uterine cavity before the contrast material is infused.

If tubal patency testing is not required but further definition of possible cavity abnormalities is sought, a simple and cheap first step is to consider saline sonohysterography. Similar to HyCoSy, this involves the insertion of a catheter (5-F) through the cervix and ultrasound examination while a small volume of normal saline is injected[33] (Box 4.3). Saline, like other clear fluids, appears black on the ultrasound screen as it is radiolucent. Even under low pressure the infusion of saline into the uterine cavity therefore separates adjacent surfaces and delineates any protrusions. Thus, a polyp or fibroid can be identified and measured and a sessile or pedunculated disposition be ascertained (Fig. 4.37A to D). A decision can then be made for definitive treatment as appropriate. The infusion of saline into the uterine cavity may also allow visualization of the Fallopian tubes but is much less reliable than

Box 4.3: Set up for contrast sonography (saline or HyCoSy)

Patient preparation:
- Screen for sexually transmitted disease (STD) and/or provide antibiotic cover
- Book to undertake during first half of menstrual cycle
- Consider a single preprocedure dose of nonsteroidal anti-inflammatory drug (NSAID) or equivalent

Office preparation:
- Ultrasound scan machine with TV probe (and abdominal probe, if available)
- Suitable scan couch with leg supports
- Clean area for equipment
- Clean drapes

Equipment:
- Sterile cleaning pack; sponge holding forceps, cotton wool balls, gloves, and Cusco's speculum (side-opening if available)
- 5-F catheter; specialized for HyCoSy, pediatric urinary catheter or other suitable sterile tubing flushed
- Connecting tubing if required
- 2 × 20 mL syringes loaded with sterile N saline
- Contrast medium as required (follow kit instructions for making up)

with contrast media which can better define the narrow lumina.

The addition of 3D rendering of this process again may facilitate visualization of an abnormality and can be a useful tool to give a patient a more "realistic" impression of their anatomy.

Doppler Ultrasound and the Endometrium

Vascular changes in the uterus follow a cyclical pattern, as might be expected with uterine artery pulsatility or resistance indices being well documented (Fig. 4.38). Lower uterine artery resistance is seen in the midluteal phase and may be lower in conception cycles. Examination of subendometrial blood flow is likely to give a more valid account of endometrial vascularization, although initial single-vessel pulsatility studies introduced inconsistencies of technique. The use of power Doppler with 3D facility and rendering (3D PD-US) increases observational validity since the modality allows for both regional analysis

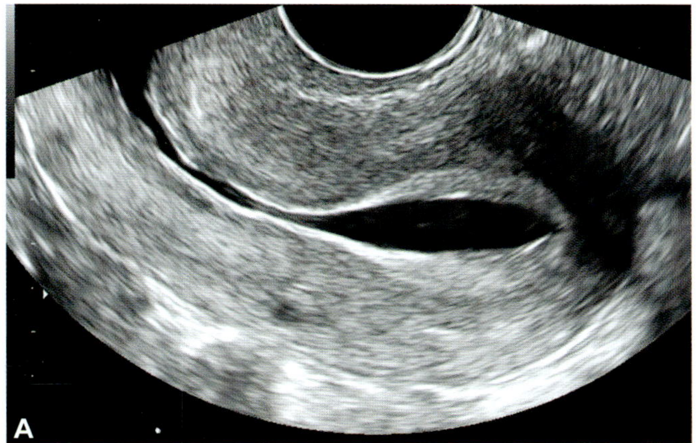

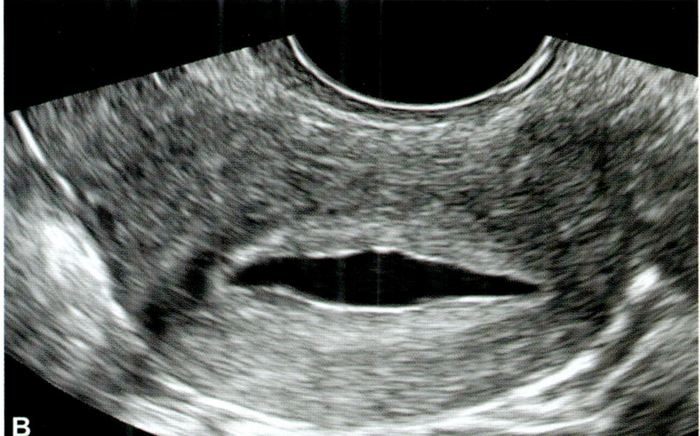

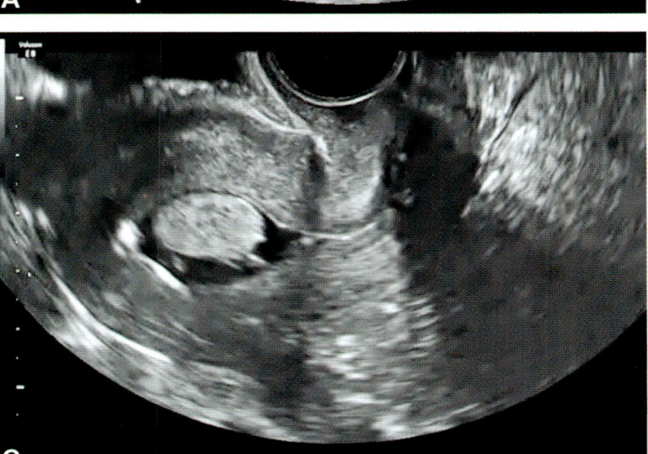

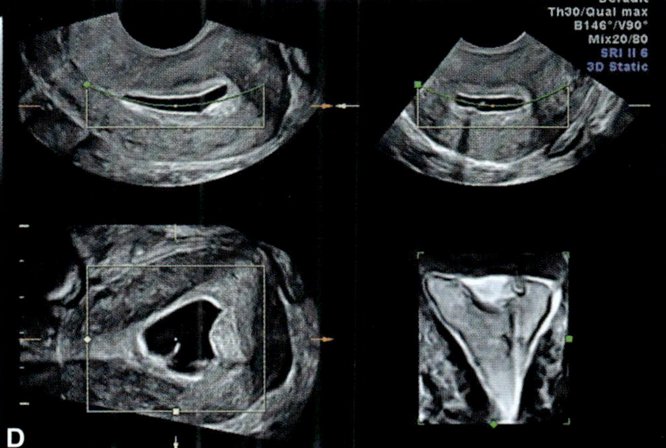

Figs. 4.37A to D: Saline infusion soongraphy: (A) and (B) normal endometrial cavity; (C) endometrial polyp; (D) 3D multiplanar view showing a fundal endometrial polyp.

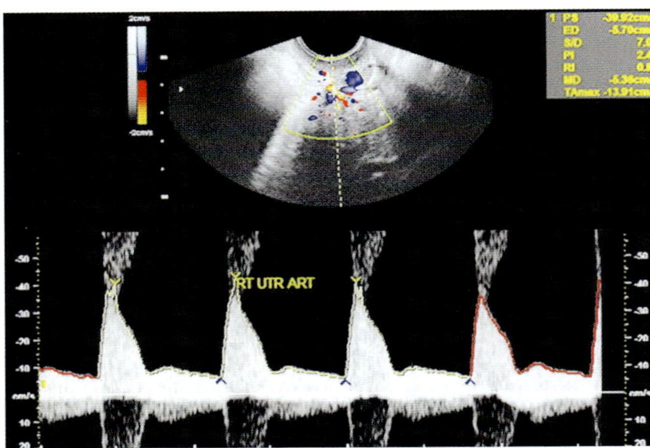

Fig. 4.38: Doppler of uterine artery.

and analysis of endometrial blood flow as a whole and is demonstrably reproducible.[34] Cyclical changes in subendometrial vascularity indices have been demonstrated[35,36] and these findings may reflect the efficacy of neovascularization occurring in the endometrium. This functional link remains hypothetical; however,[37,38] the role of 3D PD-US continues to be explored in diagnosis and management of subfertility but has yet to take its place in routine clinical settings.[39]

Color Doppler studies are of benefit in assessing intrauterine filling defects as the vascular supply pattern gives clues to the nature of attachment, for example, in defining a pedicle (Fig. 4.30) rather than sessile nature, but also distinguishing between endometrial polyps, which tend to have a single feeding vessel while fibroids tend to have a multiple vessels arranged as a rim.[40]

CONCLUSION

There is much information to be gleaned from pelvic ultrasound in relation to infertility investigation and treatment and the endometrium is a fundamental factor in fertility success. It is important therefore that along with other organs in the pelvis, the endometrium is carefully scrutinized and that findings are put into clinical context for their correct interpretation. It is important, however, that the limitations of even the most sophisticated ultrasound techniques are acknowledged such that inappropriate conclusions about endometrial function and implantation are not drawn. With the developing tools available, it is certainly possible that there may in time be a greater understanding linking ultrasound findings and endometrial function and hence there remains a need for well-designed studies to be undertaken in this field.

KEY POINTS

- It is important that the uterus is thoroughly screened in the longitudinal (sagittal) and transverse planes
- Endometrial thickness and endometrial pattern are assessed in the midsagittal plane and are the important markers of endometrial receptivity
- Endometrial thickness and texture are assessed in diagnosing endometrial pathologies
- While conventional ultrasound is useful for screening for congenital uterine anomalies, 3D ultrasound helps to classify the type of uterine anomalies
- Ultrasound helps in diagnosing and assessing number, size, and types of fibroids and polyps; and this is important in counseling women about their chances of treatment success and in triaging patients for surgery
- Studies have shown that the uterine cavity, endometrial lining, and myometrium are best visualized using sonohysterography, and that these images are further improved by the use of 3D ultrasound

REFERENCES

1. Cancer Australia. (2011). Abnormal vaginal bleeding in pre-, peri- and post-menopausal women: a diagnostic guide for general practitioners and gynaecologists. [online] Australia Government website. Available from www.canceraustralia.gov.au/publications-resources/cancer-australia-publications/abnormal-vaginal-bleeding-pre-peri-and-post.
2. Kovacs P, Matyas S, Bodas K, et al. The effect of endometrial thickness on IVF/ICSI outcome. Hum Reprod. 2003;18:2337-41.
3. Richter KS, Bugge KR, Bromer JG, et al. Relationship between endometrial thickness and embryo implantation, based on 1,294 cycles of in vitro fertilization with transfer of two blastocyst-stage embryos. Fertil Steril. 2007;87:53-9.
4. Remohi J, Ardiles G, Garcia-Velasco JA, et al. Endometrial thickness and serum oestradiol concentrations as predictors of outcome in oocyte donation. Hum Reprod. 1997;12:2271-6.
5. Bozdag G, Esinler I, Yarali H. The impact of endometrial thickness and texture on intracytoplasmic sperm injection outcome. J Reprod Med. 2009;54:303-11.
6. Weissman A, Gotlieb L, Casper RF. The detrimental effect of increased endometrial thickness on implantation and pregnancy rates and outcome in an in vitro fertilization program. Fertil Steril. 1999;71:147-9.
7. Dietterich C, Check JH, Choe JK, et al. Increased endometrial thickness on the day of human chorionic gonadotrophin

injection does not adversely affect pregnancy or implantation rates following in vitro fertilization-embryo transfer. Fertil Steril. 2002;77:781-6.
8. Yoeli R, Ashkenazi J, Orvieto R, et al. Significance of increased endometrial thickness in assisted reproduction technology treatments. J Assist Reprod Genet. 2004;21: 285-9.
9. Momeni M, Rahbar MH, Kovanci E. A meta-analysis of the relationship between endometrial thickness and outcome of in vitro fertilization cycles. J Hum Reprod Sci. 2011;4:130-7.
10. McWilliams GD, Frattarelli JL. Changes in measured endometrial thickness predict in vitro fertilization success. Fertil Steril. 2007;88:74-81.
11. Lessey BA. Assessment of endometrial receptivity. Fertil Steril. 2011;96:519-21.
12. Zohav E, Bar-Hava I, Meltcer S, et al. Early endometrial changes following successful implantation: 2 and 3-dimensional ultrasound study. Clin Exp Obstet Gynecol. 2008;35:255-6.
13. Fanchin R, Righini C, Ayoubi JM, et al. New look at endometrial echogenicity: objective computer-assisted measurements predict endometrial receptivity in in vitro fertilization-embryo transfer. Fertil Steril. 2000;74:274-81.
14. Bourgain C, Devroey P. The endometrium in stimulated cycles for IVF. Hum Reprod Update. 2003;9:515-22.
15. Shapiro BS, Daneshmand ST, Garner FC, et al. Evidence of impaired endometrial receptivity after ovarian stimulation for in vitro fertilization: a prospective randomized trial comparing fresh and frozen-thawed embryo transfers in high responders. Fertil Steril. 2011;96:516-8.
16. Singh N, Bahadur A, Mittal S, et al. Predictive value of endometrial thickness, pattern and sub-endometrial blood flows on the day of hCG by 2D Doppler in in-vitro fertilization cycles: a prospective clinical study from a tertiary care unit. J Hum Reprod Sci. 2011;4:29-33.
17. Baruffi RL, Contart P, Mauri AL, et al. A uterine ultrasonographic scoring system as a method for the prognosis of embryo implantation. J Assist Reprod Genet. 2002;19:99-102.
18. Sher G, Fisch JD. Effect of vaginal sildenafil on the outcome of in vitro fertilization (IVF) after multiple IVF failures attributed to poor endometrial development. Fertil Steril. 2002;78:1073-6.
19. Siristatidis CS, Dodd SR, Drakeley AJ. Aspirin for in vitro fertilisation. Cochrane Database Syst Rev. 2011;(8):CD0004832.
20. Afifi K, Anand S, Nallapeta S, et al. Management of endometrial polyps in subfertile women: a systematic review. Eur J Obstet Gynecol Reprod Biol. 2010;151:117-21.
21. The Royal College of Radiologists. (2006). Standards for the reporting and interpretation of imaging investigations. [online] Available from http://www.rcr.ac.uk.
22. Faivre E, Fernandez H, Deffieux X, et al. Accuracy of three-dimensional ultrasonography in differential diagnosis of septate and bicornuate uterus compared with office hysteroscopy and pelvic magnetic resonance imaging. J Minim Invasive Gynecol. 2012;19:101-6.
23. Martins WP, Raine-Fenning NJ, Leite SP, et al. A standardized measurement technique may improve the reliability of measurements of endometrial thickness and volume. Ultrasound Obstet Gynecol. 2011;38:107-15.
24. Perez-Medina T, Bajo-Arenas J, Salazar F, et al. Endometrial polyps and their implication in the pregnancy rates of patients undergoing intrauterine insemination: a prospective, randomized study. Hum Reprod. 2005;20: 1632-5.
25. Zollner U, Specketer MT, Dietl J, et al. 3D-endometrial volume and outcome of cryopreserved embryo replacement cycles. Arch Gynecol Obstet. 2012;286:517-23.
26. Schild RL, Indefrei D, Eschweiler S, et al. Three-dimensional endometrial volume calculation and pregnancy rate in an in-vitro fertilization programme. Hum Reprod. 1999;14:1255-8.
27. Kupesic S, Bekavac I, Bjelos D, et al. Assessment of endometrial receptivity by transvaginal color Doppler and three-dimensional power Doppler ultrasonography in patients undergoing in vitro fertilization procedures. J Ultrasound Med. 2001;20:125-34.
28. Yaman C, Ebner T, Sommergruber M, et al. Role of three-dimensional ultrasonographic measurement of endometrium volume as a predictor of pregnancy outcome in an IVF-ET program: a preliminary study. Fertil Steril. 2000;74:797-801.
29. Raga F, Bonilla-Musoles F, Casan EM, et al. Assessment of endometrial volume by three-dimensional ultrasound prior to embryo transfer: clues to endometrial receptivity. Hum Reprod. 1999;14:2851-4.
30. Zollner U, Zollner KP, Specketer MT, et al. Endometrial volume as assessed by three-dimensional ultrasound is a predictor of pregnancy outcome after in vitro fertilization and embryo transfer. Fertil Steril. 2003;80:1515-7.
31. Alcazar JL. Three-dimensional ultrasound assessment of endometrial receptivity: a review. Reprod Biol Endocrinol. 2006;4:56.
32. Saunders RD, Shwayder JM, Nakajima ST. Current methods of tubal patency assessment. Fertil Steril. 2011;95:2171-9.
33. Jorizzo JR, Riccio GJ, Chen MY, et al. Sonohysterography: the next step in the evaluation of the abnormal endometrium. Radiographics. 1999;19:S117-30.
34. Raine-Fenning NJ, Campbell BK, Kendall NR, et al. Endometrial and subendometrial perfusion are impaired in women with unexplained subfertility. Hum Reprod. 2004;19:2605-14.
35. Raine-Fenning NJ, Campbell BK, Clewes JS, et al. The interobserver reliability of three-dimensional power Doppler data acquisition within the female pelvis. Ultrasound Obstet Gynecol. 2004;23:501-8.
36. Jokubkiene L, Sladkevicius P, Rovas L, et al. Assessment of changes in endometrial and subendometrial volume and vascularity during the normal menstrual cycle using three-dimensional power Doppler ultrasound. Ultrasound Obstet Gynecol. 2006;27:672-9.

37. Ledee N, Chaouat G, Serazin V, et al. Endometrial vascularity by three-dimensional power Doppler ultrasound and cytokines: a complementary approach to assess uterine receptivity. J Reprod Immunol. 2008;77:57-62.
38. Siemer J, Binder H, Willeke C, et al. Three-dimensional power Doppler sonography of the (sub)endometrium and angiogenic cytokine concentrations. Reprod Biomed Online. 2008;17:249-58.
39. Ng EH, Chan CC, Tang OS, et al. The role of endometrial blood flow measured by three-dimensional power Doppler ultrasound in the prediction of pregnancy during in vitro fertilization treatment. Eur J Obstet Gynecol Reprod Biol. 2007;135:8-16.
40. Cil AP, Tulunay G, Kose MF, et al. Power Doppler properties of endometrial polyps and submucosal fibroids: a preliminary observational study in women with known intracavitary lesions. Ultrasound Obstet Gynecol. 2010;35:233-7.
41. National Institute of Clinical Excellence (NICE). Embryo transfer techniques. Fertility: assessment and treatment for people with fertility problems. Clinical Guideline No. 11. London: RCOG Press; 2004.
42. Abou-Setta AM. What is the best site for embryo deposition? A systematic review and meta-analysis using direct and adjusted indirect comparisons. Reprod Biomed Online. 2007;14:611-9.
43. Brown J, Buckingham K, Abou-Setta AM, et al. Ultrasound versus "clinical touch" for catheter guidance during embryo transfer in women. Cochrane Database Syst Rev. 2010;(1):CD006107.
44. Lesny P, Killick SR, Tetlow RL, et al. Embryo transfer—can we learn anything new from the observation of junctional zone contractions? Hum Reprod. 1998;13:1540-6.

Chapter

5

Evaluation of Tubes

Sonal Panchal

Chapter Outline

- Introduction
- Anatomy of the Fallopian Tubes
- Diagnosis of Tubal Pathologies by Ultrasound
- Tests of Tubal Patency Assessment
- Conclusion
- Key Points

INTRODUCTION

Evaluation of Fallopian tubes forms an essential part of assessment of any subfertile woman. Several investigations have been used since decades to evaluate the tubal patency. However, if the physiology of fertility is unfolded, it is evident that tuboovarian relationship and tubal function are as important as patency of the Fallopian tubes for preservation of fertility.

It is well known that ovaries are reservoirs of primordial follicles which act as precursors of fertilizable ova. Under the effect of local regulatory factors, primordial follicles in ovary undergo initial recruitment and develop into preantral and antral follicles. These antral follicles undergo cyclical recruitment under the influence of pituitary gonadotropins with one follicle selected as a dominant follicle. This follicle grows and becomes a mature ovulatory follicle that releases a mature ovum. A functioning Fallopian tube is essential to retrieve and transport the released ovum toward the uterus. Fallopian tubes are not just tubular portals, but are motile structures and have peristalsis. It is at the time of the follicular rupture that fimbrial end of the tube moves close to the ovary. The fimbrial processes cover the ovary like a ball being held in the palm.[1]

Fallopian tube plays an important role in other reproductive functions such as sperm transport and capacitation. The vital process of fertilization occurs in the tube and then the embryo is nourished and transferred to the uterus for implantation. This means it is essential that Fallopian tubes should be patent, the tuboovarian relationship should be normal, fimbrial condition should be good and accommodative to hold the ovary, and the cilia should be normal to guide the passage of ovum toward uterus and guide the passage of sperms toward the ovum.

ANATOMY OF THE FALLOPIAN TUBES

Fallopian tube extends laterally from the cornu of the uterus on each side and extend till the ovary. The tube is 10–14 cm in length and is about 1 cm in external diameter. It connects the peritoneal cavity to the endometrial cavity. The ostium of the tube is 1.5 mm in diameter at the cornual end and 3 mm in diameter at the peritoneal end. The tube is suspended by the mesosalpinx. Except for their intramural part, the tubes are covered by the peritoneum.

Fallopian tube can be divided into four anatomic regions.

1. Infundibulum is the funnel-shaped most distal end of the tube. The peritoneal ostium lies at the base of the infundibulum and is surrounded fimbriae. Fimbrial end of the tube is attached to the ovary by fimbriaca ovariaca.
2. Ampulla is about 4–6 cm in length and is the longest part of the tube. It is tortuous and has an inner diameter of 6 mm. Fertilization occurs in this region.

3. Isthmus is 2.5–4 cm part of the tube at the uterine exit of the tube. It is 1–2 mm in diameter, with thick muscular wall.
4. Interstitial or intramural segment is 1–2 cm long and constitutes the uterine-tubal junction.

TUBAL EVALUATION

The discussion in this chapter will be divided into two parts.

1. Diagnosis of tubal pathologies by ultrasound
2. Assessment of tubal patency

DIAGNOSIS OF TUBAL PATHOLOGIES BY ULTRASOUND

The tubal pathologies can be divided into:

- Inflammatory lesions
- Paratubal and fimbrial cysts
- Tubal pregnancies
- Neoplasms of the tube

Inflammatory Lesions of the Fallopian Tube: Salpingitis

Tubal inflammation may be acute or chronic. The acute form of the inflammation is usually not confined to the tubes alone, but is usually associated with inflammation in the pelvis in general and is popularly known as pelvic inflammatory disease (PID). It is common in the reproductive age group and sexually active women. Many cases may be subclinical or may have atypical presentation and therefore actual incidence is difficult to estimate.

The presentation of the disease may vary from mild pelvic pain and feeling of non–well-being to severe pelvic pain and severe systemic symptoms of infection. Chronic cases may not have any specific symptoms, though chronic pelvic pain and infertility may be commonest presentations.

The culprit microbials ascend through the cervix. The ascent of the organisms is especially facilitated by cervical instrumentation or manipulations. Though retrograde menstruation may also be the cause. However, the most supporting factor is the hormonal changes occurring during menstruation, leading to loss of bacteriostatic quality of cervical mucous and also because of break in the mechanical barrier.

Salpingitis is usually polymicrobial in origin and the organisms often found may be *Neisseria gonorrhoeae, Chlamydia trachomatis, Gardnerella vaginalis, Escherichia coli, Haemophilus influenzae*, group B beta-hemolytic streptococci, nonhemolytic streptococci, *Prevotella bivia*, Bacteroides species, Peptostreptococcus species, *Mycoplasma hominis*, and *Ureaplasma urealyticum*.

Ultrasound Diagnosis: The spectrum of ultrasound findings is wide. It may present as normal tube, thick-walled tube, hydrosalpinx, adhesions, or as tuboovarian mass.

Acute Salpingitis

In patients with acute pelvic symptoms, acute salpingitis or acute PID is suspected. Ultrasound diagnosis is difficult because fallopian tubes are not visualized normally on ultrasound. There has to be fluid in the tubal lumen or fluid outside the tube, only then can these be identified on ultrasound. Acute inflammation of the tube and pelvic organs, on ultrasound may show free fluid in pelvis, often with low-level echoes. The tubes may be seen floating in this fluid. It may show a low-resistance vascularity. The fimbrial end of the tube may show thickening (Fig. 5.1).

If this inflammatory process leads to obstruction of the tubal lumen, it may cause hydrosalpinx. Hydrosalpinx appears as an extraovarian cystic lesion in the adnexa. Its extraovarian nature can be confirmed by positive sliding organ sign (ability to slide the lesion over the ovary) or negative beak or a rim sign (beak or a rim of ovarian tissue in the margins of the lesion) (Figs. 5.2A and B).

Typically, this cystic lesion changes its shape on rotation of the probe when it is hydrosalpinx. Tubal haustra (tortuosity) may appear as incomplete septae (Figs. 5.3A and B).

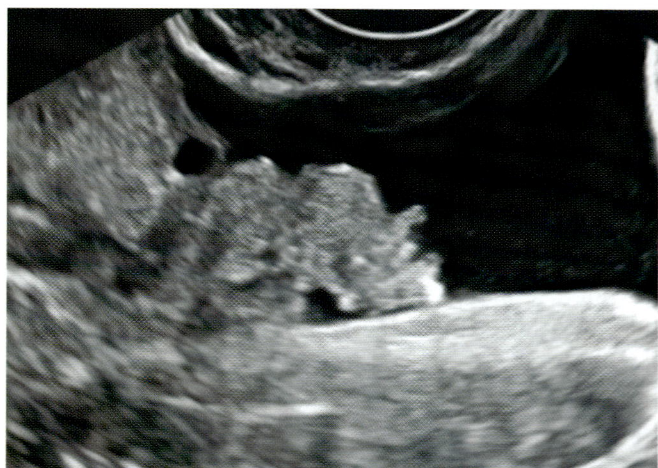

Fig. 5.1: Free fluid in pelvis with floating thick fimbrial end of fallopian tube.

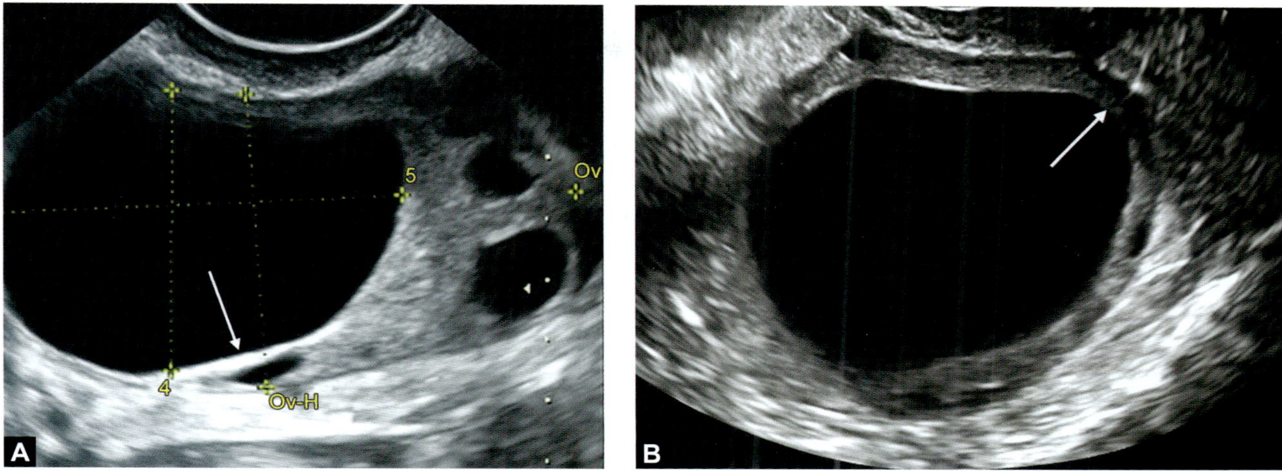

Figs. 5.2A and B: (A) Beak sign of intraovarian lesion (arrow). (B) Rim sign of ovarian tissue (arrow).

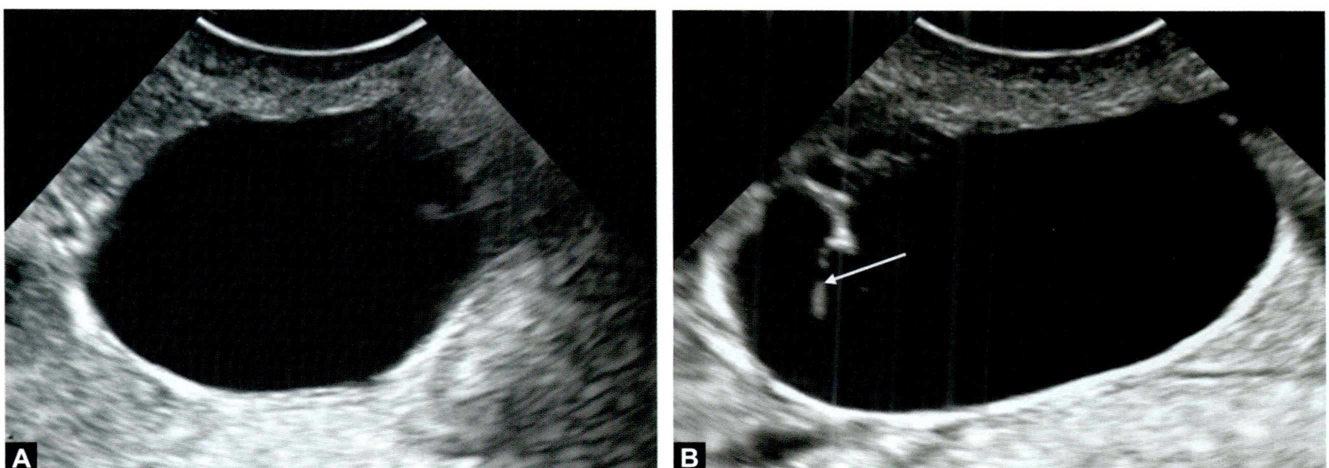

Figs. 5.3A and B: Change in shape of a cystic lesion on rotation of the probe and incomplete septum (arrow) are diagnostic of hydrosalpinx.

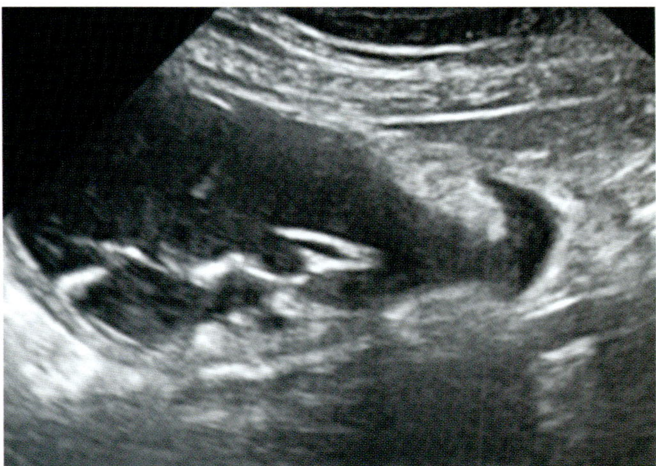

Fig. 5.4: Beak-like narrowing at one of the ends of the cystic lesion may also be indicative of a hydrosalpinx.

In case of acute inflammation, these septae are thick. Thickened haustra in transverse section of the tube may produce a cogwheel appearance. A beak-like narrowing at one of the ends of the cystic lesion may also be indicative of a hydrosalpinx (Fig. 5.4).

Hydrosalpinx may intermittently be seen in cases of partial or incomplete obstruction. In this situation, diagnosis of hydrosalpinx confirmed once is always a damaged tube. Therefore, a precise diagnosis of any cystic lesion in the adnexa is essential.

Acute salpingitis is almost always associated with oophoritis. It may be difficult to diagnose it on ultrasound. Though indicative ultrasound signs are hypoechoic ovarian stroma. Follicles may be pushed to the periphery and Doppler shows low-resistance vascularity. Local tenderness on probe pressure may also be seen.

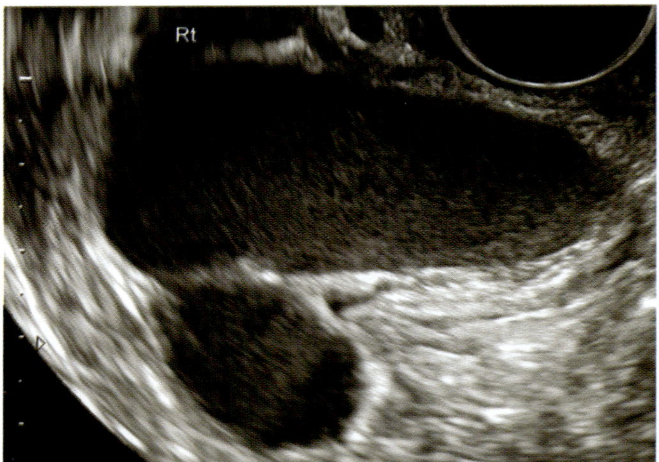

Fig. 5.5: Hydrosalpinx with low-level echogenecitites—pyosalpinx.

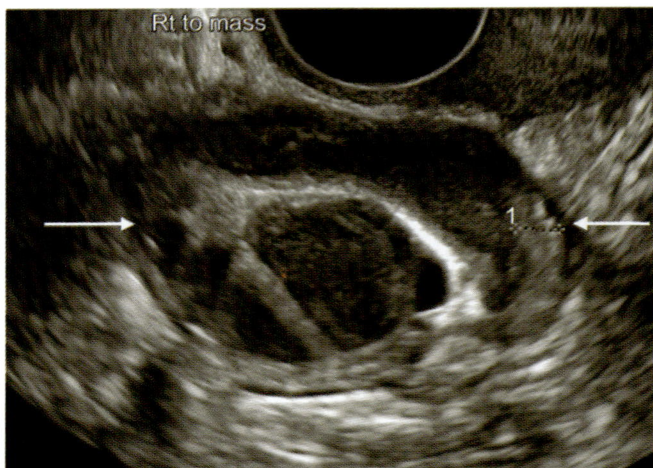

Fig. 5.6: Tuboovarian mass (arrows).

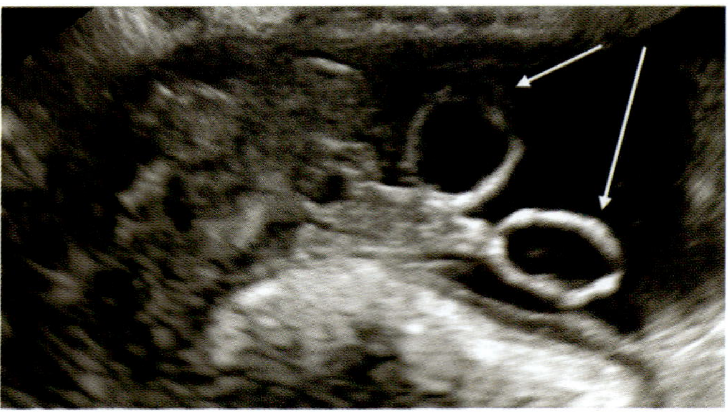

Fig. 5.7: Fimbrial cyst (arrows).

Fulminant infections may lead to purulent collection in hydrosalpinx (pyosalpinx). This typically appears as thick-walled hydrosalpinges with low-level echogenecities in the lumen (Fig. 5.5).

These may also present as tuboovarian mass, when the hydrosalpinx is seen with the ovary adherent to it, though the margins of both can be identified. In severe cases, the adherent walls may break down, when the ovarian margins cannot be identified. Ultrasound shows a complex cystic mass with thick septae and low-level echogenecities in the lumen. This is named as tuboovarian abscess.

Chronic Salpingitis

This may lead to obstructed tubes. A beaded appearance typically seen on laparoscopy is not often identifiable on ultrasound, unless there is free fluid seen in the pelvis. Though hystero-contrast sonosalpingography (HyCoSy) may demonstrate the typical appearance.

Chronic hydrosalpinx shows thin walls and haustra. Adhesions are frequently seen in chronic inflammations. Tuboovarian masses may be seen in chronic inflammations (Fig. 5.6).

Paratubal Cyst/Fimbrial Cyst

A paratubal cyst is a cystic lesion close to the tube, usually, more commonly close to the fimbrial end. It is usually unilateral and benign. On ultrasound, it appears as a thin-walled clear cystic lesion more commonly close to the fimbrial end of the tube (Fig. 5.7). It has no impact on the fertility potential of the female.

Tubal Pregnancy

It has been discussed earlier that the fertilization of the ovum occurs in the tube and the embryo travels to the endometrium in 3–4 days after fertilization. This process is facilitated by tubal peristalsis and the ciliary movements in the tubal lumen. In cases with tubal damage therefore, this transit of the embryo from the tube to the uterus is disturbed. This leads to implantation of the embryo in the tube. Though most ectopic pregnancies occur due to salpingitis or damaged tubes, in at least about 30–40% of cases, this correlation cannot be established. Hormonal dysregulation is considered as one of the possible causes in these cases.

Tubal pregnancy is the commonest of all the ectopic pregnancies. It is suspected in a patient with missed period and a serum β hCG levels of more than 1,500 IU, no intrauterine gestational sac is seen on transvaginal ultrasound scan. Clinically, it is suspected when a female with missed periods or positive urine or blood pregnancy tests complains of giddiness, sudden syncopic fall, spotting, or severe pelvic pain. Ultrasound is the modality of choice for the diagnosis of tubal pregnancy.

Ultrasound findings: These can be divided as direct signs and indirect signs.

Direct Signs of Tubal Pregnancy

In a patient with positive pregnancy test or a missed period, any adnexal mass may be indicative of an ectopic pregnancy. This mass may be isoechoic, may be isoechoic with a hyperechoic center (chorionic reaction) or may be isoechoic with the gestational sac inside (Fig. 5.8A). Gestational sac appears as an anechoic area with thick hyperechoic margins (decidual ring). Depending on the duration of the pregnancy, the gestational sac may show yolk sac or fetal pole, with or without cardiac activity. Whatever the duration of the tubal pregnancy, it always shows a low-resistance peripheral vascularity (Fig 5.8B).

Indirect Signs of Tubal Pregnancy

Adnexal signs: Active corpus luteum in the ipsilateral ovary; free fluid around the mass and in close vicinity of the ovary.

Uterine signs: Thick hyperechoic endometrium with echogenicity similar to that of decidual reaction. Though this might not be seen in all the cases. If thickening is seen, it is symmetrical. This means both the lips of the endometrium are equal in thickness (Figs. 5.9A and B)

Pseudosac: At times minimal fluid collection is seen in the endometrial cavity. This may be mistaken for a gestational

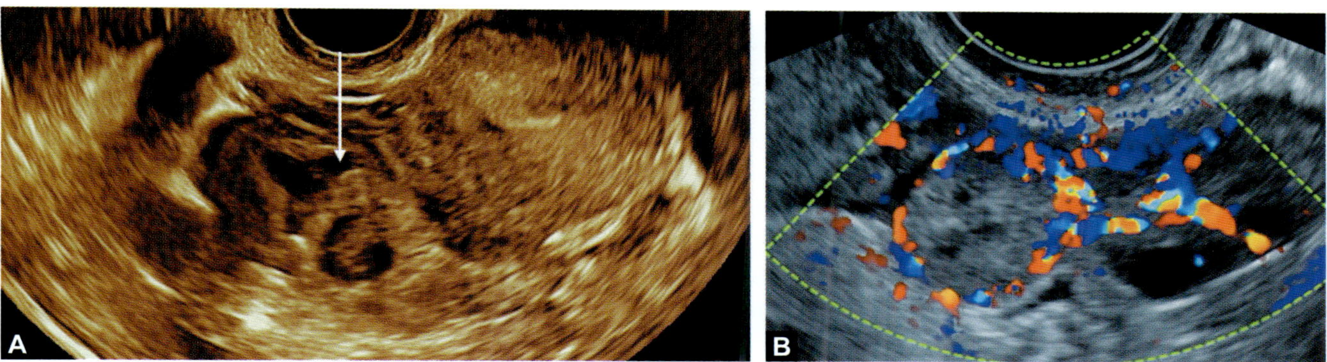

Figs. 5.8A and B: B-mode ultrasound showing adnexal mass (arrow) in the image (A) and rim of vascularity on color Doppler in the image (B).

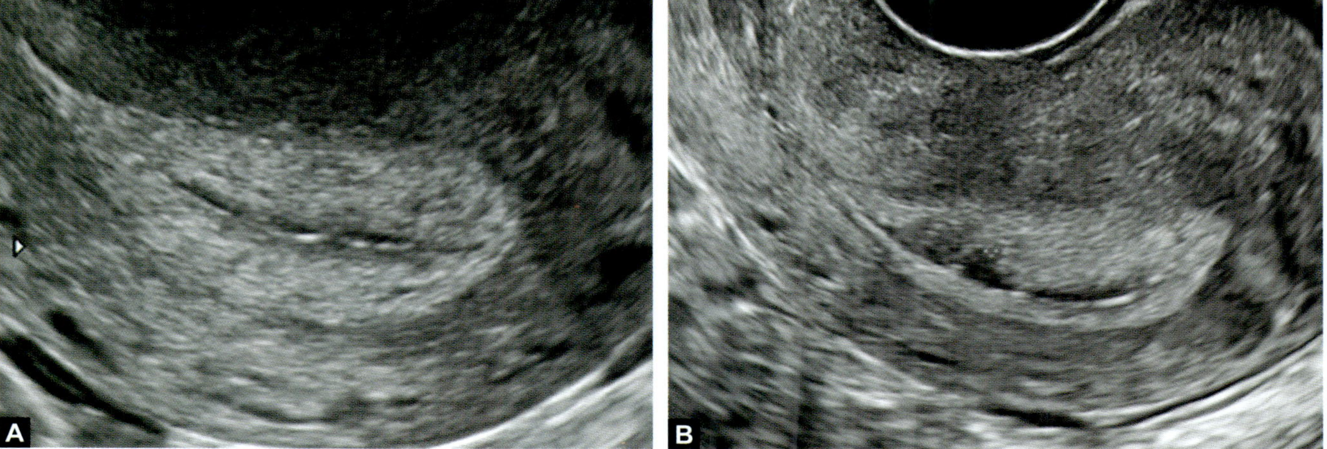

Figs. 5.9A and B: Symmetrical endometrial thickness in the image (A) is indicative of extrauterine pregnancy, whereas image (B) shows asymmetrical thickness of the anterior lip of endometrium suggestive of early intrauterine pregnancy.

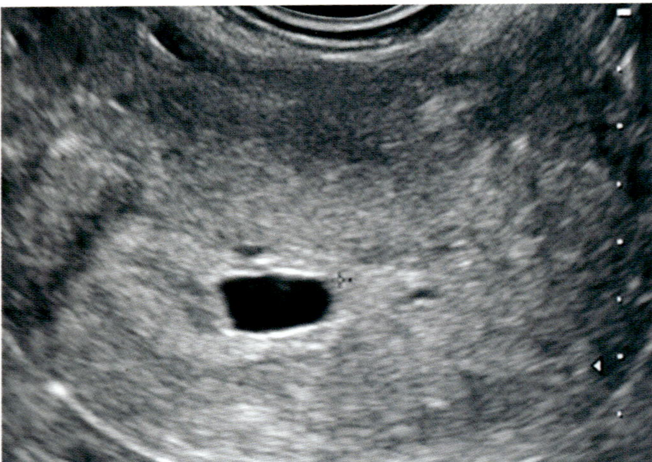

Fig. 5.10: Pseudogestational sac.

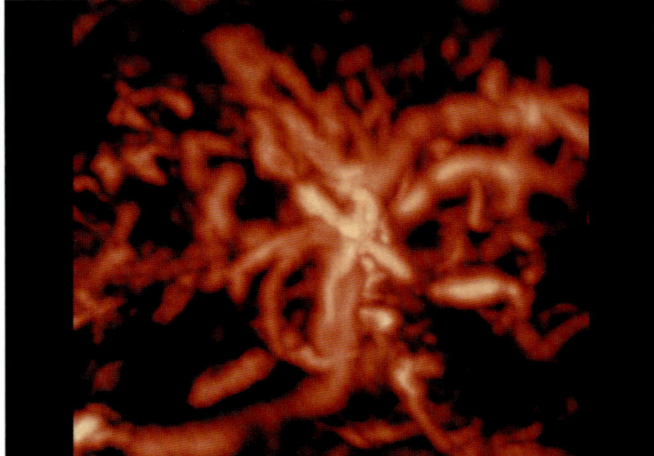

Fig. 5.11: Three-dimensional power Doppler showing typical vascular morphology of malignant lesions.

sac, but unlike a true gestational sac, this fluid filled area is central in endometrial cavity, shows no peripheral vascularity and it changes its shape with peristalsis (Fig. 5.10).

Tubal Neoplasms

These are very rare. Moreover, the histopathological diagnosis cannot be established on ultrasound. It is very difficult to establish its tubal origin. Its malignant nature can be established by its complex morphology (cystic and solid components), thick septa, and echogenic fluid. Malignant lesions may show grade 3–4 vascularity and typically has low-resistance blood flow. Three-dimensional power Doppler (3D-PD) may also show irregular vascular caliber and dichotomous branching pattern (Fig. 5.11).

TESTS OF TUBAL PATENCY ASSESSMENT

Various nonsurgical and surgical investigative modalities have been reported so far to assess Fallopian tubes. An ideal test would correctly identify all women with tubal disease with minimal false negative test results. Further, the tests should be cost-effective and less risky. While nonsurgical techniques, such as hysterosalpingography (HSG), and ultrasound-based techniques, like saline infusion sonography (SIS) and HyCoSy are less invasive and associated with less serious risks, surgical technique like laparoscopy and dye test (chromopertubation) are considered as the gold standard investigations for assessment of tubal patency and diagnosis of tubal pathology.

Hysterosalpingography

This X-ray based procedure is widely used for tubal evaluation in subfertile women who are not having any comorbidities such as PID, previous ectopic pregnancies, or endometriosis. This method is fairly accurate in detecting proximal tubal disease, safe and less expensive, and may potentially be associated with increased pregnancy rates.[2] HSG provides optimal delineation of the endometrial cavity and fallopian tubes, allowing detection of tubal patency, tubal occlusion, tubal irregularity and peritubal disease. Hysterosalpingography is generally done in the proliferative phase of the cycle in order to ensure that woman is not pregnant when the procedure is performed.

Women are generally advised to take analgesic or antispasmodic agent about 1-hour prior to the procedure to reduce lower abdominal discomfort and to avoid tubal spasm. Patient is placed in lithotomy position and aseptic precaution is essential. Testing for chlamydia and/or prophylactic antibiotic is recommended to reduce the risk of pelvic infection. Speculum is used to expose the cervix, cleaned with antiseptic solution. Anterior cervical lip is grasped with tenaculum, HSG catheter is introduced into the cervix. Radio-opaque solution is introduced through the HSG catheter into uterus. Solution is warmed to body temperature and very small amount is introduced. Under fluoroscopic guidance, filling of the uterine cavity and passage of the radio-opaque solution into the tubes and its spill from fimbrial end is observed and documented in the form of X-rays (Fig. 5.12).

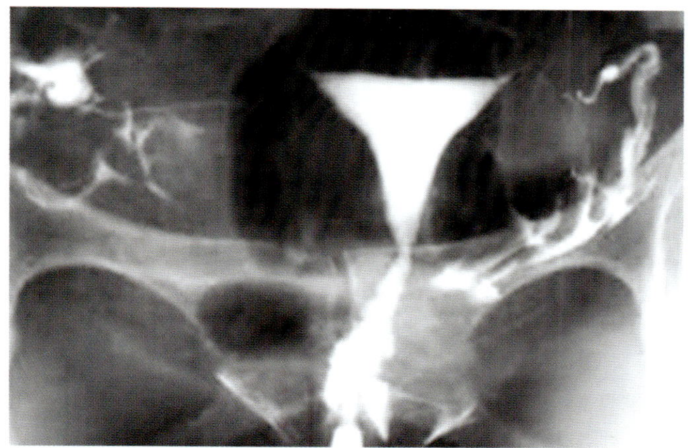

Fig. 5.12: Normal uterine cavity, tubes, and spill on HSG.

Hysterosalpingography allows to study the endometrial cavity and diagnose Müllerian abnormalities and certain endometrial lesions (Figs. 5.13A and B), in addition to its main use as assessment of the whole tube, condition of the tubal lumen and site of the block (Fig. 5.14). However, the main disadvantages are exposure to radiation and its high false negative rates.

Use of ultrasound to test tubal patency may potentially avoid the risk of radiation, while providing the necessary information as provided by HSG. While transvaginal ultrasound has now proved its place for assessment of uterus and ovaries but normal Fallopian tubes are impossible to visualize on ultrasound without any intervention. This is so because there is no tissue-fluid interface when the tubes are normal. When there is fluid in the tubal lumen or outside the tubes, they can be identified. This means that tubes can be identified on ultrasound when either there is hydrosalpinx or free fluid in pelvis as has been discussed earlier in this chapter also. Fluid can be introduced using a catheter through cervix to visualize and assess the Fallopian tubes by ultrasound. This procedure is known as saline infusion sonosalpingography. It is also named as sonohysterosalpingography as it also allows to assess the endometrial cavity.

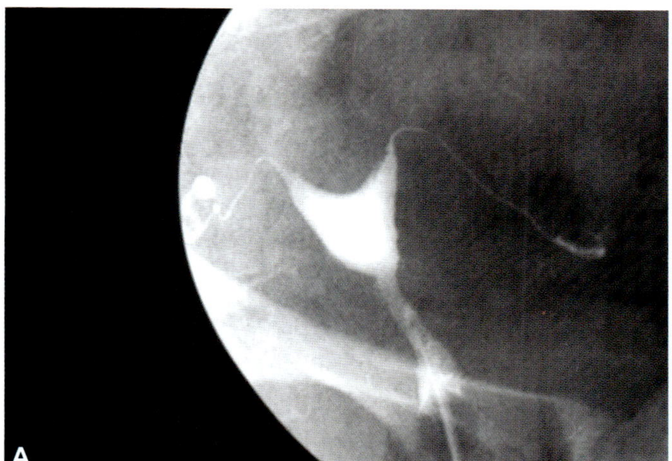

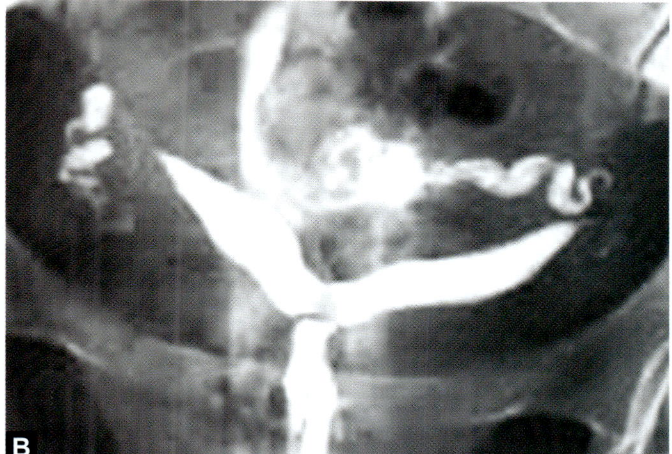

Figs. 5.13A and B: (A) Arcuate uterus with normal tubes seen on HSG. (B) Bicornuate uterus with tubes seen on HSG.

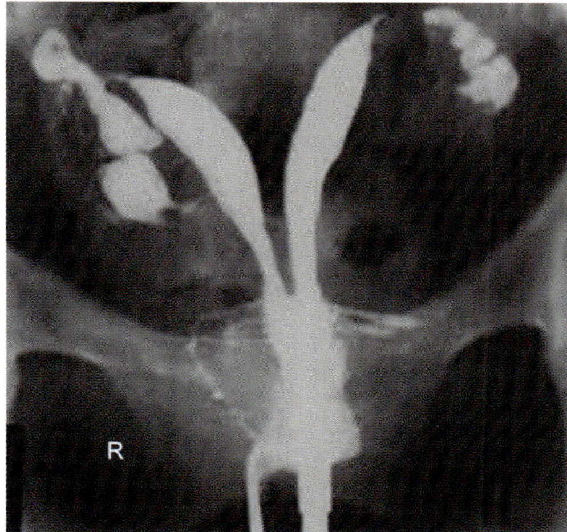

Fig. 5.14: Septate uterus with bilateral dilated distal ends of the tubes—hydrosalpinx as seen on HSG.

Sonohysterosalpingography (Saline Infusion Sonosalpingography)

Sonographic evaluation of tubes was initially described by various authors, Nanini,[3] Richman,[4] and Randolph,[5] who performed abdominal sonography following intracervical injection of fluid, but was reported first by Richman. For this procedure, 200 mL of saline was injected transvaginally. Fluid would fill-up the uterine cavity and pass through the tubes into the pelvic cavity. Rectouterine fluid on abdominal ultrasound was accepted as a criterion for patency. Tufekci reported the use of isotonic saline with transvaginal ultrasound for tubal patency in 1992.[6] Deichert was the first to report on transvaginal sonographic evaluation of tubal patency, following transcervical injection of echogenic ultrasonic contrast fluid.[7]

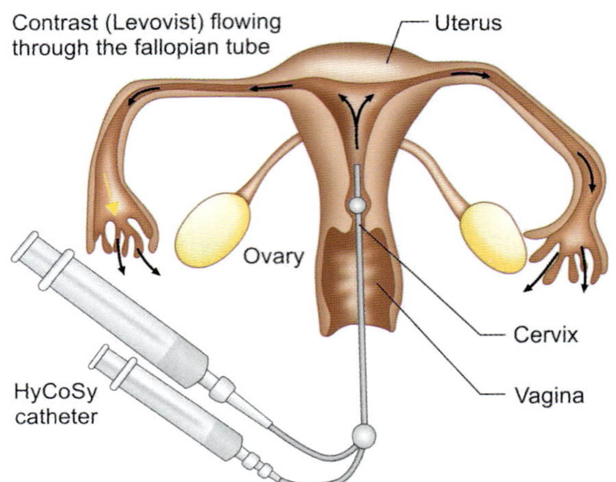

Fig. 5.15: Diagrammatic representation of saline infusion salpingography procedure.

Technique

Sonosalpingography is ideally done in mid-proliferative phase (day 6–10 of a typical 28-day cycle), after menstruation stops but before ovulation occurs, to reduce the risk of disturbing an early pregnancy. Oral analgesic, Ibuprofen 400–600 mg may be given 1–2 hours before the procedure. Preprocedural screenings for infections like chlamydia and/or prophylactic oral antibiotics are recommended. Strict asepsis is essential. A detailed transvaginal ultrasound scan is done to assess the position of pelvic organs and to rule out any pathologies, which would come in the way of the procedure. Moreover, any free fluid in pelvis is also checked for.

The probe is removed and speculum is placed in the vagina to visualize the cervix. Cervix is cleaned by an antiseptic solution. If required, cervix is fixed with tenaculum and manipulated to align it with uterus. A 5–7 Fr balloon catheter specially devised for SIS or HSG is attached to a 10-mL syringe prefilled with saline. The catheter is introduced through cervix into the uterus. Balloon is placed just beyond the internal os and is distended with 1–2 mL of distilled water or normal saline. Alternatives to this catheter are pediatric feeding tubes or small gauge Foley's catheter. Once the catheter is fixed, tenaculum and speculum are removed and transvaginal probe is introduced into the vagina for further assessment (Fig. 5.15).

Saline is injected through the catheter slowly. Scanning is done to assess the uterine cavity that is distended by saline and also passage of saline (fluid) seen through the tubes. When uterine cavity is filled with saline, any endometrial pathology can be demonstrated and diagnosed (Figs. 5.16A and B).

Spill of saline from fimbrial end is seen as fluid flows surrounding the ovary and its collection in pelvis on B-mode scanning (Fig. 5.17).

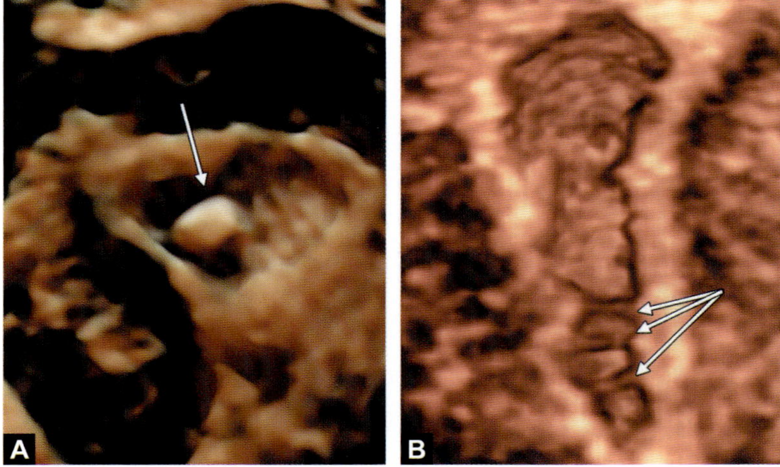

Figs. 5.16A and B: (A) Polyp on 3D saline infusion hysterography. (B) Multiple endometrial synechiea on 3D saline infusion salpingography.

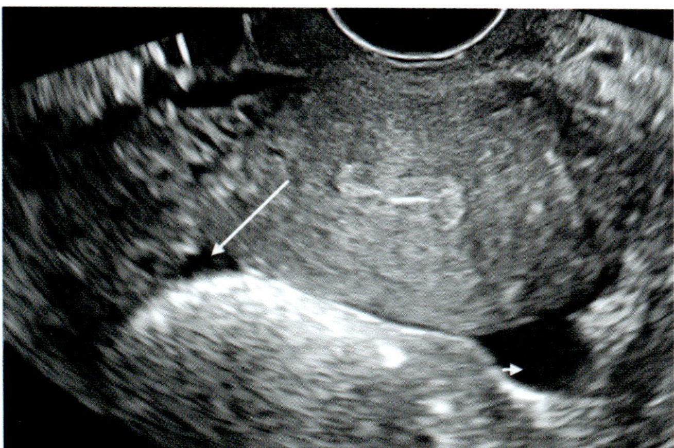

Fig. 5.17: Fluid seen around the ovary (arrow) and collecting behind the uterus (arrowhead) on saline infusion salpingography is an indication of patent tube.

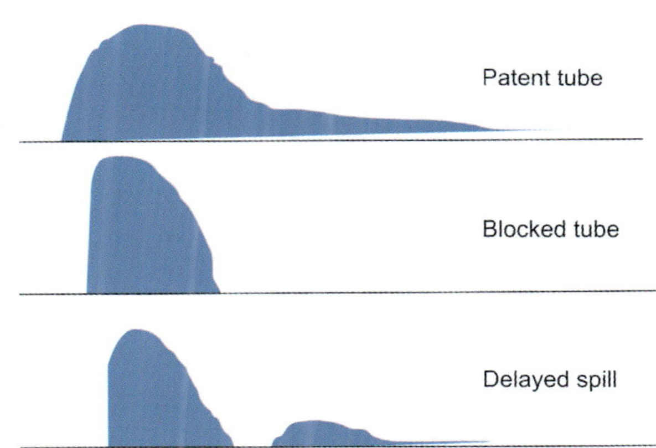

Fig. 5.18: Diagrammatic representation of the spectral pattern in normal tube, blocked tube, and partially blocked tubes.

Absence of spill may indicate blockage. However, at times when there is unilateral block, it is difficult to judge the side of block. In patients with bilateral block, distension of the uterine cavity may cause severe pain. Once the procedure is completed, the instruments are removed. Patient is informed that she might get some pelvic cramping or spotting, but is short termed and should not worry about it. The accuracy of SIS compared to chromopertubation varies from 81.82%[8] to 100%.[9,10]

The procedure is generally safe without any major complication. The risk of pelvic infection and associated peritonitis is approximately 1%. Other risks include nausea or vomiting, vasovagal syncope, and pain during or immediately after the procedure. The reported prevalence of the latter three risks combined is 8.8%.[11] Failure to perform or complete the procedure was documented in 7% in a meta-analysis of 24 studies and 2,278 procedures.[12]

The main disadvantages of the procedure though are inability to visualize the entire tubal lumen and also at times inability to establish unilateral block.

Modifications

Several modifications have been made to this basic procedure of SIS to overcome these disadvantages and improve its diagnostic accuracy as an investigative modality for tubal assessment. The reported modifications are:

- Using pulse Doppler
- Using color Doppler
- Combining air and saline

Using pulse Doppler: If examination during B-mode reveals evidence suggesting tubal occlusion or if a small segment of the tube is not visualized, a pulse Doppler examination can be performed.[13] Doppler gate is placed where the block is expected. This is exactly the point beyond which the tube is not filled with saline or color flow is not seen on injection of saline when examination is done with color Doppler. The gate is reduced to the width of the tube. Brief injections of fluid/saline lasting for 5 seconds are done while Doppler signals are observed. Patent tube is indicated by a short-filling phase with rapid, steep increase in Doppler shift followed by slow uniform fall in Doppler shift. Obstruction presents as short, steep Doppler shift with no subsequent noise signals (Fig. 5.18).

Using color Doppler: Color Doppler can be used with SIS. This is more informative when injection of saline is done selectively toward one of the tubes. Under ultrasound guidance, the tip of the catheter is placed close to either cornu, one by one. First, the color box is placed on the transverse section of the uterus. Color signals following up the uterine cavity confirm the passage of fluid in the uterus. The field of vision is immediately changed over to ovary and adnexa, by spanning the probe from transverse section of uterus, laterally. While injecting a short jet of saline, color box is placed to visualize the adnexa and ovary. Filling up of the box with color signals indicates patency of the tube and absence of such signals indicates block[14] (Figs. 5.19A and B).

Same procedure is repeated on the opposite side. In a study by Peters and Coloum of 129 infertile patients,

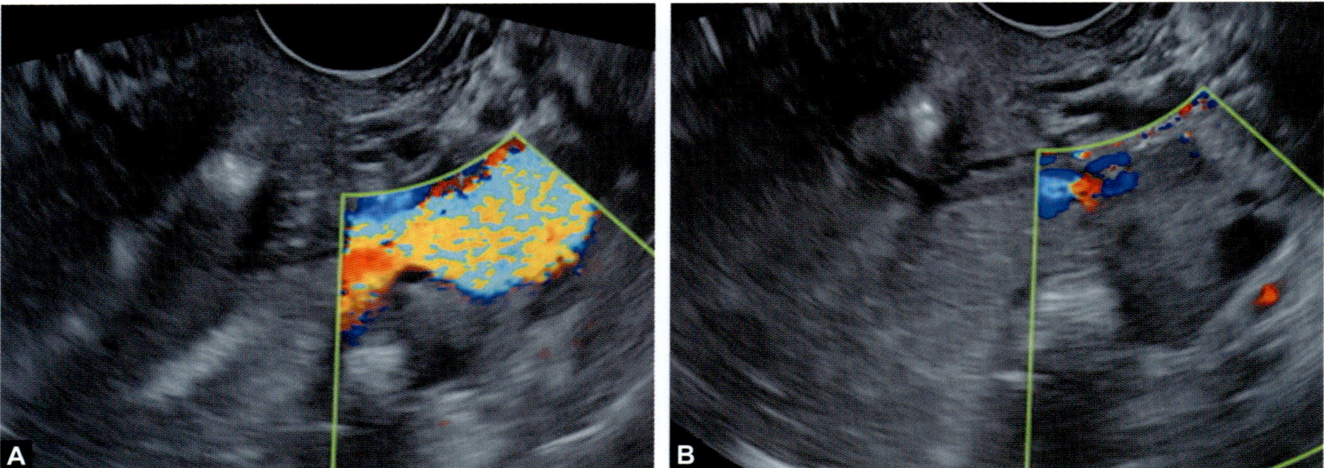

Figs. 5.19A and B: (A) Filling of the color box on injection of the saline through the catheter in the tubes indicates a patent tube. (B) Nonfilling of the color box on injection of the saline through the catheter in the tubes indicates a blocked tube.

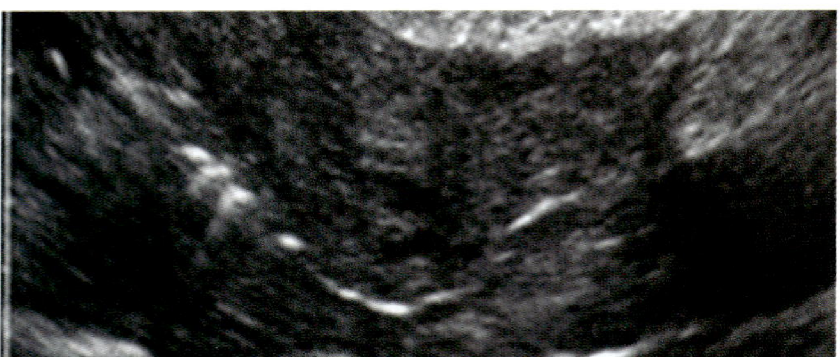

Fig. 5.20: Salpingography done with saline and air showing hyperechoic air bubbles filling up the entire tube on transverse section with tube on left side and uterus on right side on the image.

Doppler SIS showed complete agreement with HSG in 81% of cases. When compared with the gold standard test of tubal assessment, chromopertubation, Doppler SIS showed agreement in 86% of cases, while HSG agreed with chromopertubation only in 75% of cases.[14] In a small study by Kupesic et al., 91.5% agreement was seen between color Doppler sonosalpingography and chromopertubation.[9] Correlation of color Doppler sonosalpingography and HSG with chromopertubation was 81% versus 60%, respectively, in one study.[8] Sonosalpingography was 72.91% sensitive, 81.33% specific with diagnostic accuracy of 78.05%, and positive predictive value (PPV) of 71.42% for tubal pathologies according to a study by Dwivedi et al.[15] Richman and colleagues evaluated tubal patency in 36 infertile women. They compared ultrasound findings with conventional hysterosalpingogram, which had been obtained simultaneously. Ultrasound demonstrated bilateral occlusion with a sensitivity of 100% and showed tubal patency with a specificity of 96%[4]. A detailed evaluation for any pathology is important immediately prior to performing the procedure as hydrosalpinx may create turbulence in the fluid present in the tube and give a false impression of a patent tube.

Combining saline with air: When air is mixed with saline, bubbles are formed and that makes saline appear hyperechoic on ultrasound. This helps better outlining of tubal lumen. This can be done either by agitating air and saline or by injecting air after saline has been already pushed in to fill-up the uterine cavity and tubes (Fig. 5.20). The latter technique was described by Jeanty et al. and showed 79.4% agreement with results of chromopertubation, showed a sensitivity of 85.7%, and specificity of 77.2%.[16]

Hystero-Contrast-Salpingography

While intracavitary lesions are clearly delineated by anechoic media, very small hollow cavities, such as normal tubes are not always easily visualized using SIS.[17] Demonstration of the lumen of tubes requires visualization of movement of fluid using highly echogenic medium.[18] Hyperechogenic contrast medium enhances echo signals and allows detection of the flow, both by B-mode and Doppler ultrasound.

While a cheap and cost-effective option is the use of saline mixing with air, that produces a high-contrast fluid due to the presence of air bubbles. However, these bubbles stand only for a very short period and therefore tubal patency assessment may become practically difficult. Therefore, commercially available contrast media were introduced with microbubbles that can stand for a longer time. Echovist and Levovist (Schering AG, Berlin) consist of suspension of microbubbles made of special galactose microparticles. These are suspended either in galactose solution, as in Echovist or in sterile water, as in Levovist. Just before use, these solutions are prepared by mixing and vigorously shaking the microparticles with the solvent and it can stand for 5–10 minutes. These solutions completely dissolve in the body, within about 30 minutes. These can be used in all patients except those with galactosemia.

Non(embryo-)toxic gel (ExEm-gel® Gynaecologiq BV, Delft, the Netherlands), containing hydroxyethyl cellulose and glycerol, has also been used as an intrauterine medium for sonohysterography as an alternative to saline. Gel instillation offers a more stable filling of the uterine cavity. This gel and its compounds have been tested extensively and can be safely used in medicine. Gel instillation sonography has been used as an alternative to SIS in the assessment of intracavitary uterine lesions.[19,20] This gel, diluted with sterile water and mechanically mixed with air, results in "gel foam" with low viscosity.[21] The echogenic air bubbles remain suspended much longer in diluted gel than they would do in water due to the difference in viscosity. Their passage from the uterine cavity through the tubes to the abdominal cavity can be seen during ultrasound examination.

When this gel is pushed rigorously through small openings in syringes or tubes, turbulence causes local pressure drops resulting in air dissolving in the solution and yielding foam that is stable for several minutes. ExEm-gel (containing 88.25% purified water), however, is rather viscous for passing into the Fallopian tubes. Therefore 10 mL ExEm-gel is diluted with 10 mL purified water (to give mixture containing 94.12% water) and mixed to create foam. Hystero-foam-salpingography (HyFoSy) procedures may be unsuccessful, if there is difficulty inserting the catheter because of a stenotic os or if there are multiple extrusions of the gel infusion sonography (GIS) catheter or excessive backflow from a patulous os.[22]

The foam is slowly injected into the endometrial cavity through the catheter in repeated small (0.5–1 mL) boluses while observing for antegrade flow through the uterine cornua at the transverse plane using B-mode. Distal flow of contrast is followed through each tube until peritoneal spill is visualized (Fig. 5.21). It is easier to visualize spill of the foam into the peritoneal cavity after locating the ovaries.[23,24] The foam usually maintains its echogenicity long enough to allow acquisition of 3D volume images.

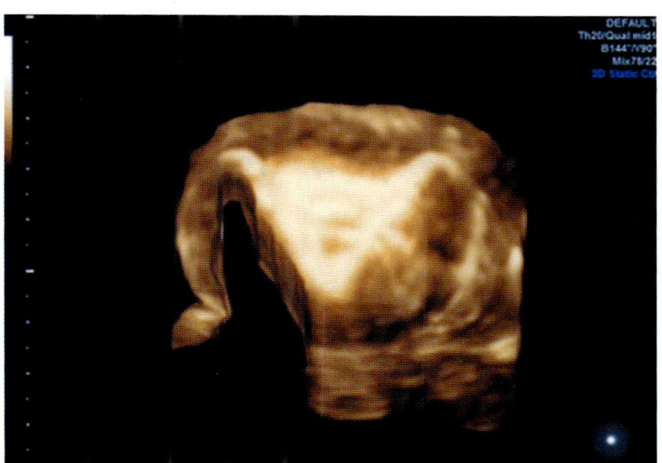

Fig. 5.21: Patent normal fallopian tube as seen on HyFoSy.

The mixture at this ratio created foam is sufficiently stable to show echogenicity for at least 5 minutes and sufficiently fluidy to pass through patent tubes. The viscosity of this foam is comparable with that of Echovist.

Contrast agent that is more easily available in most countries is SonoVue (Bracco). This contrast agent consists of sodium hexafluoride microparticles in normal saline. For assessment of tubal status, 1 mL of SonoVue is diluted with 4 mL of normal saline and is agitated to create foam for injection into the uterus. This contrast is safe for tubal patency assessment, as it is approved for intravascular use also. It is used as an ultrasound contrast agent for vascular studies and for diagnosis of malignancy.

This contrast appears hyperechoic on ultrasound and therefore is called positive contrast. The scanning technique is the same as that for SIS. Using positive contrast, it is possible to delineate the whole tube along with the uterine cavity even on B-mode scanning. This method of tubal evaluation is called HyCoSy. There are ultrasound equipments with contrast mode (contrast tuned imaging technology based on harmonics). Combination of a second-generation contrast medium with contrast-coded imaging (CCI), which discriminates the harmonic response of contrast microbubbles from ultrasound echoes of surrounding tissues, is very helpful for clearer visualization of the fluid passage throughout the tubes. Recently, high accuracy (90%) of automated 3D-CCI HyCoSy in detecting tubal patency has been reported[25] (Figs. 5.22A and B).

Hystero-contrast sonosalpingography has several advantages over SIS in that it helps clearer visualization of uterine cavity, better assessment of tubal lumen and

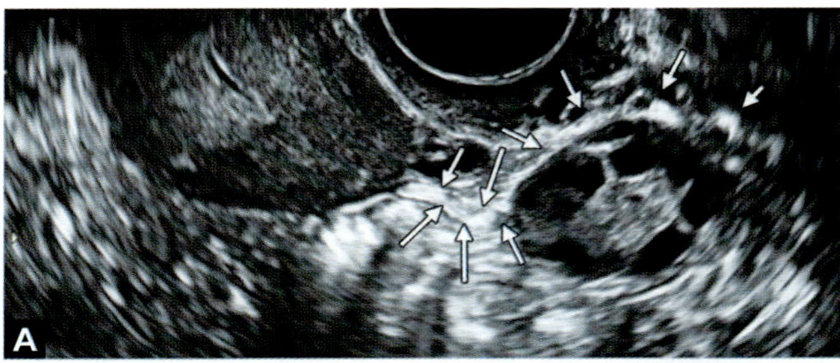

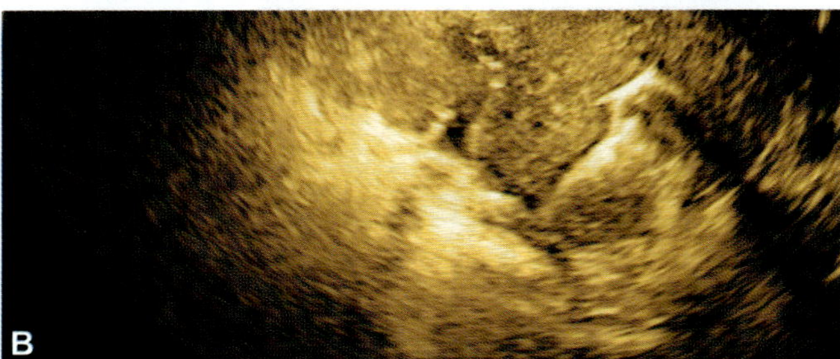

Figs. 5.22A and B: (A) Contrast as it fills up the tube, the entire tubal lumen becomes hyperechoic—as seen on B-mode. (B) Contrast mode shows the normal tube filled with positive contrast.

fimbriae, clearer visualization of spill, and a more exact localization of site of block. However, it is important to mention here that though for tubal patency evaluation, positive contrast is much better than the negative contrast (saline), positive contrast being echogenic, actually obscures the endometrial lesions like polyps and synechiea.

Using Contrast Mode with Positive Contrast

This actually makes it easier to view the spill from the fimbrial end, if the tube is patent. If the tube is not patent, the contrast column in the tube can identify the site of block.

Technique

The procedure technique for HyCoSy is same as for SIS (Box 5.1). As delineation of the tube is better with HyCoSy, total amount of contrast needed is as less as 2–3 mL per tube. For diagnosis of tubal patency, two to three observation phases per tube are needed, with an observation period of continuous flow of about 10 seconds. Visualization of long segments of tube beyond intramural part of the tube usually indicates patency, although whole tube must be observed and spill should be confirmed. Appearance or increase in the fluid in pouch of Douglas may be an indirect sign of tubal patency, same as for SIS.

How Efficient is HyCoSy?

Hystero-contrast-sonosalpingography with contrast is more efficient than with saline solution in determining Fallopian tube patency and is as efficient as HSG and can be used instead of HSG for screening infertile patients.[26] In a diagnostic accuracy study of HyCoSy performed with air and saline (Hydro-HyCoSy) and with contrast media (SonoVue-HyCoSy) considering HSG and/or chromopertubation as reference tests, SonoVue-HyCoSy has been found to be more accurate than SIS for the assessment of Fallopian tubes.[27] While the sensitivity, specificity, PPV, and negative predictive value (NPV) of SIS were 91%, 71%, 55%, and 95%, respectively; they were 87%, 84%, 69%, and 94%, respectively for SonoVue-HyCoSy. The diagnostic accuracy of SIS and of SonoVue-HyCoSy was 77% and 85%, with a Cohen's kappa of 0.52 and 0.66, respectively. In another small study comparing HyCoSy and chromopertubation, there was a high degree of correlation in assessing

Box 5.1: Hystero-contrast-sonosalpingography—preparation and procedure

- Premedication with ibuprofen 1–2 hours prior to procedure
- Ensure patient has had infection (e.g. chlamydia) screening and/or prophylactic antibiotics prescribed
- Lithotomy like position of patient
- Preprocedure detailed pelvic (transvaginal) scan is done to rule out pathologies
- Speculum is inserted and cervix may need to be fixed with tenaculum
- 5–7 Fr ballooned catheter is introduced in cervix with balloon placed above the internal os
- Speculum and tenaculum removed. Transvaginal ultrasound probe inserted
- Contrast mode is activated on the ultrasound machine
- Contrast is prepared by dissolving in the solvent and diluted with saline
- Recheck location of both ovaries so that the operator is aware of the position to check for the fimbrial spill of the contrast
- Obtain transverse section of uterus demonstrating both cornua
- Contrast is slowly injected as scanning is done to image the cornu of uterus and ovary together
- Passage of contrast is followed from cornu of uterus to fimbrial end of the tube
- Once visualized one side, quickly move the probe to the other side to confirm bilateral spill
- Balloon is deflated and catheter is removed

tubal patency, with sensitivity, specificity, PPV, and NPV of 100%, 55.6%, 80%, and 100%, respectively.[28]

One study[29] reported that SonoVue® (Bracco) was more accurate than saline and air medium, especially in the reduction of false occlusion results. Another study,[26] which compared Infoson® (MBI) with saline, found that Infoson®-enhanced HyCoSy provided a significantly larger number of correct diagnoses than saline HyCoSy with an accuracy comparable to that of HSG.

Hystero-contrast-sonosalpingography is accurate in determining tubal patency and evaluating the uterine cavity and can supplant HSG as the first-line diagnostic test in an infertility work-up.[30] Compared to conventional HSG, HyCoSy provides a simultaneous ultrasound evaluation of pelvis and a more cost-effective evaluation of tubal pathology and can be successfully used as a first-line noninvasive screening method.[31] In spite of all the advantages, a recent systematic review[32] found no benefit of commercially available hyperechogenic contrast agents over saline solution in diagnosing tubal patency.

In spite of all advantages, Balen et al. found that both SIS and HyCoSy are insufficiently accurate and inferior to HSG.[33] They quoted a false positive rate of 9% and false negative rate of 20% for HyCoSy. This is because Fallopian tubes are tortuous and usually not confined to a single plane. Moreover, distal parts of the tube may be obscured by bowel gas.

Both false patency and false occlusion results can occur with HyCoSy, irrespective of the type of contrast medium used. One meta-analysis[34] on HyCoSy with Echovist® (Schering AG) reported a false occlusion rate of 10.3% and false patency rate of 6.7%. False patency results from HyCoSy can arise in the following situations. First, bilateral cornual block can result in back pressure of Echovist® within the uterine cavity with intravasation into the extrauterine vessels and mimic tubal filling. Second, Echovist® can track along the pouch of Douglas from a patent tube to the other side, giving the impression of bilateral tubal patency.[35] These problems should be minimized with careful ultrasound technique and can theoretically also occur with HyFoSy. On the other hand, false occlusion results are more difficult to correct and may be unavoidable. It is easier to diagnose tubal patency than it is tubal occlusion by HyCoSy.

There are many factors that can give rise to a false occlusion result. First, the tubal lumen may be temporarily occluded by a mucous plug, blood clot, myometrial spasm, or mucosal edema.[26,27,36-38] The proximal segment being the narrowest part of the fallopian tube is especially prone to this resulting in a diagnosis of a cornual block. Second, technical difficulty can arise from multiple reasons. Contrast leakage or cervical stenosis can occur resulting in failure to achieve adequate pressure of hydrotubation.[35]

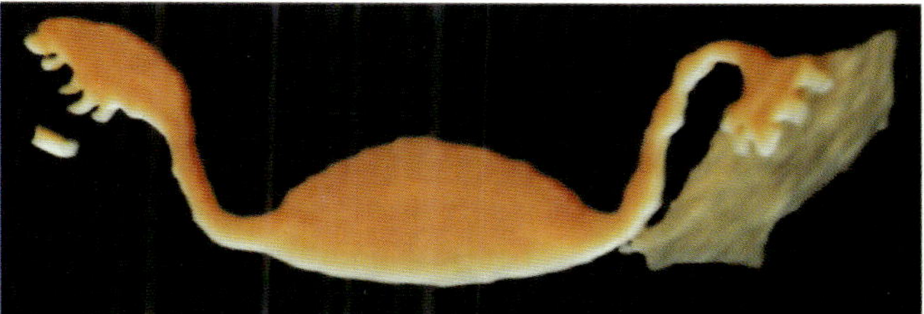

Fig. 5.23: Three-dimensional-HyCoSy, showing endometrial cavity and both the tubes with fimbrial ends.

Modifications

Additional use of pulsed wave Doppler in HyCoSy can be used as a supplement to gray-scale imaging to improve the diagnostic accuracy in cases of suspected tubal occlusion, and in patients in whom intratubal flow was demonstrated only over a short distance.[10] Three-dimensional power Doppler helps to visualize the whole tube and spill[36] (Fig. 5.23). This technique has shown to be superior to conventional HyCoSy with free spill from Fallopian tubes was demonstrated in 91% of tubes using 3D-PD as compared to only 46% by conventional HyCoSy and the contrast agent required was almost half for 3D-PD in one study.[36] There are several advantages with 3D-HyCoSy techniques. It allows simultaneous visualization of the uterine cavity and whole tube, short procedure time and reduced patient discomfort, requirement of less amount of contrast and storage of the 3D volume, which allows off-line review and reassessment.

Technique of Three-Dimensional HyCoSy

SonoVue (Bracco) is used as the contrast agent. Patient preparation, catheter placement and preparation of contrast media are done according to the method described earlier for 2D-HyCoSy. Procedure is performed using a 3D ultrasound machine, with contrast mode. A high-frequency transvaginal volume probe (6–9 MHz) is used for pelvic evaluation.

The transvaginal probe is positioned to visualize the transverse section of the uterus and, if possible, both ovaries laterally. The CCI mode is then started, causing the view of the pelvis to become completely anechoic. In CCI, the ultrasound machine emits a beam at a selected frequency and receives a narrow band of harmonic signal, avoiding overlap between the tissue and the contrast response. The image displayed is based only on harmonic signals produced by contrast-medium microspheres; broadband ultrasonic signals from surrounding tissue are filtered out completely.[38,39]

Using CCI technology during HyCoSy, the intrauterine injection of ultrasound contrast medium in a completely anechoic pelvis was visualized as hyperechoic fluid, seen first in the uterus, then in the tube if it was proximally patent and, finally, as it spilled into the abdominal cavity if the tube was completely patent distally. As the contrast is slowly injected through the balloon catheter into the uterus, transvaginal probe is so oriented that uterine cornu and ovaries are seen on the same plane. Having defined the contrast filling in the tubes, 3D is switched on and volumes are acquired for each side independently.

The sonographic volume acquisition is done with sweep angle, as wide as possible to include the uterus in transverse section and both ovaries laterally (maximum 120°). If it is not possible to accommodate both the ovaries together in a single image, volume of one side may be taken at a time. The contrast medium is hyperechogenic allowing the tubal course and shape to be studied and more than one 3D volume acquisition to be performed. Multiple volumes may be acquired as the contrast is being injected.

Rendering is done in front back viewing direction. Surface-enhanced mode is used. Threshold is set to make the contrast path more clearly visible. Magicut (electronic scalpel) is then used to cut all shadows other than the contrast path. Then high-definition (HD) live rendering mode is switched on and direction of the light is adjusted to visualize the fimbriae and spill to its best. After the final picture is ready, both the halves are matched and put together to make a complete picture of uterus and both tubes (Figs. 5.24A to C).

In a series of 65 subfertile women in whom we performed 3D-HyCoSy followed by a laparoscopy and dye test to evaluate the diagnostic accuracy, the results of 3D-HyCoSy were consistent with that of laparoscopy except in two women.[40] One of these two patients had unilateral tubal block on HyCoSy, but the tube was patent on laparoscopy with injection of the methylene blue dye with

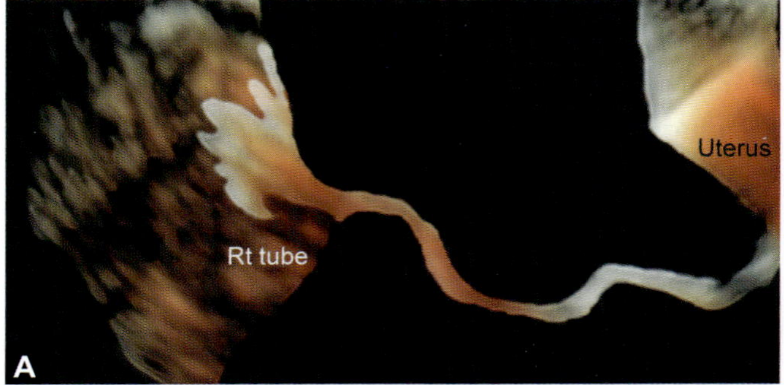

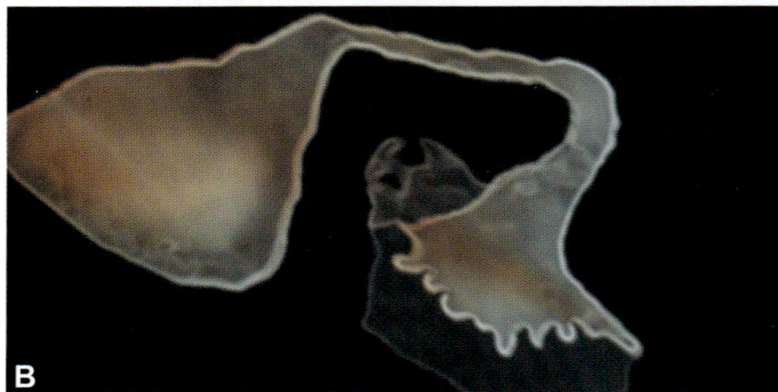

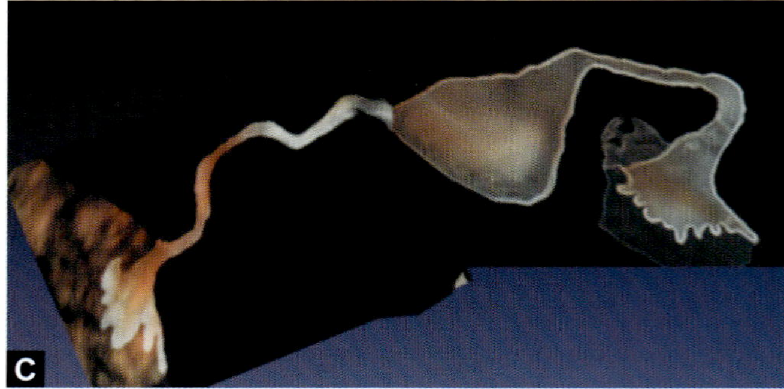

Figs. 5.24A to C: Individual left and right lateral 3D-HyCoSy and the reconstructed complete image of uterus and both the tubes.

pressure. In the other patient, the fimbrial end of the tube was not clearly visualized on 3D-HyCoSy and was thought to be blocked, but on laparoscopy, the distal tubal portion was buried behind the ovary due to endometriosis and the tube was patent. This technique is more informative and reliable than two-dimensional (2D) HyCoSy. Whole extent of the tubal lumen and fimbrial condition can be visualized (Figs. 5.25 to 5.28).

Relation of fimbrial end of tube to ovary can also be defined. Large studies have reported that 3D-HyCoSy is highly accurate with 100% sensitivity, 67% specificity, 89% PPV, and 100% NPV for tubal patency and concordance

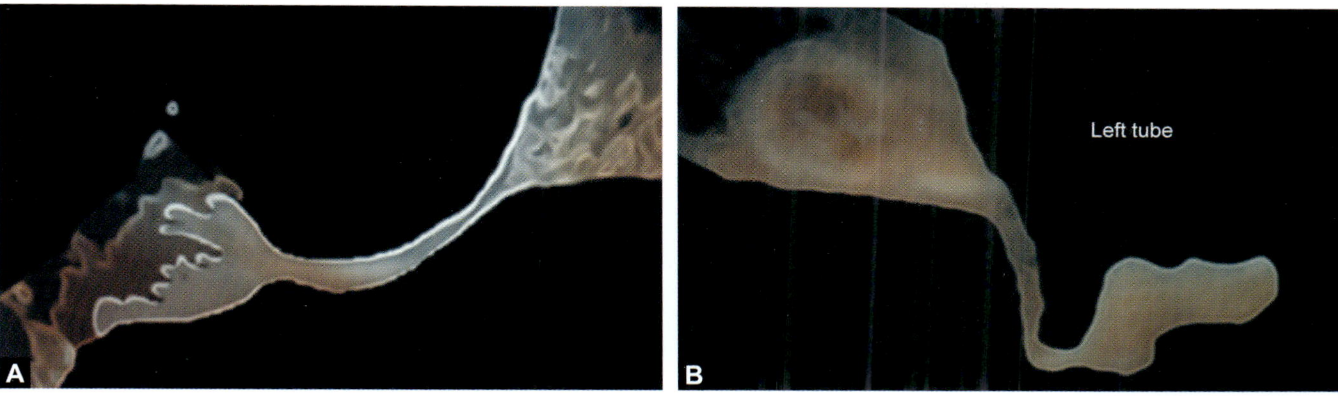

Figs. 5.25A and B: (A) Normal tube. (B) Distal hydrosalpinx.

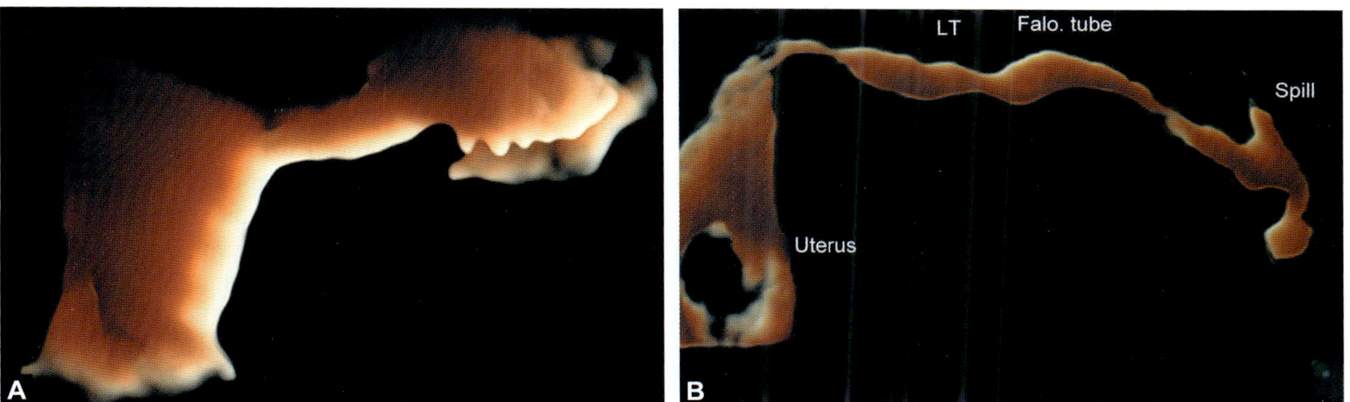

Figs. 5.26A and B: (A) Dilated tube-hydrosalpinx with pruned fimbria. (B) Chronically inflamed beaded tube.

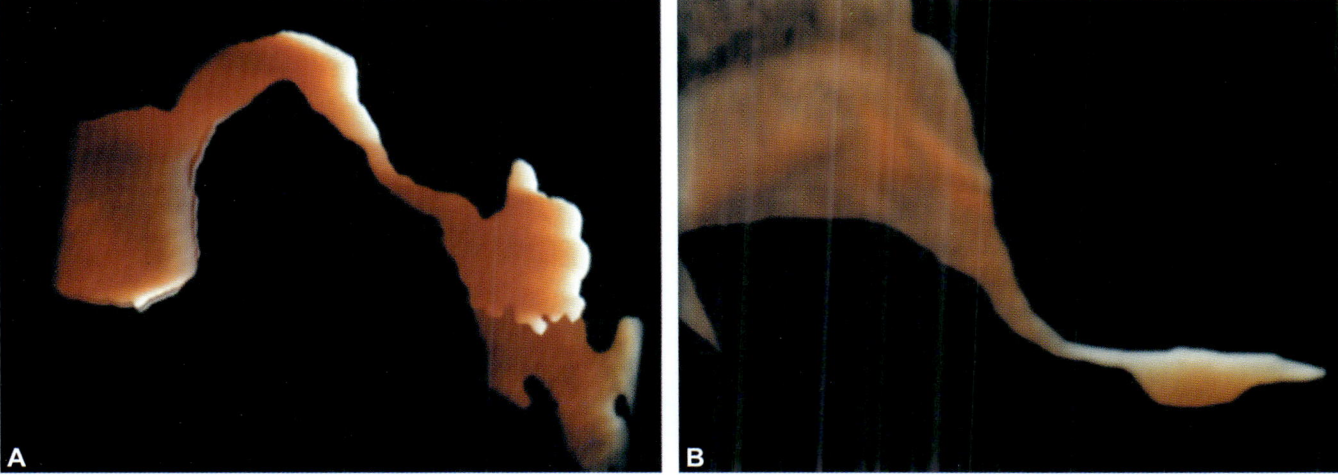

Figs. 5.27A and B: (A) Proximally dilated tube with distal pruned fimbria. (B) Blocked tube.

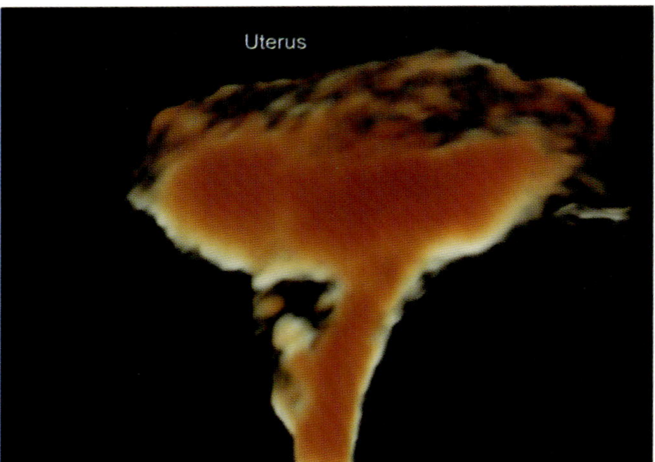

Fig. 5.28: Bilateral blocked tubes.

rate with laparoscopy of 91%.[41] In a study by Kupesic et al., 3D-HyCoSy (sensitivity, specificity, PPV, and NPV of 97.9%, 100%, 97.9%, and 100%, respectively) was found to be marginally superior to 2D-HyCoSy (sensitivity, specificity, PPV, and NPV of 93.6%, 97.3%, 98.2%, and 97.3%, respectively) for tubal assessment.[42]

A recent systematic review[43] reported that 3D-HyCoSy shows high diagnostic accuracy with a pooled sensitivity of 98% and pooled specificity of 90%. Three-dimensional-HyCoSy offers several advantages over 2D-HyCoSy. Three-dimensional volume acquisition and reconstruction of the multiplanar tubal anatomy allows easy visualization of the contrast medium flow throughout the entire tubal length. This reduces false patency and uncertain results due to difficulty tracing the course of convoluted tubes with 2D-HyCoSy. As static images of the tube are captured in an automated process, the procedure is less operator dependent, with no need for difficult probe movements and the captured images can be stored for later review. Since image reconstruction can be performed offline, the procedure time is shorter and less contrast is required, which may help to reduce pain. Nevertheless, 3D-HyCoSy should be regarded as complementary and cannot fully replace 2D-HyCoSy. The main limitations of 3D technology are that of cost, availability, and inability to visualize the real-time passage of contrast medium through the fallopian tubes.[43,44]

Automated 3D volume acquisition permits visualization of the tubes in the coronal view and of the tubal course in 3D space, and should allow less-experienced operators to evaluate tubal patency status relatively easily.

Because of good degree of statistical comparability and concordance of conventional HyCoSy with HSG and laparoscopy and dye test, National Institute for Health and Clinical Excellence (NICE) has recommended HyCoSy as a suitable outpatient procedure for tubal patency assessment in women who are not known to have any comorbidity such as PID, previous ectopic pregnancy, or endometriosis.[26,45] Hystero-contrast-sonosalpingography is well-tolerated by women and associated risks are minimal with the risk of pelvic infection is less than or equal to 1%.

CONCLUSION

Tubal evaluation is essential in subfertile patients. Ultrasound is the modality of choice for diagnosis of tubal pathologies like salpingitis, hydrosalpinx, and tuboovarian masses. Hysterosalpingography has been used for a long time for assessment of tubal patency. Saline infusion sonography has been proved to be fairly reliable technique for tubal evaluation. Its diagnostic accuracy can be improved by the use of pulse Doppler and color Doppler. Introduction of ultrasound contrast media and HyCoSy has improved the visibility of the tubal lumen. Hystero-contrast sonosalpingography is as efficient as HSG in assessing tubal patency and has the advantage of simultaneous pelvic evaluation for pelvic pathology and ovarian reserve. Hystero-contrast sonosalpingography can, therefore, be considered as first-line investigative tool in low-risk women who are not known to have any reproductive comorbidities. Hystero-contrast sonosalpingography combined with 3D ultrasound has the ability to increase the diagnostic accuracy, but this technique is not widely used because of limited availability of 3D ultrasound. While laparoscopic chromopertubation is the gold standard investigative modality for tubal assessment, its use can be restricted to selective group of women as most women could have less invasive ultrasound methods to assess tubal patency.

KEY POINTS

- Evaluation of Fallopian tubes is an essential part of subfertility investigation
- Assessment of fimbrial health is as important as assessment of patency of the tubes
- Laparoscopy and dye test (chromopertubation) is the gold standard investigation for assessment of tubal patency and pathology, but is reserved for high-risk

women in whom reproductive comorbidity is suspected and for those in whom tubal block is suspected on HSG or HyCoSy

- Less invasive investigative tools like X-ray-based HSG and ultrasound-based SIS and HyCoSy are recommended as the first-line investigation for tubal patency assessment in women at low risk for reproductive pathologies like PID or endometriosis
- The role of SIS as a primary investigative tool to assess tubal patency is limited due its low accuracy, but modified SIS by using saline mixed with air or with Doppler application can increase its diagnostic accuracy
- Hystero-contrast-sonosalpingography is as efficient and accurate as HSG in evaluating tubal patency and has the advantage of simultaneous evaluation for pelvic pathology and ovarian reserve
- Modified HyCoSy with application of 3D-PD (3D-HyCoSy) and postprocessing software techniques allows simultaneous visualization of uterine cavity and Fallopian tubes and may potentially increase the diagnostic accuracy. However, it is not used widely due to its limited availability

REFERENCES

1. Gordts S, Campo R, Rombauts L, et al. Endoscopic visualization of the process of fimbrial ovum retrieval in the human. Hum Reprod. 1998;13(6):1425-8.
2. Johnson N, Vandekerckhove P, Watson A, et al. Tubal flushing for subfertility. Cochrane Database Syst Rev. 2002;(3):CD003718.
3. Nanini R, Chelo E, Branconi F, et al. Dynamic echohysteroscopy: a new diagnostic technique in the study of female infertility. Acta Eur Fertil. 1981;12(2):165-71.
4. Richman TS, Viscomi GN, deChurney A, et al. Fallopian tubal patency assessed by ultrasound fluid injection. Work in progress. Radiology. 1984;152(2):507-10.
5. Randolph JF, Ying YK, Maier DB, et al. Comparison of real time ultrasonography, hysterosalpingography and laparoscopy/hysteroscopy in the evaluation of uterine abnormalities and tubal patency. Fertil Steril. 1986;46(5):828-32.
6. Tüfekçi EC, Girit S, Bayirli MD, et al. Evaluation of tubal patency by transvaginal sonosalpingography. Fertil Steril. 1992;57(2):336-40.
7. Deichert U, Schlief R, van de Sandt M, et al. Transvaginal hysterosalpingo-contrast sonography (HyCoSy) compared with conventional tubal diagnostics. Hum Reprod. 1989;4(4):418-24.
8. Stern J, Peters AJ, Coulam CB. Color Doppler ultrasonography assessment of tubal patency: a comparison study with traditional techniques. Fertil Steril. 1992;58(5):897-900.
9. Kupesic S, Kurjak A. Gynecological vaginal sonographic interventional procedures—what does color add? Gynecol Perinatol. 1994;3:57-60.
10. Deichert U, Schlief R, van de Sandt M, et al. Transvaginal hysterosalpingo-contrast sonography for the assessment of tubal patency with gray scale imaging and additional use of pulsed wave Doppler. Fertil Steril. 1992;57(1):62-7.
11. Dessole S, Farina M, Rubattu G, et al. Side effects and complications of sonohysterosalpingography. Fertil Steril. 2003;8(3):620-4.
12. de Kroon CD, de Bock GH, Dieben SW, et al. Saline contrast hysterosonography in abnormal uterine bleeding: a systematic review and meta-analysis. BJOG. 2003;110(10):938-47.
13. Deichert U, van de Sandt M. Transvaginal hysterosalpingo-contrast sonography (Hy-Co-Sy). The assessment of tubal patency and uterine abnormalities by contrast enhanced sonography. Advances in Echo-Contrast. 1993;2:55-8.
14. Peters AJ, Coulam CB. Hysterosalpingography with color Doppler sonography. Am J Obstet Gynecol. 1991;164 (6 Pt 1):1530-2.
15. Dhar Dwivedi AN, Jain M, Tripathi S, Garg S, Jain S. Diagnostic accuracy of sonosalpingography for assessing tubal pathology in women with secondary infertility taking laparoscopy as gold standard. Surg Sci. 2012;3:414-7.
16. Jeanty P, Besnard S, Arnold A, et al. Air-contrast sonohysterography as a first step assessment of tubal patency. J Ultrasound Med. 2000;19(8):519-27.
17. Davison GB, Leeton J. A case of female fertility investigated by contrast-enhanced echo-gynecography. J Clin Ultrasound. 1988;16(1):44-7.
18. Bonilla-Musoles F, Simón C, Serra V, et al. An assessment of hysterosalpingosonography as a diagnostic tool for uterine cavity defects and tubal patency. J Clin Ultrasound. 1992;20(3):175-81.
19. Van den Bosch T, Betsas G, Van Schoubroeck D, et al. Gel infusion sonography (GIS) in the evaluation of the uterine cavity. Ultrasound Obstet Gynecol. 2009; 4:711-4.
20. Werbrouck E, Veldman J, Luts J, et al. Detection of endometrial pathology using saline infusion sonography (SIS) versus gel instillation sonography (GIS): a prospective cohort study. Fertil Steril 2011;95:285-8.
21. Emanuel MH, van Vliet M, Weber M, Exalto N. First experiences with hysterosalpingo-foam-sonography (HyFoSy) for office tubal patency testing. Hum Reprod. 2012;27:114-7.
22. Lim SL, Jung JJ, Yu SL, Rajesh H. A comparison of hysterosalpingo-foam sonography (HyFoSy) and hysterosalpingo-contrast sonography with saline medium (HyCoSy) in the assessment of tubal patency. Eur J Obstet Gynecol Reprod Biol. 2015;195:168-72.
23. Emanuel MH, Exalto N. First experiences with hysterosalpingo-foam sonography (HyFoSy) for office tubal patency testing. Hum Reprod. 2012;27(1):114-7.
24. Van Schoubroeck D, Van den Bosch T, Meuleman C, Tomassetti C, D'Hooghe T, Timmerman D. The use of a

new gel foam for the evaluation of tubal patency. Gynecol Obstet Invest. 2013;75(3):152-6.
25. Zhou L, Zhang X, Chen X, et al. Value of three-dimensional hysterosalpingo-contrast sonography with SonoVue in the assessment of tubal patency. Ultrasound Obstet Gynecol. 2012;40:93-8.
26. Boudghene FP, Bazot M, Robert Y, et al. Assessment of fallopian tube patency by HyCoSy: comparison of a positive contrast agent with saline solution. Ultrasound Obstet Gynecol. 2001;18(5):525-30.
27. Lanzani C, Savasi V, Leone FP, et al. Two-dimensional HyCoSy with contrast tuned imaging technology and a second generation contrast media for assessment of tubal patency in an infertility program. Fertil Steril. 2009;92(3):1158-61.
28. Tanawattanachaeron S, Suwajanakorn S, Uerpairojkit B, et al. Transvaginal hystero-contrast sonography (HyCoSy) compared with chromolaparoscopy. J Obstet Gynaecol Res. 2000;26(1):71-5.
29. Lanzani C, Savasi V, Leone FP, Ratti M, Ferrazzi E. Two-dimensional HyCoSy with contrast tuned imaging technology and a second-generation contrast media for the assessment of tubal patency in an infertility program. Fertil Steril. 2009;92(3):1158-61.
30. Lucaino DE, Exacoustos C, Johns DA, et al. Can hysterosalpingo-contrast sonography replace hysterosalpingography in confirming tubal blockage after hysteroscopic sterilization and in the evaluation of the uterus and tubes in infertile patients? Am J Obstet Gynecol. 2011;204(1):79.el-5.
31. Korell M, Seehaus D, Strowitzki T, et al. Radiologic versus ultrasound fallopian tube imaging. Painfulness of the examination and diagnostic reliability of hysterosalpingography and hysterosalpingo-contrast-ultrasonography with echovist 200. Ultraschall Med. 1997;18(1):3-7.
32. Maheux-Lacroix S, Boutin A, Moore L, et al. Hysterosalpingosonography for diagnosing tubal occlusion in subfertile women: a systematic review with meta-analysis. Hum Reprod. 2014;29(5):953-63.
33. Balen FG, Allen CM, Gardener JE, et al. 3-dimensional reconstruction of ultrasound images of the uterine cavity. Br J Radiol. 1993;66(787):588-91.
34. Holz K, Becker R, Schurmann R. Ultrasound in the investigation of tubal patency. A meta-analysis of three comparative studies of Echovist-200 including 1,007 women. Zentralbl Gynakol. 1997;119(8):366-73.
35. Watrelot A, Hamilton J, Grudzinskas JG. Advances in the assessment of the uterus and fallopian tube function. Best Pract Res Clin Obstet Gynaecol. 2003;17(2):187-209.
36. Sladkevicius P, Ojha K, Campbell S, Nargund G. Three-dimensional power Doppler imaging in the assessment of Fallopian tube patency. Ultrasound Obstet Gynecol. 2000;16(7):644-7.
37. Exacoustos C, Di Giovanni A, Szabolcs B, Binder-Reisinger H, Gabardi C, Arduini D. Automated sonographic tubal patency evaluation with three-dimensional coded contrast imaging (CCI) during hysterosalpingo-contrast sonography (HyCoSy). Ultrasound Obstet Gynecol. 2009;34(5):609-12.
38. Exacoustos C, Zupi E, Szabolcs B, et al. Contrast-tuned imaging and second-generation contrast agent SonoVue: a new ultrasound approach to evaluation of tubal patency. J Minim Invasive Gynecol. 2009;16(4):437-44.
39. Testa AC, Timmerman D, Van Belle V, et al. Intravenous contrast ultrasound examination using contrast-tuned imaging (CnTI) and the contrast medium SonoVue for discrimination between benign and malignant adnexal masses with solid components. Ultrasound Obstet Gynecol. 2009;34:699-710.
40. Panchal S, Nagori CB. Imaging techniques for assessment of tubal status: JHRS. 2014;7(1):2-12.
41. Chan CC, Ng EH, Tang OS, et al. Comparison of three-dimensional hysterosalpingo-contrast-sonography and diagnostic laparoscopy with chromopertubation in the assessment of tubal patency for the investigation of subfertility. Acta Obstet Gynecol Scand. 2005;84(9): 909-13.
42. Kupesic S, Plavsic BM. 2D and 3D hysterosalpingo-contrast-sonography in the assessment of uterine cavity and tubal patency. Eur J Obstet Gynecol Reprod Biol. 2007;133(1):64-9.
43. Alcázar JL, Martinez-Astorquiza Corral T, Orozco R, Dominguez-Piriz J, Juez L, Errasti T. Three-dimensional hysterosalpingo-contrast-sonography for the assessment of tubal patency in women with infertility: a systematic review with meta-analysis. Gynecol Obstet Invest. 2016;81(4):289-95.
44. Badawy SZA, Spirt BA. Ultrasound-guided fallopian tube catheterization. In: Rizk B, Puscheck EE (Eds). Ultrasonography in Gynecology, 1st edition. Cambridge, UK: Cambridge University Press; 2014. pp. 285-6.
45. Dijkman AB, Mol BW, van der Veen F, et al. Can hystero-salpingo-contrast-sonography replace hysterosalpingography in the assessment of tubal subfertility? Eur J Radiol. 2000;35(1):44-8.

Chapter 6

Assessment of Ovarian Reserve

Kannamannadiar Jayaprakasan

Chapter Outline

INTRODUCTION

Ovarian reserve is defined as the quantity and quality of the primordial follicular pool remaining within the ovaries at any given time.[1] Ovarian reserve is a measure of ovarian ageing as it diminishes with age.[2,3] The gradual decline in ovarian reserve dictates the onset of several age-related reproductive events including shortening of the length of the menstrual cycle, menstrual irregularity[4,5] and, finally, the menopause.[6] The associated and well-known age-related decrease in fertility[7,8] is also primarily related to declining ovarian reserve rather than uterine ageing as evident by the equivalent pregnancy rates seen in women of all ages undergoing assisted reproduction treatment (ART) with oocyte donation from younger women.[9,10] Ovarian reserve, therefore, clearly reflects the fertility potential of a woman and strongly influences the possibility of conception either spontaneously or in conjunction with fertility treatment. Women with decreased ovarian reserve may also be at an increased risk of experiencing adverse reproductive events such as miscarriage,[11] aneuploidy,[12] multiple pregnancy,[13] and preeclampsia.[14]

Careful evaluation of subfertile women for signs of reduced ovarian reserve by reliable tests at the outset will help the clinician provide appropriate counseling of the couple about their realistic chances of conception, both spontaneously and after treatment, and may facilitate the choice of treatment for that individual couple. The evaluation of ovarian reserve is now an integral part of the pretreatment assessment of a woman about to undergo ART, and is generally recommended for all women planning in vitro fertilization (IVF). The aim is to identify those women likely to respond poorly, who have a low chance of success and are more likely to have their treatment cycle cancelled, and those prone to ovarian hyperstimulation syndrome (OHSS), which is associated with significant morbidity and potential mortality. An accurate assessment of ovarian reserve and a prediction of ovarian response are important as they allow the treatment protocol to be tailored to the individual, thus potentially increasing the number of oocytes retrieved without risking an exaggerated response. Furthermore, ovarian reserve assessment is increasingly being requested and performed in young patients with cancer prior to and following adjuvant treatment in order to predict the degree of potential impact of chemotherapy and radiotherapy on their reproductive life span. Girls and young women affected with cancer who wish to have children in the future could be advised on their fertility options, which include a rapid cycle prior to cancer treatment, fertility preservation, or no action dependent on their ovarian reserve which can be used to guide them and the treating physicians.

OVARIAN RESERVE TESTS

While chronological age is a marker of ovarian reserve, there is a considerable interindividual variation in quantitative and qualitative ovarian reserve as indicated by histological studies demonstrating a variable number of primordial follicle cohort within the ovaries at any given age,[15,16] and in the clinically evident variability in response to gonadotropin stimulation and live birth rates following IVF in women of the same age group.[17] Several ultrasound and endocrine markers of ovarian reserve based on the mechanism of ovarian ageing have been identified and proposed for the prediction of fertility. Primarily, all of these tests aim to estimate the number of gonadotropin-responsive or "selectable follicles," which are assumed to be reflective of primordial follicle population. Two key challenges in assessing the predictive ability of these markers are the population in whom the predictive evaluation should be performed and the outcome against which the markers need to be evaluated.[18,19] While the ideal population to be assessed is general women wishing to delay conception, studies are invariably conducted on those women attending the infertility clinic and those undergoing IVF. The IVF population offers an ideal clinical group in which a defined clinical outcome directly relating to ovarian reserve, but not influenced by male factor, can be evaluated as it provides a quantitative assessment of the number of eggs retrieved and poor ovarian response to gonadotropin stimulation or cycle cancellation due to inadequate follicle development, both of which are closely linked to the likelihood of the desired outcome namely live birth.[18]

The reported endocrine markers of ovarian reserve include factors produced by the developing follicles, such as anti-Müllerian hormone (AMH), inhibin B, estradiol, and the hormone under the inhibitory control of the latter two factors, follicle-stimulating hormone (FSH). There are various ultrasound markers which include the total antral follicle count (AFC), ovarian volume, and ovarian vascularity. The sensitivities, specificities, and predictive values of these tests have been evaluated in many studies by correlating the test results with the number of oocytes retrieved, the poor or exaggerated ovarian response to controlled ovarian stimulation, and pregnancy or live birth rates following during IVF.[1]

Ultrasound Markers

Over the last two decades, various ultrasound markers have been investigated to evaluate their role in the prediction of ovarian reserve. The three most common markers that have been specifically addressed are ovarian volume, AFC, and ovarian stromal blood flow. Most investigators have used conventional two-dimensional (2D) ultrasound to assess ovarian morphology and quantify these ovarian reserve variables. The introduction of three-dimensional (3D) ultrasound, quantitative 3D power Doppler angiography (3D-PDA), and automated volume measurements [sonography-based automatic volume count (SonoAVC: GE Healthcare)] has enabled clinicians and researchers to use these advanced ultrasound modalities with a view to improve the predictive accuracy of ultrasound assessment of ovarian reserve.

Ovarian Volume

The first ultrasound marker of ovarian reserve to be evaluated was ovarian volume.[20] It can easily be measured from 2D ultrasound images, using the principle of the volume calculation of an ellipsoid using the formula: length × width × depth × ft/6 (Figs. 6.1A and B) or with 3D ultrasound and associated softwares. The commonly used method to calculate ovarian volume from 3D ultrasound ovarian volume dataset is "rotational" method possible through Virtual Organ Computer-Aided Analysis (VOCAL™: GE Healthcare), which also generates a 3D model of the ovary (Figs. 6.2A to D). The technique involves manual delineation of the ovary in the multiplanar display that shows the three perpendicular planes characteristic of 3D ultrasound. VOCAL allows rotation of the 3D dataset about a central axis through a number of predefined rotation steps.[21] The most appropriate rotation step for its use in a clinical or research setting recommended is 9° as it provides the best compromise between reliability, validity, and time taken for measurement. While the volume measurements using 3D technique have been shown to be statistically more reproducible than 2D measurements, the degree of reproducibility between observers with 3D US is extremely high.[21]

The role of ovarian volume as a marker of reserve has been evaluated in many studies with conflicting results. The rationale of using ovarian volume as an ovarian reserve marker is that the volume reflects the size of total follicle population remaining within the ovary which was confirmed in a histological study.[22] Syrop et al. found a reduction in estradiol levels, the number of oocytes collected and pregnancy rates correlated with decreasing ovary volume in women undergoing assisted reproduction cycles,[20] and Bowen et al. found a significant correlation between

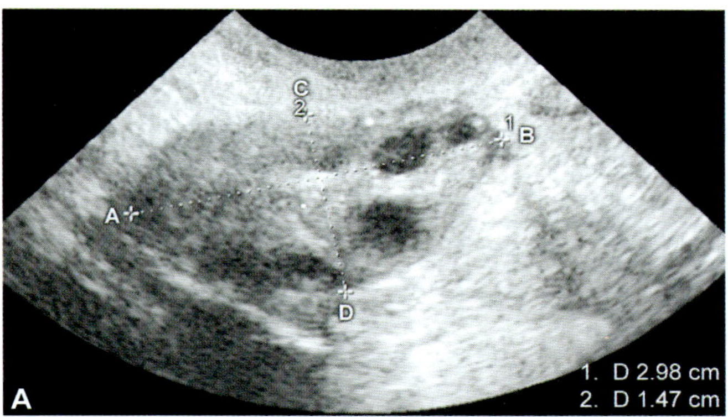

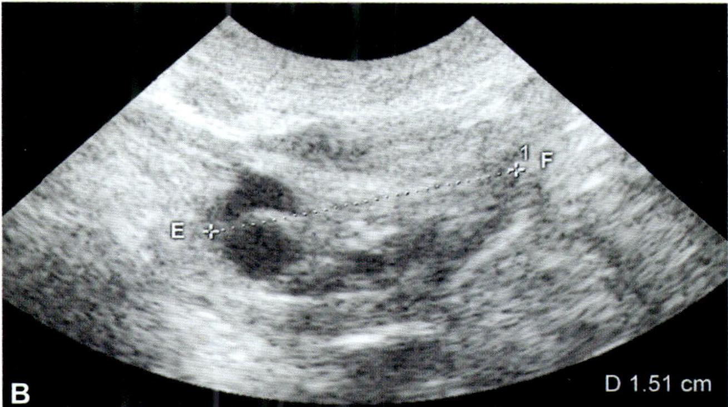

Figs. 6.1A and B: Two-dimensional method of volume calculation. Volume is measured using an ellipsoid formula: length × width × depth × $\pi/6$. (A) Longitudinal diameter (A-B) and anteroposterior diameter (C-D) are measured in the longitudinal plane. (B) Transverse diameter (E-F) is measured in the transverse plane.

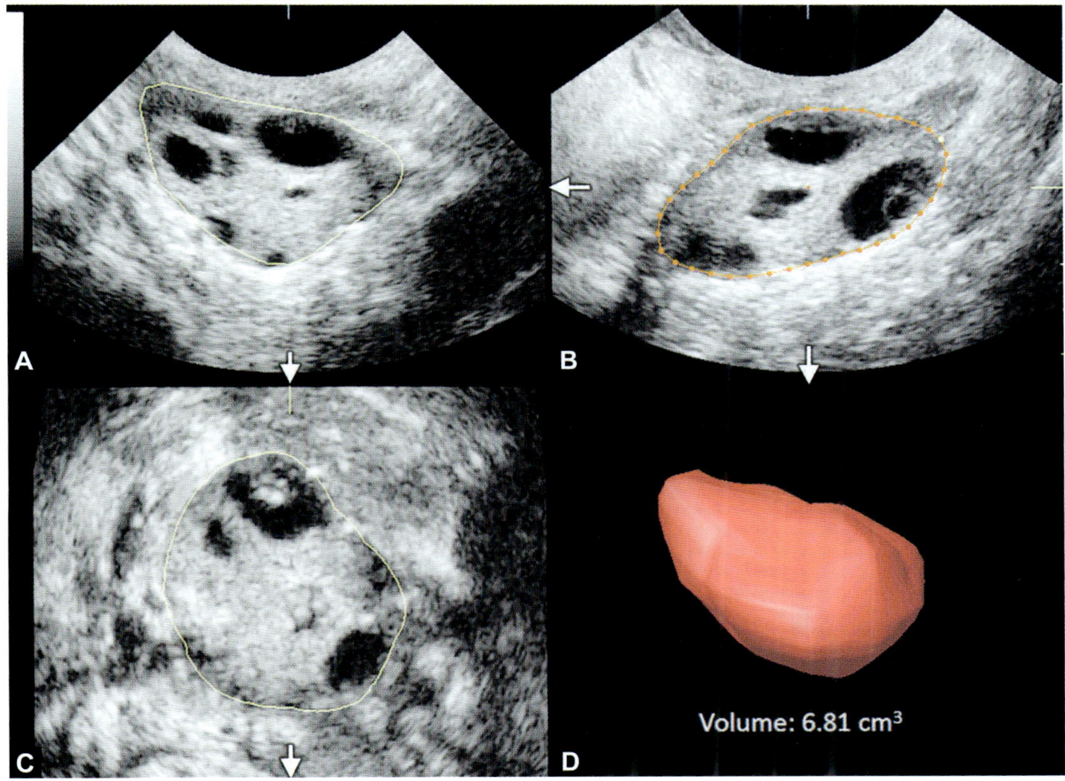

Figs. 6.2A to D: Three-dimensional method of volume calculation: VOCAL. The measurement is performed in the B-plane by outlining the ovarian cortex manually. The ovarian dataset has been rotated 180° through twenty 9° rotation steps about a central vertical axis denoted by the blue arrow in the B-plane. The resultant 3D model of the ovary is shown in (D). (*Abbreviation:* 3D, three-dimensional; VOCAL, Virtual Organ Computer-Aided Analysis)

reduced ovarian volume, increasing age and FSH levels.[23] Schild et al. examined the role of ovarian volume measurements made using pretreatment 3D datasets in 152 IVF cycles and found no relation to IVF outcome other than a nonsignificant trend to smaller ovarian measurements in the conception group.[24] Subgroup analysis comparing absolute ovarian size revealed a pregnancy rate of only 6.7% in patients with a minimum unilateral ovarian volume of no more than 3 cm^3, which represented a single standard deviation below the mean, compared with 21.9%

in patients with a minimum ovarian volume of more than 3 cm^3. However, other studies have not seen such significant differences in ovarian volume between normal and poor responders in women aged less than 37 years[25] or in women at high risk for cancellation of assisted reproduction cycles.[26] While the value of ovarian volume on its own in predicting poor ovarian response is limited, ovarian volume measurement in women with or without polycystic ovaries may be a useful tool for predicting excessive response to ovarian stimulation.[27] An ovarian volume of more than 10 cm^3 in the absence of a dominant follicle or cyst of more than 10 mm is diagnostic of a polycystic ovary[28] itself is a risk factor for excessive ovarian response and OHSS.

A systematic review of all the relevant high-quality studies concluded that ovarian volume, as an individual marker of ovarian reserve and predictor of response to stimulation, has minimal clinical application.[1] Further, the use of ovarian volume as a marker in routine clinical practice is limited if there is a cyst or a large follicle in the ovary as it will falsely increase the baseline ovarian volume. The value of ovarian volume as a prognosticator of ovarian response is limited in certain other clinical situations such as in polycystic ovary syndrome (PCOS) women who have an increased ovarian volume due to a possible increase in the ovarian stroma and in women who had ovarian surgery, which may decrease ovarian volume without reducing the follicular pool;[29] although recent evidence suggests surgery may have a detrimental effect on ovarian reserve and the number of follicles.

Antral Follicle Count

The different types of growing follicles seen within the ovaries, depending on the stages of development, include primordial follicles, early growing follicles, antral follicles, and preovulatory follicles. While the ovarian reserve is principally composed of primordial or resting follicles, early growing follicles, which measure less than 1–2 mm in diameter, are composed of large primary, secondary, and preantral follicles, which grow at a slow rate in response to local regulatory factors, with endogenous FSH playing a permissive role. A small proportion of follicles develop into antral follicles of that measure 2 mm or more in diameter, which are highly sensitive and responsive to FSH and are commonly termed "selectable follicles" therefore. Larger antral follicles measuring 5–10 mm are gonadotropin-dependent. The number of "selectable" gonadotropin-responsive (2–5 mm) and gonadotropin-dependent (5–10 mm) follicles present in the ovaries is believed to reflect the number of remaining primordial follicles and, thus, the ovarian reserve. Further, the number of selectable follicles, that are available to recruit, determines the ovarian response to controlled ovarian stimulation during IVF. Antral follicles of at least 2 mm will be readily seen on transvaginal ultrasound and the AFC measured using ultrasound is considered as a good predictor of ovarian reserve and ovarian response to gonadotropin stimulation during IVF treatment.[1]

The number of gonadotropin responsive antral follicles detected by transvaginal ultrasound has been evaluated in the general subfertility population and in women undergoing ART, as a measure of ovarian ageing. The correlation between the number of antral follicles with a diameter up to 10 mm measured during the early follicular phase and reproductive ageing has been investigated in a cohort of 162 regularly cycling women of 25–46 years of age with proven fertility.[30] The AFC (r = –0.67) showed a higher correlation with chronological age than the total ovarian volume (r = –0.29) and there was a decline in the mean number of antral follicles of 8.2% (95% CI: 5.2–11.2%) per chronological year. This was evident when the range of follicles across different age groups was evaluated with the number of follicles ranging from 7 to 22 at the age 30 and between 2 and 7 by 40 years of age. There was a biphasic pattern of decline in AFCs with a mean yearly decline of 4.8% before the age of 37 years compared to 11.7% thereafter. This finding was concordant with the age-related decline in primordial follicles as noted in the classical histological study of the ovaries obtained during autopsy or surgery in premenopausal women.[6] When the histological data were restricted to the women of the same age group of this study as in the study by Scheffer et al., the disappearance rate of primordial follicles was similar before 37 years at 4.0% per year but higher at 23% after this age. Even though this study is limited by its cross-sectional study design, the data indicate that AFC, which is thought to be reflective of the primordial follicle population, is a marker of ovarian ageing.

Tomas et al. were the first to report the role of AFC in predicting the ovarian response during IVF treatment.[31] The number of antral follicles measuring 2–5 mm was measured using conventional 2D transvaginal ultrasound, performed after pituitary downregulation in 166 women undergoing their first cycle of IVF treatment. Based on the total number of antral follicles, the women were divided into those with inactive ovaries that contained less than 5 follicles, those with normal ovaries containing 5–15 follicles, and those with polycystic-like ovaries (PCO) with more than 15 follicles. Despite a similar total gonadotropin dose for ovarian stimulation in all three groups, there was a significant difference in the mean number of oocytes retrieved (5.4 ± 2.5; 7.4 ± 4.5; and 10.5 ± 5.1, respectively; $P = 0.006$), which was directly related to the number of antral follicles ($r^2 = 0.131$; $P < 0.001$). While the ovarian volume was correlated with the AFC ($r^2 = 0.097$; $P < 0.001$), it had no relationship to the number of oocytes retrieved. The authors concluded that the number of small follicles observed before the ovarian stimulation was a better predictor of IVF outcome than ovarian volume or age alone.

Subsequently, many studies have evaluated the predictive ability of AFC in assessing ovarian response and conception following IVF treatment. A significant correlation between the number of antral follicles with diameters measuring between 2 and 10 mm,[32] or 2 and 6 mm,[33] or 2 and 8,[34] or 2 and 5 mm,[35,36] as assessed by both conventional 2D[37,38] and 3D[39,40] transvaginal ultrasound, and the number of oocytes retrieved has been observed. However, the relationship between AFC and conception following IVF has been poor in most of these studies. This has been confirmed in a meta-analysis,[1] which concluded the performance of AFC in the prediction of poor response in IVF was adequate and better than the widely used "ovarian reserve" marker, the basal FSH level, although its performance for predicting conception is poor. The optimum cut-off levels of AFC (2–10 mm in diameter) with the maximum sum of sensitivity and specificity for the prediction of poor ovarian response are reported as 10.[32] Further reports indicated that AFC is equal to AMH, the best endocrine marker of ovarian reserve, in predicting poor ovarian response, but both AFC and AMH are poor predictors of pregnancy rates following IVF treatment.[32,41] This suggests that the ovarian reserve markers including AFC are able to quantify the quantity better than the quality of the remaining follicle pool.

Recent studies incorporating a large number of IVF cycles have reported that AFC is a significant predictor of live birth rates.[42,43] Table 6.1 illustrates the probabilities of live birth at different AFC thresholds based on the data collected from a single tertiary fertility unit in the United Kingdom (UK),[43] while the data need to be validated externally before applying these results for counseling couples in other clinics. The significant predictive ability of AFC to estimate live births observed in larger studies may be related to its significant ability to predict the number of oocytes retrieved during IVF, which is strongly correlated with live birth rate independent of age.[19]

Antral follicle count has also been considered as the most significant predictor of the development of OHSS and ovarian hyper-response in women undergoing IVF treatment. The optimum cut-off[7] levels with the maximum sum of sensitivity and specificity for the prediction of exaggerated response is 22,[44] which seems more in keeping with the normal ranges defined by the Rotterdam consensus on the ultrasonographic diagnostic criteria for the PCO, which by definition represents the upper extreme of normality. A meta-analysis by Broer et al. confirmed that the predictive ability of AFC for exaggerated ovarian response is equivalent to AMH, which is the best endocrine marker in predicting exaggerated ovarian response.[45]

While the AFC is confirmed to be one of the two best available predictors of ovarian reserve, there is a wide variation in terms of the technique of measurements, the timing of AFC measurement in relation to menstrual cycle and phase of IVF treatment (pretreatment or after downregulation) and the size of antral follicle cohort that are included in the total AFC. The AFC can be measured using conventional 2D or 3D ultrasound (Figs. 6.3A to D) with an acceptably high level of clinical agreement.[46,47] Recent developments have seen the introduction of a 3D automated technique; SonoAVC, which allows a semiautomated analysis of the antral follicle population (Figs. 6.4A to D).[48] Although 3D ultrasound and SonoAVC have been shown to offer a significant advantage over 2D imaging in terms of measurement reliability of AFC, the predictive ability of AFC for ovarian response during IVF has been similar with all the measurement methods. Further, there are limitations with routine use of 3D ultrasound and SonoAVC with its relatively higher cost limiting widespread uptake particularly if its use is limited to the field of reproductive medicine. It has, therefore, generally been agreed that the use of real-time 2D ultrasound imaging is adequate for measurement and counting of antral follicles in routine clinical practice.[49] Antral follicle count is best performed in the early follicular phase of the menstrual cycle (days 2–5) to minimize the effect of intracycle fluctuations and reduce the likelihood of incorrectly including coexisting ovarian cysts or the corpus luteum in the AFC. Further, this helps to schedule all pretreatment assessment concurrently as it is widespread clinical practice to perform standard baseline endocrine assays such as basal FSH and luteinizing hormone (LH) levels in the

Table 6.1: Performance of AFC at different cut-off levels as a predictor of treatment outcome during ART in a tertiary fertility unit in the United Kingdom (1,012 cycles); the overall prevalence (pretest probability) of live birth, poor ovarian response, and cycle cancellation in the whole study population correspond to 35.5%, 11.9%, and 5%

AFC cut-off	*(n) subjects*	*Probability of live birth (%)*	*Probability of poor ovarian response (%)*	*Probability of cycle cancellation (%)*
≤3	3	0	67	30
≤4	20	5	67	30
≤5	46	6.5	57	24
≤6	70	7	57	24
≤7	116	16	50	21
≤8	145	20	44	17
≤9	186	22.5	38	15
≤10	235	23	35	14
≤11	286	26	33	13
≤12	334	27	28	11
≤13	391	27	26	10
≤14	433	28	24	10
≤15	488	29	22	9
≤16	528	30	21	8
≤17	580	31	19	7
≤18	622	31	18	7
≤19	654	32	17	7
≤20	687	33	17	7
<21	720	32	16	6
≤22	734	32	16	6
≤23	754	32	15	6
≥24	250	39	1.6	

AFC, antral follicle count

Note: Poor response is defined as cycle cancellation due to inadequate follicular response or retrieval of less than three oocytes.

early follicular phase. Use of gonadotropin-releasing hormone (GnRH) agonist therapy as part of the conventional "long" downregulation protocol does not influence the AFC, which has a similar accuracy for the prediction of ovarian response regardless of whether the assessment is performed before treatment is commenced or after downregulation.[50] However, assessment prior to treatment has an additional advantage in that it provides an opportunity for a pretreatment evaluation of pelvis to screen for pathology such as a hydrosalpinx, endometrial polyp, uterine anomaly, submucosal fibroid, or an endometriotic cyst all of which have been shown to have an adverse effect on IVF outcome and are amenable to surgery.

As discussed before, there is limited consensus on which follicles should be included in the total AFC, and the current evidence base includes studies using follicles measuring 2–5, 2–6, 2–8, or 2–10 mm in diameter. Manual measurement of the number and diameter of each and

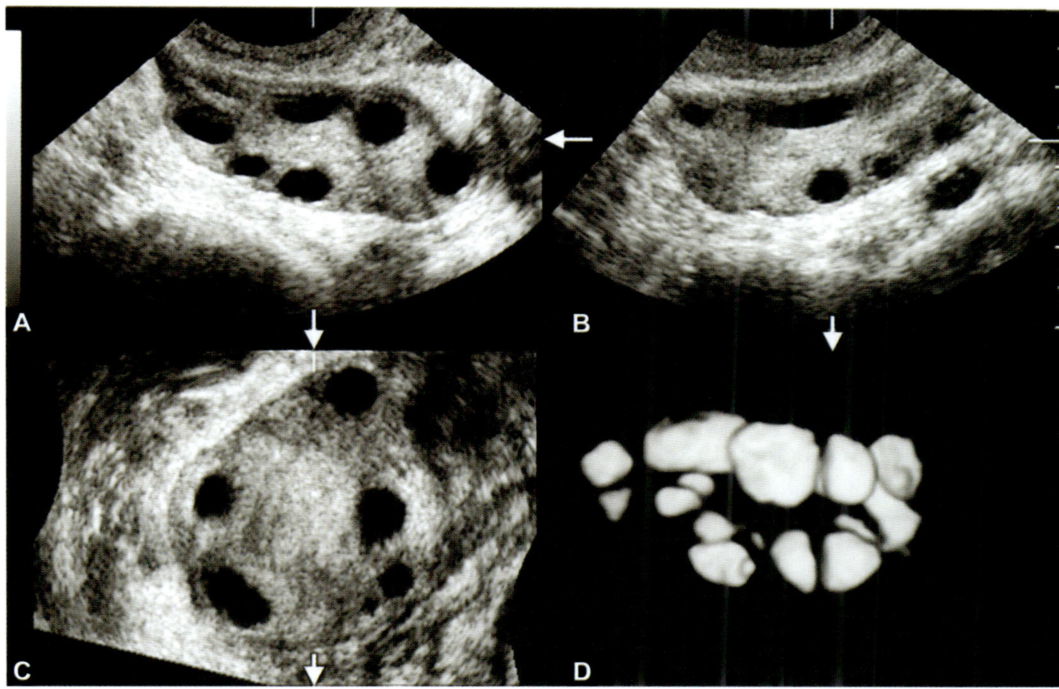

Figs. 6.3A to D: Three-dimensional multiplanar display of the ovary showing antral follicles. Three mutually related orthogonal image planes at 90° to one another are shown. (A) Longitudinal view or A-plane, (B) transverse view or B-plane, and (C) coronal view or C-plane. Antral follicles are clearly visualized with the application of "inversion mode" to a 3D ultrasonographic dataset, which allows immediate demonstration of antral follicles within an ovary (D). (*Abbreviation:* 3D, three-dimensional)

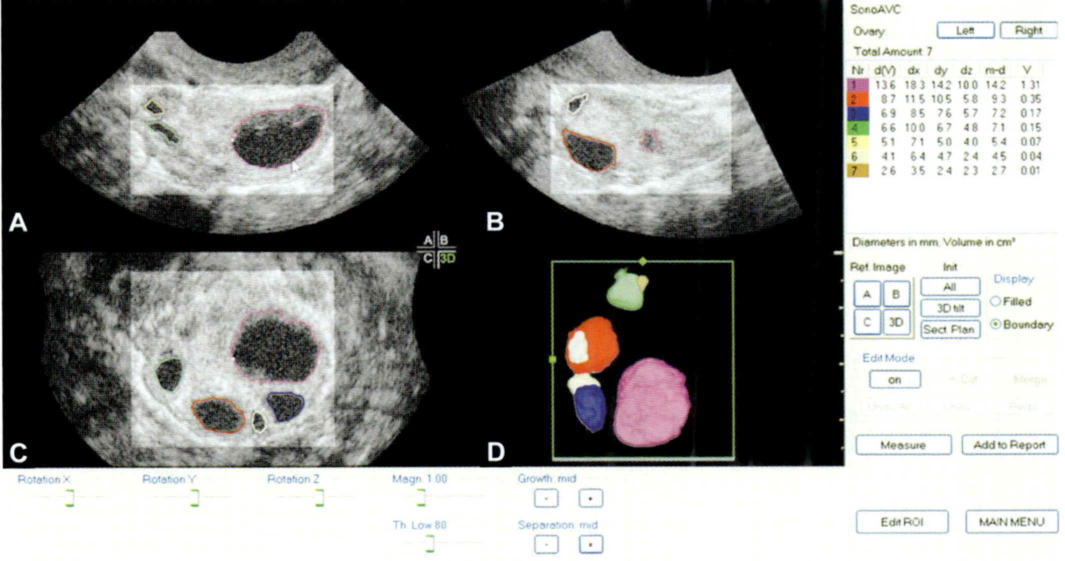

Figs. 6.4A to D: (A to D) Semiautomated AFC made using SonoAVC: It identifies the follicles and color codes each follicle differently. It also provides an automated assessment of the number of follicles with their size and volume. This ovary has one follicle above 10 mm which needs to be excluded from the total AFC. (*Abbreviation:* AFC, antral follicle count; SonoAVC, sonography-based automatic volume count)

every antral follicle, especially the smaller ones, is labor intensive and not straightforward. A recent study utilizing SonoAVC for automated antral follicle measurements reported the number of antral follicles measuring 2–6 mm is the most reflective of the quantitative status of ovarian reserve as this follicular cohort is most closely related to serum AMH levels, and is the best predictor of ovarian response as assessed by the number of mature oocytes retrieved at egg collection.[51] However, the predictive ability of this cohort of antral follicles is equivalent to that of total follicle counts made using cohorts of 2–5, 2–8, and 2–10 mm for the prediction of poor ovarian response, the most clinically useful information required prior to enrolling a woman into IVF treatment program. This is possibly because of the fact that the total follicle count is largely defined by the number of smaller antral follicles measuring 2–6 mm anyway as these follicles accounted for 76% and 70% of the total number of antral follicles measuring 2–8 and 2–10 mm, respectively, in one study.[51] In order to avoid the time-consuming process of measuring each and every follicle, it is recommended that counting all identifiable antral follicles of 2–10 mm in diameter would provide the most practical method for assessment of AFC in day-to-day clinical practice.

While the biological variation in the number of antral follicles between cycles has been reported,[52] the predictive value of AFCs demonstrated minimal intercycle variation.[53] The intercycle variability was greater[52] as was the interobserver variability[54] at higher AFCs and this indicates that the cycle variability may partly be due to the variation in the reproducibility between the observers. When the impact of intercycle variability on the response to gonadotropin stimulation in two consecutive IVF cycles was evaluated, there was no difference in ovarian response or cycle cancellation rates between the low and high AFC cycles in an individual.[52] The variability was relatively low in older women and women with a low AFC. This finding is clinically valuable as little difference in AFCs between cycles is expected once a woman was predicted to have low ovarian reserve due to a reduced AFC.[55] A study, utilizing 3D ultrasound to limit the observer variation in measurement reproducibility, reported minimal variation in AFC between cycles with a mean interval of 5.4 ± 1.2 months.[56] This observation obviates the need for repeating follicle count to predict ovarian response in women undergoing repeated IVF cycles, if the subsequent treatment cycle is performed within 6 months of the initial assessment.

In summary, AFC can be performed in the early follicular phase using conventional 2D ultrasound and using a high-resolution transvaginal ultrasound transducer of a minimum frequency of 7 MHz, which allows clear visualization of 2 mm follicles. Antral follicle cohort of 2–10 mm in diameter can be included in the total AFC. A systematic approach should be adopted for AFC assessment, which should ideally be performed by an appropriately trained person. A practical approach to measure the number of antral follicles in the ovary is described in Box 6.1.

Ovarian Blood Flow

Various endocrine and paracrine factors are involved in the complex process of ovarian folliculogenesis.[57] An

Box 6.1: A systematic approach to count antral follicles

1. Transvaginal ultrasound scan using high-resolution transducer of at least 7 MHz frequency
2. Women should empty their bladder prior to ultrasound assessment
3. Identify the ovary
4. Perform a sweep through the ovary in longitudinal and transverse planes to identify the follicles and to rule out any pathology
5. Keep the ovary in its longitudinal plane and decide on the direction of the sweep to measure and count follicles
6. Measure the largest follicle in two dimensions
   - If the largest follicle is less than or equal to 10 mm in diameter:
     - Start to count from outer ovarian margin of the sweep to the opposite margin
     - Consider every round or oval transonic structure within the ovarian margins to be a follicle
     - Repeat the procedure in the contralateral ovary
     - Combine the number of follicles in each ovary to obtain the total AFC
   - If the largest follicle is more than 10 mm in diameter:
     - Measure all the other larger follicles sequentially in the order of reducing size until a follicle with a diameter of 10 mm is identified
     - Perform a total count (as described) regardless of follicle diameter
     - Subtract the number of follicles of more than 10 mm from the total follicle count

adequate ovarian blood supply is essential to its normal function and may influence the endocrine and paracrine signals that effect the growth and development of follicles.[58] It has been suggested that an increased ovarian blood flow may lead to a higher delivery of gonadotropins and other growth factors to the granulosa-theca cell complex of the developing follicles resulting in a multifollicular response to ovarian stimulation during ART.[59,60] Other studies, although cross sectional in nature, have reported an age-related decline in ovarian stromal vascularity in both fertile and subfertile populations.[40,61,62] Ultrasound assessment of ovarian blood flow may be helpful in predicting the response to controlled ovarian stimulation during ART. Due to the anatomical difficulty in visualizing the infundibulopelvic-ovarian vessels, and in order to standardize measurements, a main artery in the ovarian stroma is generally examined to elicit flow velocity wave forms, which are assumed to be representative of the total ovarian vascular dynamics.[63]

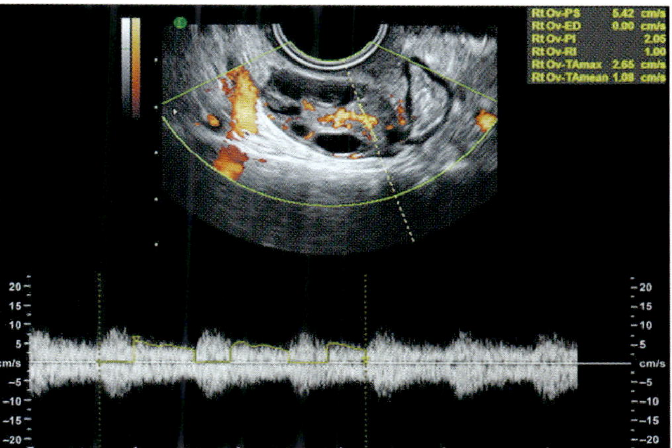

Fig. 6.5: Two-dimensional pulse wave Doppler of ovary: Doppler gate is applied to the prominent ovarian stromal vessel to obtain blood flow velocity wave form which is used to analyze blood flow velocity and resistance indices.

With the conventional 2D pulse wave Doppler technique, the arteries within the ovarian stroma are visualized with the color Doppler technique, ensuring that no artery near the surface is measured. The blood flow velocity waveforms are obtained by placing the Doppler gate over the colored areas and activating the pulsed Doppler function. No correction is usually made for the angle of insonation in the vessels of the ovarian stroma because it cannot be detected for smaller vessels. However, the highest achievable signals are sought. Blood flow velocity waveforms illustrating the frequency and intensity of the shifted Doppler frequencies are demonstrated (Fig. 6.5). Optimal flow velocity waveforms with maximum Doppler shift are selected for analysis. Peak systolic velocity (PSV) and measures of impedance to blood flow [pulsatility index (PI) and resistance index (RI)] are measured.

With 3D-PDA, a 3D ovarian volume dataset with power Doppler signals can be obtained. Power Doppler setting should be kept optimum so as to offer the best compromise between small ovarian vessel detection and artifact, and these are kept constant for each and every patient for a meaningful comparison to be possible. As discussed before, ovarian volume is measured from the 3D power Doppler dataset of the ovary by using VOCAL through the manual delineation of the ovarian cortex in the transverse or longitudinal plane as the volume was rotated about a central axis through a number of rotation steps. Quantification of power Doppler information within the resultant 3D ovarian model (Fig. 6.6) can be performed using the "histogram facility." Three indices of vascularity are generated: (1) the vascularization index (VI), which represents the ratio of power Doppler information within the total dataset relative to both color and gray information; (2) the flow index (FI), which is proportional to the power Doppler signal intensity (Figs. 6.7A and B); and (3) the vascularization flow index (VFI), which reflects a combination of the two. These indices are generally thought to indicate the degree of vascularity and the volume flow rate within the ovaries.

Zaidi et al. were the first group to evaluate the correlation between ovarian stromal blood flow and follicular response in an IVF program.[59] They measured the ovarian stromal PSV and PI in 105 women in the early follicular phase and found that poor responders, defined as those who developed six or less follicles at the time of oocyte retrieval, had a significantly lower mean ovarian PSV, but no difference in PI, when compared with normal responders. The adjusted odds of a poor response increased significantly by an estimated 22% per 1 cm/s decrease in velocity. While most subsequent work based on 2D pulse-wave Doppler assessment of individual ovarian stromal vessels—based on 2D pulse-wave Doppler assessment of individual vessels—showed a significant correlation between the absolute velocity and impedance to blood flow and ovarian response in terms of the number of oocytes retrieved,[63,64] although recent studies utilizing larger population did not reveal an association between blood flow indices and ovarian response during IVF.[65]

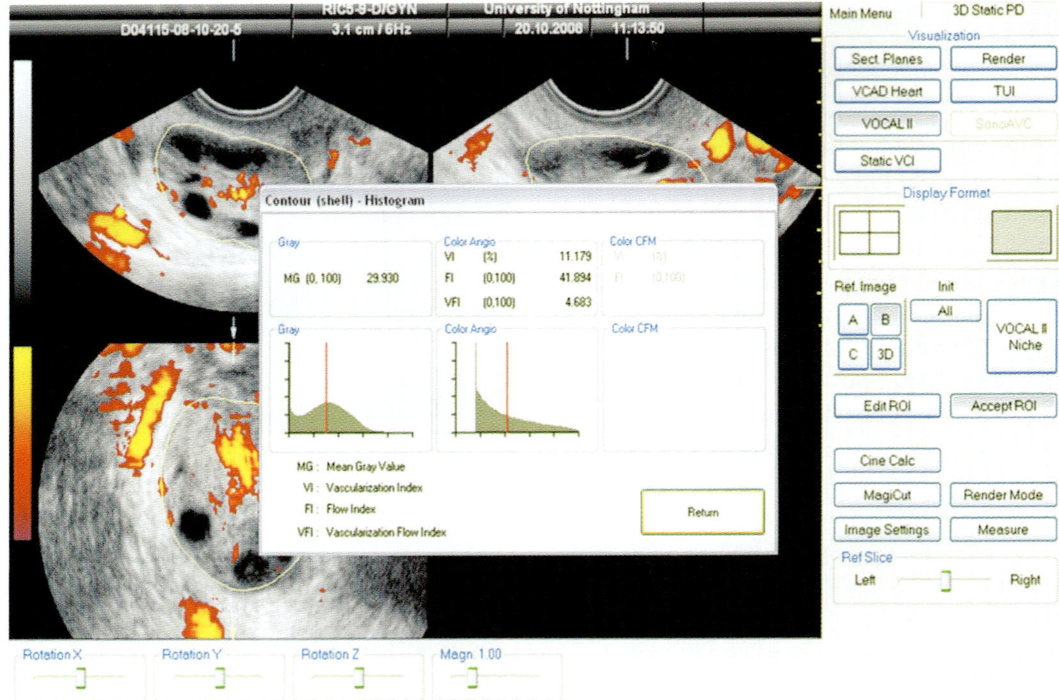

Fig. 6.6: Three-dimensional power Doppler assessment of ovarian vascularity: The power Doppler information within the defined 3D model of the ovary (using VOCAL) is quantified using the histogram facility. Three vascular indices: VI, FI, and VFI are demonstrated. (*Abbreviation:* 3D, three-dimensional; FI, flow index; VFI, vascularization flow index; VI, vascularization index; VOCAL, Virtual Organ Computer-Aided Analysis)

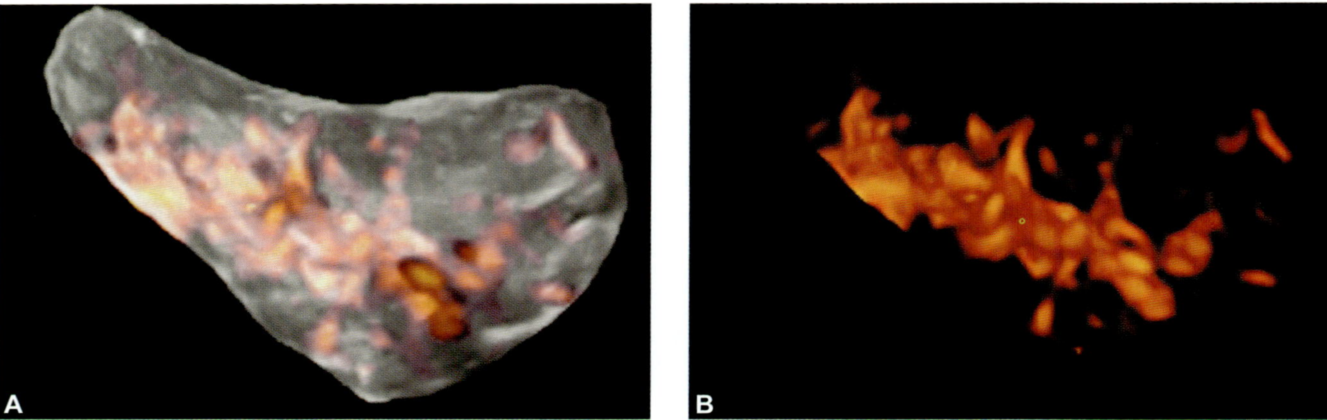

Figs. 6.7A and B: (A) Both gray-scale and Doppler information are shown in the 3D "glass body" model of an ovary. The VI represents the proportion of power Doppler information within this defined volume relative to both color and gray information providing an indication of the degree of vascularity. (B) The same ovary is shown but with the gray-scale information removed. The FI represents the mean power Doppler signal intensity within the dataset and reflects the volume flow rate. (*Abbreviation:* 3D, three-dimensional; FI, flow index; VI, vascularization index)

More recently, work has been done utilizing 3D ultrasound and power Doppler angiography allowing the demonstration and quantification of the total blood flow within ovaries. Kupesic et al. used 3D-PDA to evaluate ultrasound-derived ovarian predictors of ovarian response and outcome in 56 women with normal basal serum FSH concentrations (<10 mIU/mL) undergoing their first cycle of IVF.[66] Multiple regression analysis of the six most predictive variables—including the peak estradiol on the day of human chorionic gonadotropin (hCG) administration, total ovarian volume, total ovarian stromal area, age, and total AFC—revealed ovarian FI to be the second best predictor of the number of mature oocytes collected and pregnancy, followed by the ovarian stromal FI after AFC. However, most subsequent larger studies did not find a strong relationship between 3D power Doppler indices and poor ovarian response or exaggerated ovarian response or pregnancy during IVF.[39,44,67,68] It appears to be the role of ovarian 3D vascular indices as an independent predictor of ovarian reserve is limited and its use should be restricted as a research tool until convincing evidence for its routine clinical use is reported.

CONCLUSION

Antral follicle count is the most significant predictor of ovarian reserve and ovarian response among the ultrasound markers; although decreased ovarian volume (<3 cm^3) and reduced stromal blood flow are also implicated for poor treatment outcome during IVF treatment. While the antral follicle cohort of 2–6 mm reflects the most "functional quantitative ovarian reserve," it is recommended to include follicles of 2–10 mm in the total AFC as it is practically easier to count those follicle pool, majority of which comprises of 2–6 mm follicles anyway, without compromising the predictive accuracy. The total AFC can be measured using 2D or 3D ultrasound with an acceptably high level of agreement both between and within observers. A total follicle count of 10 and 22 is generally considered as the optimum cut-off levels for the prediction of poor and exaggerated ovarian response, respectively. The AFC measurement can be performed either in the early follicular phase of the cycle before treatment begins or after downregulation with similar predictive accuracy. However, assessment prior to treatment has an additional advantage in that it provides an opportunity for a pretreatment evaluation of pelvis to screen for pathology. Antral follicle count and AMH are currently the two best predictors of ovarian reserve among all the endocrine and ultrasound markers and are equally predictive of both poor and exaggerated ovarian response during IVF treatment. Antral follicle count is currently considered the ovarian reserve test of choice in routine clinical practice, as it is easy to perform while there is limited availability of AMH assays. The new development in automated assessment of follicle count using SonoAVC is promising and has the potential to improve the reproducibility and accuracy of AFC measurements.

KEY POINTS

- Ovarian reserve is a marker of ovarian ageing
- Careful evaluation of ovarian reserve will help the clinician to provide appropriate counseling of the couple about their realistic chances of conception, both spontaneously and after treatment, and may facilitate the choice of treatment for that individual couple
- The commonly used ultrasonographic markers of ovarian reserve are AFC, ovarian volume, and ovarian blood flow
- Ovarian volume:
    - While a unilateral ovarian volume of less than 3 cm^3 is regarded as a cut-off value, indicating reduced chances of conception after ART, its routine clinical application in predicting IVF outcome is limited
- Antral follicle count:
    - The total AFC is made by counting the number of antral follicles measuring 2–10 mm in both ovaries
    - The AFC may be considered as the test of choice in assessment of diminished ovarian reserve
    - Antral follicle count of 10 and 22 is considered as the optimum cut-off levels for the prediction of poor and exaggerated ovarian response, respectively
    - The recently introduced 3D automated technique, SonoAVC, allows a semiautomated analysis of the AFC
- Ovarian blood flow:
    - The role of ovarian blood flow in the prediction of ovarian reserve and ovarian response remains controversial

REFERENCES

1. Broekmans FJ, Kwee J, Hendriks DJ, et al. A systematic review of tests predicting ovarian reserve and IVF outcome. Hum Reprod Update. 2006;12(6):685-718.
2. Gougeon A. Ovarian follicular growth in humans: ovarian ageing and population of growing follicles. Maturitas. 1998;30(2):137-42.
3. Baird DT, Collins J, Egozcue J, et al. Fertility and ageing. Hum Reprod Update. 2005;11(3):261-76.
4. Treloar AE, Boynton RE, Behn BG, et al. Variation of the human menstrual cycle through reproductive life. Int J Fertil. 1967;12(1 Pt 2):77-126.
5. Treloar AE. Menstrual cyclicity and the pre-menopause. Maturitas. 1981;3(3-4):249-64.
6. Faddy MJ, Gosden RG, Gougeon A, et al. Accelerated disappearance of ovarian follicles in mid-life: implications for forecasting menopause. Hum Reprod. 1992;7(10):1342-6.
7. van Noord-Zaadstra BM, Looman CW, Alsbach H, et al. Delaying childbearing: effect of age on fecundity and outcome of pregnancy. BMJ. 1991;302(6789):1361-5.

8. Menken J, Trussell J, Larsen U. Age and infertility. Science. 1986;233(4771):1389-94.
9. Van Voorhis BJ. Clinical practice. In-vitro fertilization. N Engl J Med. 2007;356(4):379-86.
10. Navot D, Drews MR, Bergh PA, et al. Age-related decline in female fertility is not due to diminished capacity of the uterus to sustain embryo implantation. Fertil Steril. 1994;61(1):97-101.
11. Trout SW, Seifer DB. Do women with unexplained recurrent pregnancy loss have higher day 3 serum FSH and estradiol values? Fertil Steril. 2000;74(2):335-7.
12. Freeman SB, Yang Q, Allran K, et al. Women with a reduced ovarian complement may have an increased risk for a child with Down syndrome. Am J Hum Genet. 2000;66(5):1680-3.
13. Lambalk CB, De Koning CH, Braat DD. The endocrinology of dizygotic twinning in the human. Mol Cell Endocrinol. 1998;145(1-2):97-102.
14. Woldringh GH, Frunt MH, Kremer JA, et al. Decreased ovarian reserve relates to pre-eclampsia in IVF/ICSI pregnancies. Hum Reprod. 2006;21(11):2948-54.
15. Gougeon A, Ecochard R, Thalabard JC. Age-related changes of the population of human ovarian follicles: increase in the disappearance rate of non-growing and early-growing follicles in aging women. Biol Reprod. 1994;50(3):653-63.
16. Hansen KR, Knowlton NS, Thyer AC, et al. A new model of reproductive aging: the decline in ovarian non-growing follicle number from birth to menopause. Hum Reprod. 2008;23(3):699-708.
17. Arslan M, Bocca S, Mirkin S, et al. Controlled ovarian hyperstimulation protocols for in vitro fertilization: two decades of experience after the birth of Elizabeth Carr. Fertil Steril. 2005;84(3):555-69.
18. Maheshwari A, Bhattacharya S, Johnson NP. Predicting fertility. Hum Fertil (Camb). 2008;11(2):109-17.
19. Sunkara SK, Rittenberg V, Raine-Fenning N, et al. Association between the number of eggs and live birth in IVF treatment: an analysis of 400 135 treatment cycles. Hum Reprod. 2011;26(7):1768-74.
20. Syrop CH, Willhoite A, Van Voorhis BJ. Ovarian volume: a novel outcome predictor for assisted reproduction. Fertil Steril. 1995;64(6):1167-71.
21. Raine-Fenning NJ, Campbell BK, Clewes JS, et al. The interobserver reliability of ovarian volume measurement is improved with three-dimensional ultrasound, but dependent upon technique. Ultrasound Med Biol. 2003;29(12):1685-90.
22. Lass A, Silye R, Abrams DC, et al. Follicular density in ovarian biopsy of infertile women: a novel method to assess ovarian reserve. Hum Reprod. 1997;12(5):1028-31.
23. Bowen S, Norian J, Santoro N, et al. Simple tools for assessment of ovarian reserve (OR): individual ovarian dimensions are reliable predictors of OR. Fertil Steril. 2007;88(2):390-5.
24. Schild RL, Knobloch C, Dorn C, et al. The role of ovarian volume in an in vitro fertilization programme as assessed by 3D ultrasound. Arch Gynecol Obstet. 2001;265(2):67-72.
25. Elgindy EA, El-Haieg DO, El-Sebaey A. Anti-Müllerian hormone: correlation of early follicular, ovulatory and midluteal levels with ovarian response and cycle outcome in intracytoplasmic sperm injection patients. Fertil Steril. 2008;89(6):1670-6.
26. McIlveen M, Skull JD, Ledger WL. Evaluation of the utility of multiple endocrine and ultrasound measures of ovarian reserve in the prediction of cycle cancellation in a high-risk IVF population. Hum Reprod. 2007;22(3):778-85.
27. Lass A, Vassiliev A, Decosterd G, et al. Relationship of baseline ovarian volume to ovarian response in World Health Organization II anovulatory patients who underwent ovulation induction with gonadotropins. Fertil Steril. 2002;78(2):265-9.
28. Balen AH, Laven JS, Tan SL, et al. Ultrasound assessment of the polycystic ovary: international consensus definitions. Hum Reprod Update. 2003;9(6):505-14.
29. Nahum R, Shifren JL, Chang Y, et al. Antral follicle assessment as a tool for predicting outcome in IVF—is it a better predictor than age and FSH? J Assist Reprod Genet. 2001;18(3):151-5.
30. Scheffer GJ, Broekmans FJ, Dorland M, et al. Antral follicle counts by transvaginal ultrasonography are related to age in women with proven natural fertility. Fertil Steril. 1999;72(5):845-51.
31. Tomas C, Nuojua-Huttunen S, Martikainen H. Pretreatment transvaginal ultrasound examination predicts ovarian responsiveness to gonadotrophins in in-vitro fertilization. Hum Reprod. 1997;12(2):220-3.
32. Jayaprakasan K, Campbell B, Hopkisson J, et al. A prospective, comparative analysis of anti-Mullerian hormone, inhibin-B, and three-dimensional ultrasound determinants of ovarian reserve in the prediction of poor response to controlled ovarian stimulation. Fertil Steril. 2010;93(3):855-64.
33. Haadsma ML, Bukman A, Groen H, et al. The number of small antral follicles (2–6 mm) determines the outcome of endocrine ovarian reserve tests in a subfertile population. Hum Reprod. 2007;22(7):1925-31.
34. Sharara FI, McClamrock HD. Antral follicle count and ovarian volume predict IVF outcome. Fertil Steril. 2000;74:S176.
35. Bancsi LF, Broekmans FJ, Eijkemans MJ, et al. Predictors of poor ovarian response in in vitro fertilization: a prospective study comparing basal markers of ovarian reserve. Fertil Steril. 2002;77(2):328-36.
36. Chang MY, Chiang CH, Hsieh TT, et al. Use of the antral follicle count to predict the outcome of assisted reproductive technologies. Fertil Steril. 1998;69(3):505-10.
37. Hsieh YY, Chang CC, Tsai HD. Antral follicle counting in predicting the retrieved oocyte number after ovarian hyperstimulation. J Assist Reprod Genet. 2001;18(6):320-4.
38. Ng EH, Yeung WS, Ho PC. The significance of antral follicle count in controlled ovarian stimulation and intrauterine insemination. J Assist Reprod Genet. 2005;22(9-10):323-8.

39. Ng EH, Tang OS, Chan CC, et al. Ovarian stromal vascularity is not predictive of ovarian response and pregnancy. Reprod Biomed Online. 2006;12(1):43-9.
40. Kupesic S, Kurjak A, Bjelos D, et al. Three-dimensional ultrasonographic ovarian measurements and in vitro fertilization outcome are related to age. Fertil Steril. 2003;79(1):190-7.
41. Broer SL, Mol BW, Hendriks D, et al. The role of anti-Mullerian hormone in prediction of outcome after IVF: comparison with the antral follicle count. Fertil Steril. 2009;91(3):705-14.
42. Holte J, Brodin T, Berglund L, et al. Antral follicle counts are strongly associated with live-birth rates after assisted reproduction, with superior treatment outcome in women with polycystic ovaries. Fertil Steril. 2011;96(3):594-9.
43. Jayaprakasan K, Chan Y, Islam R, et al. Prediction of in vitro fertilization outcome at different antral follicle count thresholds in a prospective cohort of 1,012 women. Fertil Steril. 2012;98(3):657-63.
44. Jayaprakasan K, Jayaprakasan R, Al-Hasie HA, et al. Can quantitative three-dimensional power Doppler angiography be used to predict ovarian hyperstimulation syndrome? Ultrasound Obstet Gynecol. 2009;33(5):583-91.
45. Broer SL, Dolleman M, Opmeer BC, et al. AMH and AFC as predictors of excessive response in controlled ovarian hyperstimulation: a meta-analysis. Hum Reprod Update. 2011;17(1):46-54.
46. Jayaprakasan K, Walker KF, Clewes JS, et al. The interobserver reliability of off-line antral follicle counts made from stored three-dimensional ultrasound data: a comparative study of different measurement techniques. Ultrasound Obstet Gynecol. 2007;29(3):335-41.
47. Deb S, Jayaprakasan K, Campbell BK, et al. Intraobserver and interobserver reliability of automated antral follicle counts made using three-dimensional ultrasound and SonoAVC. Ultrasound Obstet Gynecol. 2009;33(4):477-83.
48. Raine-Fenning N, Jayaprakasan K, Clewes J, et al. SonoAVC: a novel method of automatic volume calculation. Ultrasound Obstet Gynecol. 2008;31(6):691-6.
49. Broekmans FJ, de Ziegler D, Howles CM, et al. The antral follicle count: practical recommendations for better standardization. Fertil Steril. 2010;94(3):1044-51.
50. Jayaprakasan K, Hopkisson JF, Campbell BK, et al. Quantification of the effect of pituitary down-regulation on 3D ultrasound predictors of ovarian response. Hum Reprod. 2008;23(7):1538-44.
51. Jayaprakasan K, Deb S, Batcha M, et al. The cohort of antral follicles measuring 2–6 mm reflects the quantitative status of ovarian reserve as assessed by serum levels of anti-Müllerian hormone and response to controlled ovarian stimulation. Fertil Steril. 2010;94(5):1775-81.
52. Hansen KR, Morris JL, Thyer AC, et al. Reproductive aging and variability in the ovarian antral follicle count: application in the clinical setting. Fertil Steril. 2003;80(3):577-83.
53. Bancsi LF, Broekmans FJ, Looman CW, et al. Impact of repeated antral follicle counts on the prediction of poor ovarian response in women undergoing in vitro fertilization. Fertil Steril. 2004;81(1):35-41.
54. Scheffer GJ, Broekmans FJ, Bancsi LF, et al. Quantitative transvaginal two- and three-dimensional sonography of the ovaries: reproducibility of antral follicle counts. Ultrasound Obstet Gynecol. 2002;20(3):270-5.
55. Elter K, Sismanoglu A, Durmusoglu F. Intercycle variabilities of basal antral follicle count and ovarian volume in subfertile women and their relationship to reproductive aging: a prospective study. Gynecol Endocrinol. 2005;20(3): 137-43.
56. Jayaprakasan K, Campbell B, Hopkisson J, Clewes J, Johnson I, Raine-Fenning N. Establishing the intercycle variability of three-dimensional ultrasonographic predictors of ovarian reserve. Fertil Steril. 2008 Dec;90(6):2126-32.
57. McGee EA, Hsueh AJ. Initial and cyclic recruitment of ovarian follicles. Endocr Rev. 2000;21(2):200-14.
58. Redmer DA, Reynolds LP. Angiogenesis in the ovary. Rev Reprod. 1996;1(3):182-92.
59. Zaidi J, Barber J, Kyei-Mensah A, et al. Relationship of ovarian stromal blood flow at the baseline ultrasound scan to subsequent follicular response in an in vitro fertilization program. Obstet Gynecol. 1996;88(5):779-84.
60. Zaidi J, Campbell S, Pittrof R, et al. Ovarian stromal blood flow in women with polycystic ovaries: a possible new marker for diagnosis? Hum Reprod. 1995;10(8):1992-6.
61. Pan HA, Cheng YC, Li CH, et al. Ovarian stroma flow intensity decreases by age: a three-dimensional power Doppler ultrasonographic study. Ultrasound Med Biol. 2002;28(4): 425-30.
62. Ng EH, Chan CC, Yeung WS, et al. Effect of age on ovarian stromal flow measured by three-dimensional ultrasound with power Doppler in Chinese women with proven fertility. Hum Reprod. 2004;19(9):2132-7.
63. Bassil S, Wyns C, Toussaint-Demylle D, et al. The relationship between ovarian vascularity and the duration of stimulation in in-vitro fertilization. Hum Reprod. 1997;12(6):1240-5.
64. Engmann L, Sladkevicius P, Agrawal R, et al. Value of ovarian stromal blood flow velocity measurement after pituitary suppression in the prediction of ovarian responsiveness and outcome of in vitro fertilization treatment. Fertil Steril. 1999;71(1):22-9.
65. Ng EH, Tang OS, Chan CC, et al. Ovarian stromal blood flow in the prediction of ovarian response during in vitro fertilization treatment. Hum Reprod. 2005;20(11):3147-51.
66. Kupesic S, Kurjak A. Predictors of IVF outcome by three-dimensional ultrasound. Hum Reprod. 2002;17(4):950-5.
67. Mercé LT, Barco MJ, Bau S, et al. Prediction of ovarian response and IVF/ICSI outcome by three-dimensional ultrasonography and power Doppler angiography. Eur J Obstet Gynecol Reprod Biol. 2007;132(1):93-100.
68. Jayaprakasan K, Al-Hasie H, Jayaprakasan R, et al. The three-dimensional ultrasonographic ovarian vascularity of women developing poor ovarian response during assisted reproduction treatment and its predictive value. Fertil Steril. 2009;92(6):1862-9.

Chapter

7

Ovarian Pathology

Ouma Pillai, Kamal Ojha

Chapter Outline

INTRODUCTION

One the most common requests for transvaginal ultrasound (TVS) is imaging of the ovaries. This request may be for a number of reasons, but scanning ovaries is an integral part of evaluation of subfertile women. While transabdominal ultrasound provides good information on the exact anatomical relationship of the pelvic organs,[1] its low resolution makes fine detailing of the ovary extremely difficult. A TVS with a high-frequency transducer is the tool of choice for imaging the female pelvis and for fine detailing of the ovary. Minute structures of up to 1–2 mm can be detected in the ovaries. There are a number of studies, which have also demonstrated good detection rates of postmenopausal ovaries by TVS, which are usually significantly smaller and devoid of follicles as compared to women of reproductive years.

Elective TVS should be ideally done in the early follicular phase of the menstrual cycle, when the ovary will not contain structures such as the corpus luteum, which would skew the overall size of the organ.

HOW TO SCAN AND LOOK FOR OVARIES?

Normal ovaries in women of reproductive years are somehow easier to detect due to the fact that they have markers such as follicles and corpus luteum. Systematic approaches of identifying ovaries and scanning through ovaries have been described in detail in Chapter 2. To image the ovary, the probe is usually rotated anticlockwise and directed toward the side wall until the iliac vein comes into view and then the probe is slowly moved up until the ovaries are located just above. The examination should begin with a TVS probe, performed with an empty bladder.[2]

Ovaries in women who have had a hysterectomy are difficult to detect on TVS because of the change of anatomy, whereby the space occupied by the uterus has now been replaced by bowel. However, the same technique is applied whereby the iliac vein is located first, and the adnexa is spanned in an up and down motion of the hand while the probe is in the transverse position (anticlockwise rotation of 90°). If there is difficulty in doing so, a hand can be gently placed on the patient's abdomen, in the region of the ovary and pressure is gently applied to locate the ovary. This helps in moving the bowel away and bringing the ovary closer to the probe hence good resolution.

NORMAL PHYSIOLOGY

The menstrual cycle results in the preparation of the endometrium for implantation, the production of a ripe fertilization-competent ovum at ovulation, and either the endometrial implantation and support of the developing zygote if fertilization occurs or the shedding of the endometrial lining and unfertilized ovum in the menstrual blood flow if it does not. The menstrual cycle is normally approximately 1 month long, although cycle length may vary between 21 and 35 days, without associated pathology. It is regulated at the endocrine level by the cyclical release of follicle stimulating hormone (FSH) and luteinizing hormone (LH) from the anterior pituitary. Follicle stimulating hormone and LH govern the ovarian biosynthesis of steroid hormones, primarily estradiol (E2) and progesterone (P).

The menstrual cycle is divided into a proliferative or follicular phase, commonly of 7–21 days (depending on the time required for follicular maturation), a secretory phase of relatively constant in length (14 days), and a menstrual phase of 5–7 days. The ovaries, uterus, and cervix all undergo substantial changes during the cycle, as detailed in the following text for a typical 28-day cycle. Ultrasound appearance of ovaries varies depending on the time of menstrual cycle, when scan is performed.

Days 1–5: Onset of vaginal menstrual bleeding during which the secretory endometrial mucosa degenerates, sloughs off and is shed in the menstrual blood flow. The endometrium in the early follicular phase is thin with no obvious basal layer. The ovary is best imaged by TVS in the early follicular phase as there will be follicular recruitment and they are still small. They will not likely to be mistaken for pathology at this stage and it is a good time to assess the antral follicles count for ovarian reserve.

Days 5–14: The follicular phase continues until ovulation takes place. Increasing levels of pituitary FSH stimulate the development and maturation of a cohort of follicles. One dominant follicle then acquires granulosa cells which then respond to the LH surge. The dominant follicle itself synthesizes increasing amounts of E2. Estradiol production rises steeply from day 10 and reaches a peak on day 13, the concurrent rise in LH leading to ovulation. The uterine endometrium proliferates throughout the follicular phase, under the influence of E2, to provide a highly vascularized surface receptive to the fertilized ovum. The cervix remains small and closed by highly viscous mucus.

On ultrasound, the endometrium appears echogenic and thickened. It has the typical triple-layer appearance, which is associated with the presence of a dominant follicle. The follicle grows in size and is hypoechoic as it contains fluid. Blood flow with Doppler is not significantly increased around the follicle. It will reach up to 18–20 mm approximately in diameter before rupturing to release an oocyte.

Day 14: Ovulation occurs and the ovum (egg) is released from its follicle and enters the fimbria of the fallopian tube. During ovulation, the cervical mucus becomes less viscous and the os cervix enlarges, allowing sperm to pass through. These changes could be observed on ultrasound in the cervical canal. The corresponding change on the endometrium is loss of the triple-layer appearance, and the follicle appears to have a collapsed appearance, unlike the cystic appearance prior to ovulation.

Days 14–28: The luteal phase begins as the corpus luteum that develops from the now empty Graafian follicle and starts to produce progesterone. In response, the endometrium differentiates to perform a secretory function. The effect of progesterone on the endometrium is maximal around day 22 in a regular cycle, when the embryo, if fertilization occurs, results in implantation. If fertilization has not occurred, E2 and P begin to inhibit the release of hypothalamic gonadotropin releasing hormone (GnRH), which leads to degeneration of the corpus luteum. The resulting rapid drop in serum E2 and P levels cause constriction of the endometrial blood vessels and endometrial ischemia; the uterine mucosa is shed and this begins another menstrual bleed.

The ultrasound features of a corpus luteum shows an echogenic irregular solid or cystic structure which has increased vascularity observed with power Doppler flows.

CORPUS LUTEUM

Ultrasound images of a corpus luteum will change on a daily basis as it fills with fluid, blood, clot and then shrinks to form the corpus albicans. The corpus luteum may have an anechoic center (Fig. 7.1) or a typical "spider web" appearance if it contains a clot. It can also be solid, being mistaken for a neoplastic lesion. The image can be further investigated with the use of Doppler. Link this with physiology description of vascularity changes within the corpus luteum in the luteal phase, a typical "halo" appearance (Fig. 7.2) or "ring of fire" is seen due to the vascularity

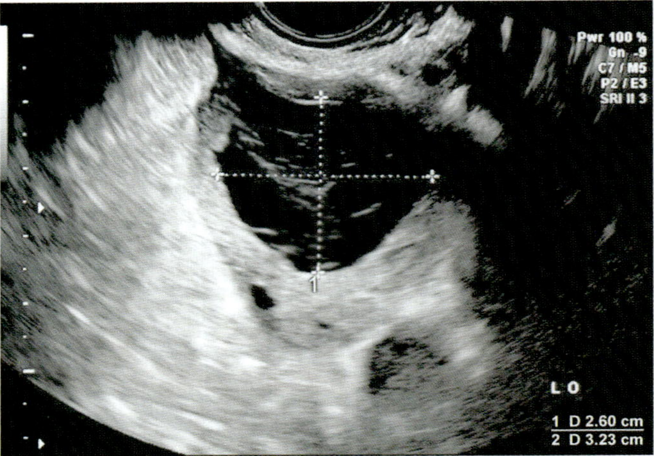

Fig. 7.1: This figure shows a cystic corpus luteum on the ovary.

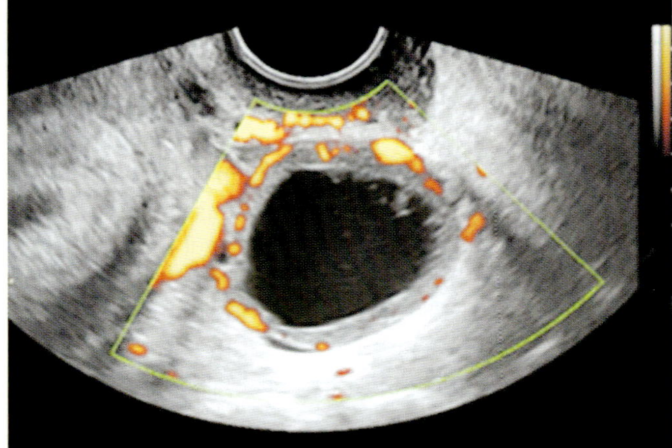

Fig. 7.2: Doppler reveals vascularity around the corpus luteum, demonstrating the "halo" sign.

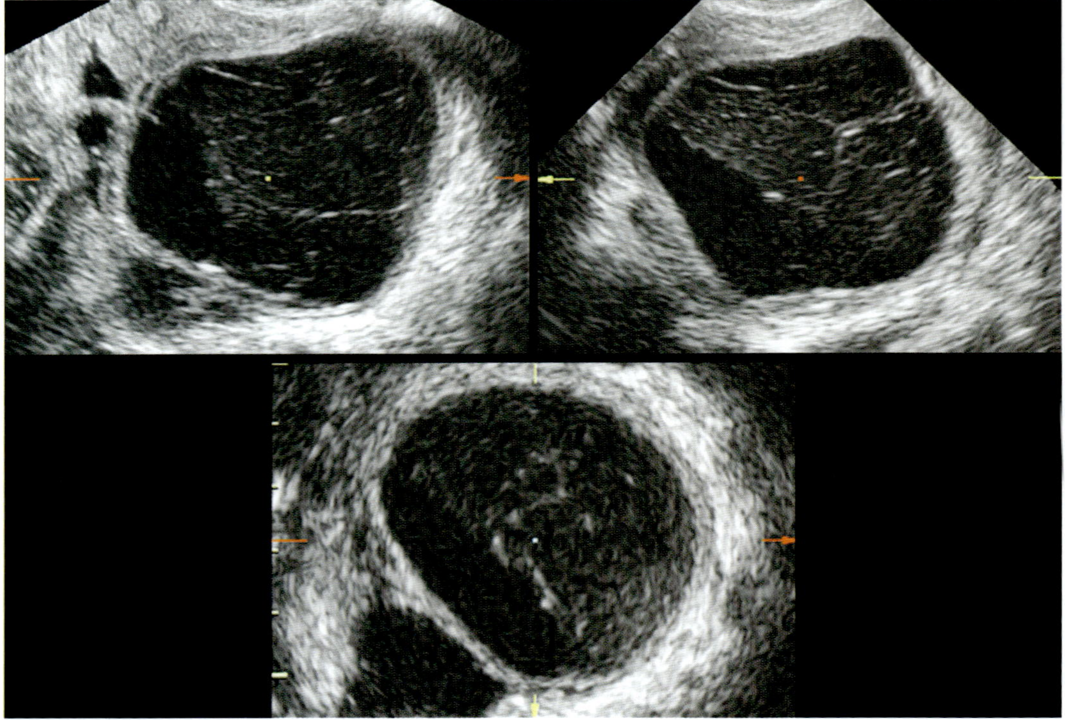

Fig. 7.3: A 3D multiplanar view of a hemorrhagic corpus luteum. Note lacy pattern inside the cyst.

around the structure. It can also be surrounded by a hyperechoic ring, which may persist long after the corpus luteum has involuted. It is important thus to know the time of the menstrual cycle that the scan is performed. These features disappear as the menstrual cycle starts again. A corpus luteum will typically measure 2–3 cm in diameter. However, in case of corpus luteal hemorrhage the size could be larger with a lacy pattern (Fig. 7.3), it may be associated with pain and treatment generally is conservative rarely requiring laparoscopic hemostasis. The corpus luteum will be hypoechoic or the center will appear black if filled with fluid. If it contains blood, it can have typical

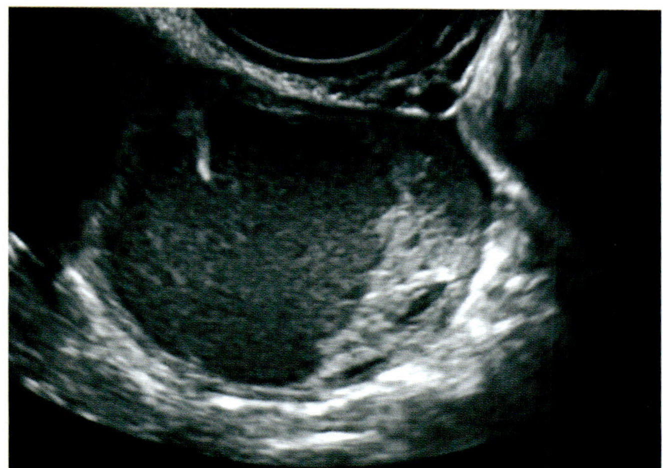

Fig. 7.4: A hemorrhagic cyst with an organized clot.

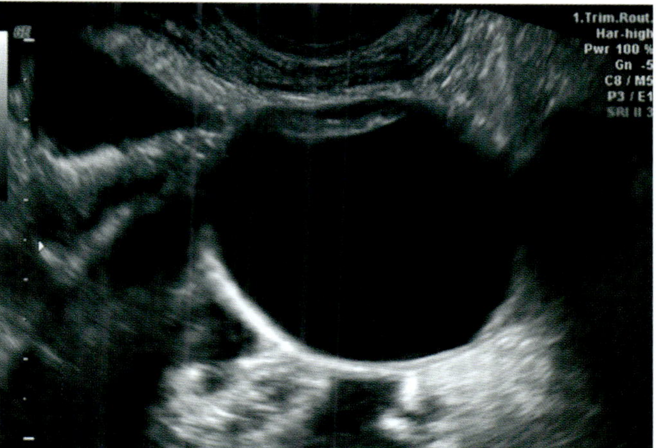

Fig. 7.5: A hypoechogenic simple cyst on the right ovary filled with fluid, having smooth and regular capsule with no hyperechoic contents.

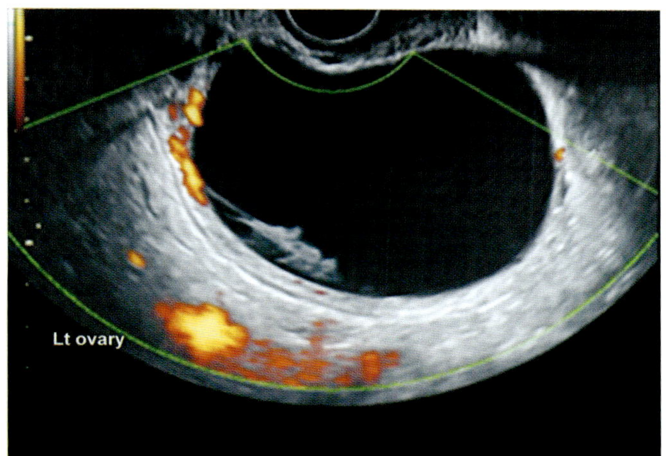

Fig. 7.6: The cyst wall shows minimal vascularity on Doppler studies.

spider web appearance and will be hyperechoic if it contains an organized clot (Fig. 7.4), which is resolving.[3]

FUNCTIONAL OVARIAN CYST

The functional cyst is the most common ovarian lesion found in the reproductive years. They are usually unilocular, anechoic with thin smooth inner and outer walls (Fig. 7.5). They will measure between 2 and 6 cm. Doppler application reveals scanty vascularity around the cyst (Fig. 7.6). Most will resolve spontaneously and patients are best managed by a rescan after 2–3 cycles on days 5–10. If there is no suppression, hormonal suppression with the combined oral contraceptive pill (COCP) can be attempted.[3]

POLYCYSTIC OVARIAN SYNDROME

Polycystic ovarian syndrome (PCOS) is the most common cause of medically treatable infertility and is the cause of anovulation in more than 70% of cases.[4] Therefore, it is an important condition to diagnose in the assessment for subfertile women. The diagnosis of PCOS not only carries important long-term health implications such as increased metabolic risks but also helps to guide appropriate management fertility treatment. During controlled ovarian stimulation, women with PCOS are at an increased risk of developing excessive ovarian responsiveness to gonadotrophins and are therefore more prone to develop ovarian hyperstimulation syndrome (OHSS),[5] which is associated with significant morbidity and even mortality.[6] An accurate diagnosis of PCOS allows the clinician to formulate an optimal ovarian stimulation protocol aiming for multifollicular response without compromising women's safety.[7]

The diagnosis of PCOS has been controversial for long period, despite its clinical relevance. The diagnostic criteria were first reported during the first international conference on PCOS at the National Institutes of Health (NIH) in the United States in 1990 and three key features of PCOS were generally agreed: chronic anovulation, hyperandrogenism (clinical or laboratory evidence), and the absence of other endocrine disorders (e.g. congenital adrenal hyperplasia, hyperprolactinemia, or thyroid abnormalities).[8] This consensus aimed to identify the core group of PCOS women with the most significant features of the disease and the greatest metabolic risks. However, these diagnostic criteria have not addressed the heterogeneity of the syndrome where the associated clinical features, such as menstrual disturbance, obesity, and hyperandrogenism manifesting as hirsutism or acne, vary considerably between women.[9] Moreover, the appearance of polycystic ovaries on ultrasonography was not included in the definition despite this feature being mandatory in many centers.[10] However, in all subsequent definitions of PCOS, both the Rotterdam criteria (2003) and the Androgen Excess Society (AES) criteria (2006), added the sonographic appearance of polycystic ovaries allowing some flexibility in the diagnosis.[11,12]

Various parameters have been proposed to morphologically define polycystic ovary (PCO) by ultrasound, but there have been no consensus about their diagnostic values. The classical description of PCO is that of enlarged ovaries containing an increased number of small follicles encircling the ovarian cortex together with an increased bright echogenic stroma (Figs. 7.7A and B).[13] In the Rotterdam criteria, the distribution of follicles and a description of the stroma have not been included in the definition of PCO. Presence of 12 or more follicles measuring 2–9 mm in diameter in a single ovary and/or an increased ovarian volume greater than 10 cm^3 (Figs. 7.7B and 7.8) indicates that the ovary is polycystic.[14] In the Rotterdam guidelines, the calculation of ovarian volume is based on conventional ultrasound measurements. Assuming the ovary is ovoid, ovarian volume is calculated using ellipsoid formula, $0.523 \times D1 \times D2 \times D3$, where D1, D2, and D3 represent maximal longitudinal, anteroposterior, and transverse diameter, respectively (*see* Chapter 6, Figs. 6.1A and B). However, many polycystic ovaries are irregular in shape and the geometric assumption cannot be applied to the irregularly shaped ovarian stroma. Volume estimation of irregular ovaries can be made using 3D ultrasound and are more reliable and valid.[15,16] There are various ways to derive volume measures but rotational method through the VOCAL-imaging program (Virtual Organ Computer-Aided Analysis™) has been commonly used (*see* Chapter 6, Figs. 6.2A to D). Three-dimensional ultrasound also permits a unique measurement of stromal volume through the calculation and subtraction of total follicular volume from total ovarian volume.[17]

The Rotterdam criteria on US diagnosis of PCO has been criticized especially because of the technical improvement in ultrasound resolution with use of the latest generation of devices with maximum probe frequencies >8 MHz. This applies mainly to follicle count, while the threshold for ovarian volume does not appear to be influenced by the technical improvement of ultrasound. With the new appliances, the threshold of 12 follicles per ovary leads to an artificial overestimation of the PCO prevalence in the general population. It was proposed to use a threshold to 25 with new US machines.[18] It must be emphasized, however, that this threshold of 25 corresponds to the 95th percentile of the populations of "normal" women. While Ant-Mullerian Hormone (AMH) may be a good substitute for US criteria for PCO, an international consensus is needed to use the proposed follicle number threshold or AMH in the routine clinical practice.

While echogenic stroma is not considered in the currently used definition of PCO, researchers have suggested stromal hypertrophy seen on ultrasound is correlated with serum androgen levels and fasting insulin levels.[19]

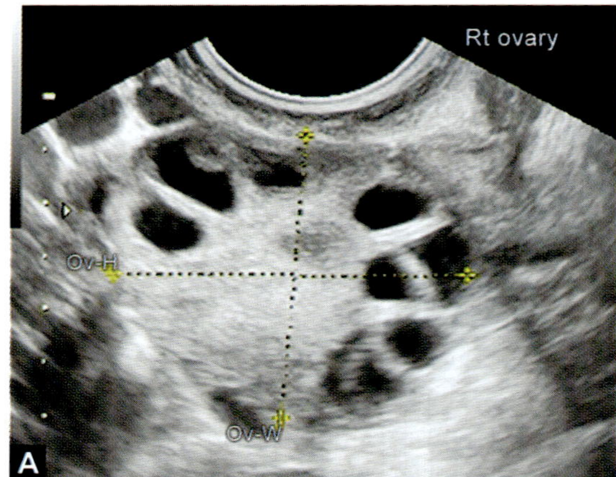

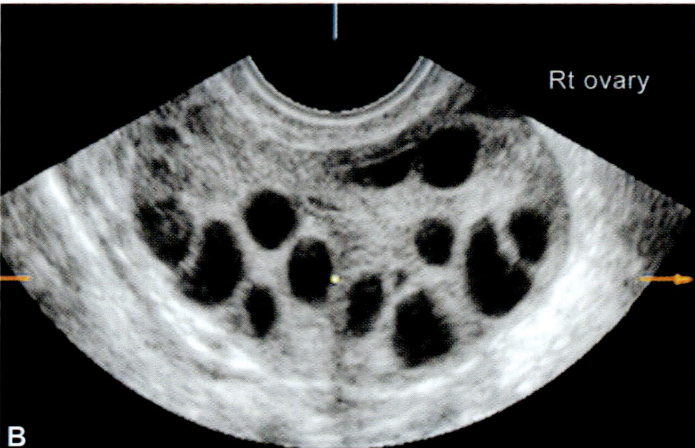

Figs. 7.7A and B: Polycystic ovarian syndrome with peripheral distribution of follicles around echogenic stroma and (A) generalized distribution of follicles (B).

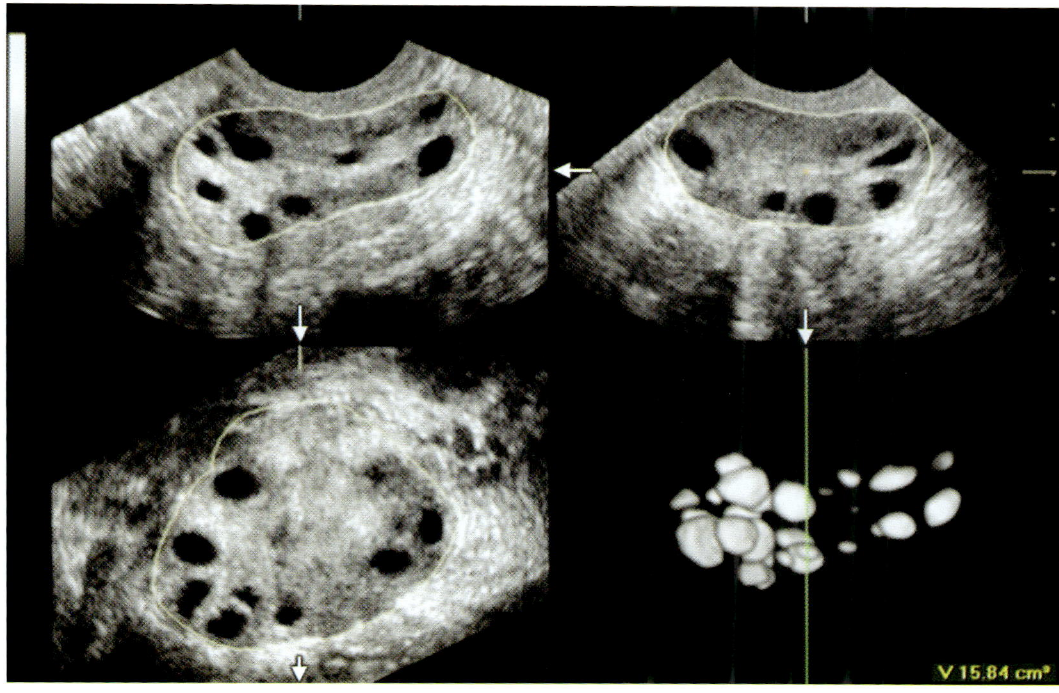

Fig. 7.8: A 3D multiplanar view of polycystic ovary with inversion mode demonstrating multiple antral follicles (lower right picture). The ovary is enlarged and contains multiple follicles which are scattered all around the ovary. The ovarian volume as measured using VOCAL shows 15.84 mL.

With the conventional two-dimensional (2D) ultrasound scan, the degree of echogenicity of the ovarian stroma is usually assessed subjectively and this is open to observer bias especially when other features of PCOS have already been seen. With the advances in ultrasound software, the echogenicity of the ovarian stroma can be determined objectively by measuring the intensity level of the ultrasound pixels within the stroma displayed on then sonographic image. The mean echogenicity of a given area can then be calculated. While the degree of stromal echogenicity does not differ significantly between women with PCOS and controls, the stromal index, defined as the ratio of mean stromal echogenicity to mean echogenicity of the entire ovary, is significantly higher in women with PCOS.[20] These findings are thought to relate to the increased volume of ovarian stroma relative to a lower mean echogenicity of the entire ovary due to increased number of follicles. Three-dimensional ultrasound provides an alternative way to examine stromal echogenicity objectively through the assessment of the mean grayness of the ovary, which represents the mean tissue intensity or echogenicity in the region of interest.[17] Current evidence shows no differences in stromal echogenicity measured using 3D ultrasound between the polycystic ovary and control groups.

The apparent stromal hypertrophy seen in women with polycystic ovaries may relate to increased vascularity within the ovarian stroma. Ovarian vascularity can be assessed subjectively through the application of color or power Doppler maps to a single plane to examine the flow pattern or objectively by measuring flow velocity and the resistance to flow through pulsed-wave Doppler on a single vessel. It has been observed that pulsatility index and resistance index of both ovarian artery and stromal artery were significantly lower in women with PCOS,[21] but this was not supported by other investigators.[22] Quantitative 3D power Doppler angiography facilitates the assessment of total blood flow within the defined volume of interest, allowing the objective assessment of total vascular flow within an organ or a specified volume of tissue (Fig. 7.9).[23] The data on ovarian blood flow quantified using 3D power Doppler in polycystic ovary are conflicting.[24,25]

HYPERSTIMULATED OVARIES

This is a result of ovulation induction in the context of assisted reproductive treatment. Patients have enlarged ovaries with multiple follicles or corpora lutea, there may be associated ascites. The ovaries are so enlarged and may

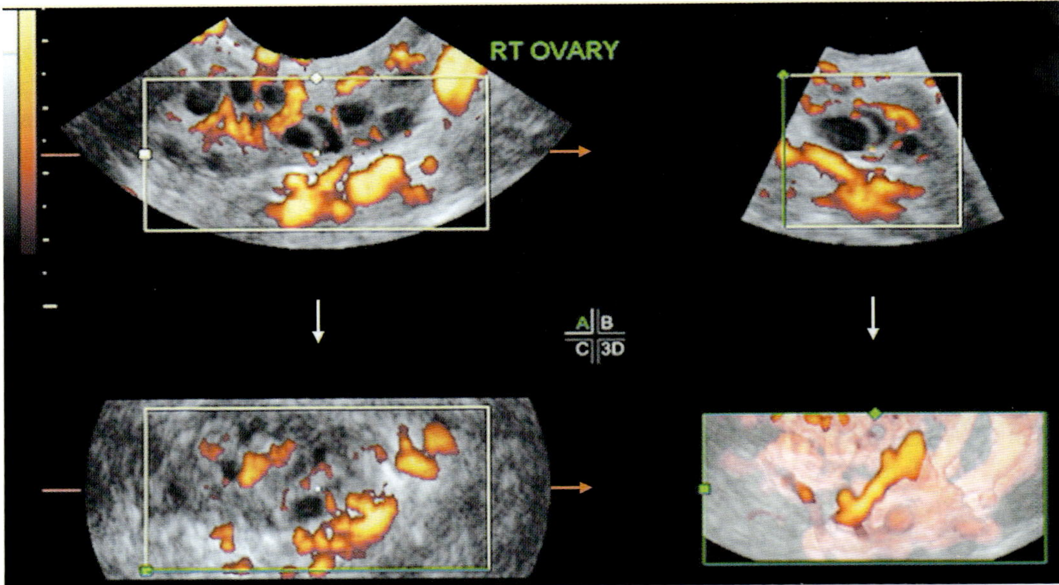

Fig. 7.9: A 3D power Doppler imaging of a polycystic ovary demonstrating stromal vascularity.

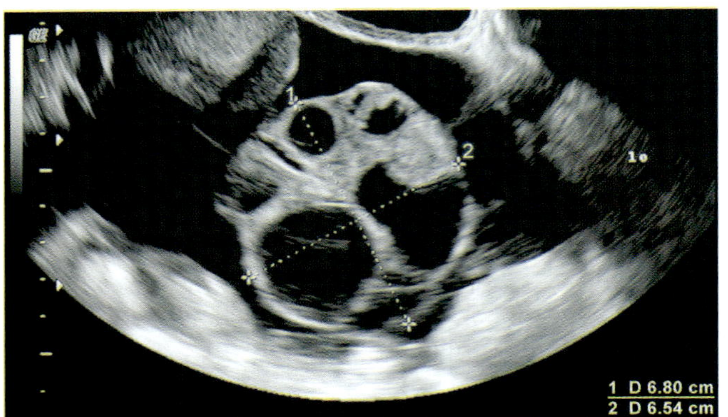

Fig. 7.10: An enlarged ovary with stimulated large follicles. The ovary is free floating in free fluid.

be displaced, it is sometimes better to use the abdominal transducer to visualize the whole ovaries. They generally respond to conservative treatment and very rarely they may present with torsion (Fig. 7.10).

OVARIAN TORSION

This condition usually involves both the ovary and Fallopian tube. The torted ovary is a very difficult diagnosis to make using the TVS. However, the ovary is usually enlarged with a hyperechoic hilus, the follicles may be pushed to the surface and there is no visible blood flow. The patient is also very tender during the procedure. The diagnosis relies primarily on clinical signs and symptoms. The ultrasound scan can only support the clinical diagnosis. This is further detailed in Chapter 11.

The ultrasound features that may help in identifying cases with ovarian torsion (Chapter 11 Fig 2 A-C)

- ovarian edema, usually manifesting as hypoechoic or heterogeneous central stroma with several small peripherally located follicles
- ovarian enlargement relative to the contralateral unaffected ovary
- an ovarian cyst or mass
- an abnormal ovarian location, in the midline, anterior to, or above the uterus or in the Pouch of Douglas
- abnormal ovarian blood flow, defined as the lack of venous and arterial flow or detection of only arterial flow on Doppler evaluation
- the presence of free fluid in the Douglas pouch or around the affected ovary;
- evidence of a distended fallopian tube The diagnostic accuracy for ovarian torsion using US is of 74.6%.[26]

Abnormal ovarian blood flow and the presence of free fluid were the most diagnostically accurate when compared to isolated sonographic signs (positive predictive values, 80.0% and 89.2%, respectively; negative predictive values, 46.2% and 46.2%). Using combinations of sonographic signs yielded higher specificity and positive predictive values and lower sensitivity and negative predictive values for ovarian torsion. The absence of typical sonographic signs does not rule out ovarian torsion, especially when the clinical presentation is suggestive. Basing assessments on multiple sonographic signs, including Doppler evaluation, increases the diagnostic accuracy.

CYSTADENOMA

These are the most common cystic structure found in the postmenopausal women but can be seen some time in women of reproductive age. These can either be of the serous (Fig. 7.11) or mucinous (Fig. 7.12) type. They can measure up to 5 cm, be multiloculated and have septae that emanate radially. They usually are persistent through a number of cycles.

It is difficult to differentiate between the two types except that mucinous cysts can emanate low-level echoes while serous cysts are anechoic. The serous type can contain a septae that emanate out from a common point in the ovarian stoma. They do not have shadowing and color Doppler will show minimal flow in the septa (Fig. 7.13).

ENDOMETRIOMA

Often referred as chocolate cysts, these have typical appearances with a thick wall, often septated, may have solid component and have mixed echogenicity. They are similar to hemorrhagic corpus luteum if they are small but unlike the latter they do not have a rich vascular supply in the wall. Follow-up follicular phase scan usually shows a persistent hemorrhagic structure. The typical description is a "ground glass" appearance (Fig. 7.14). Rarely an endometrioma can

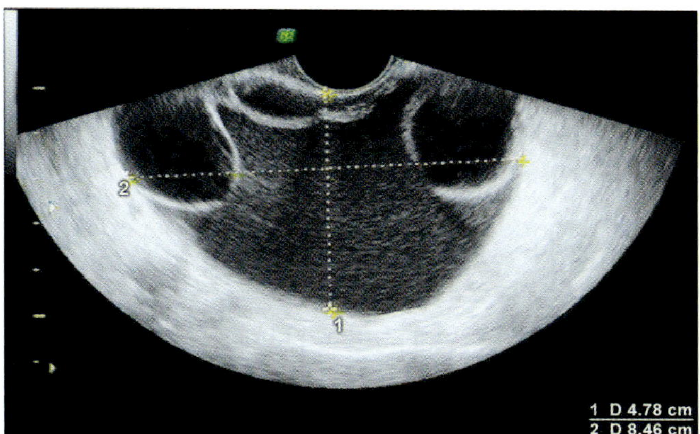

Fig. 7.11: A benign cystadenoma of the ovary. The content is mainly hypoechogenic fluid. The capsule is regular and the cyst contains some septae which are thin and regular too.

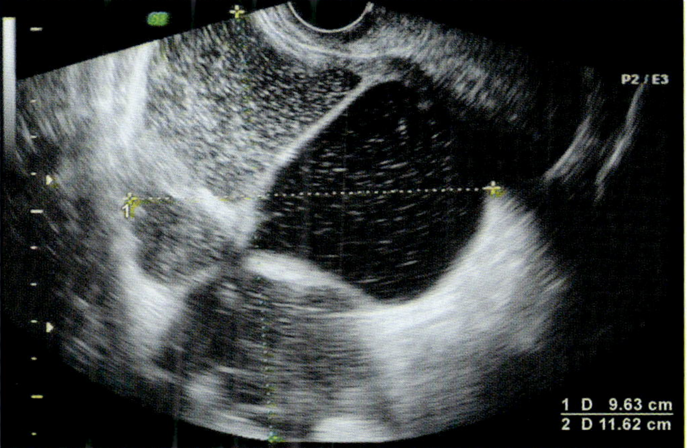

Fig. 7.12: A septated mucinous cystadenoma. The capsule wall is regular with thin septae.

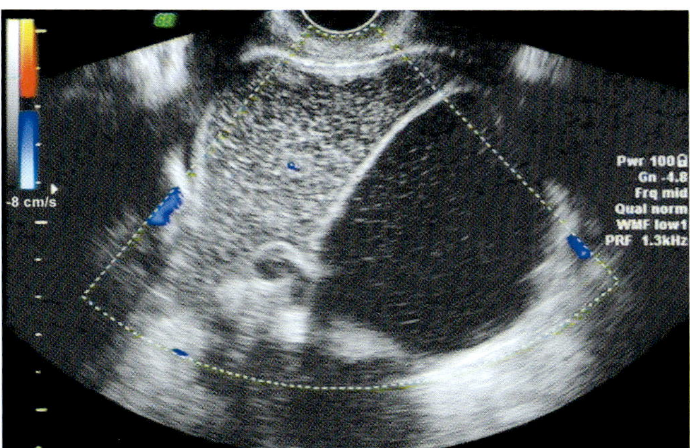

Fig. 7.13: No relevant flow is demonstrated on Doppler imaging.

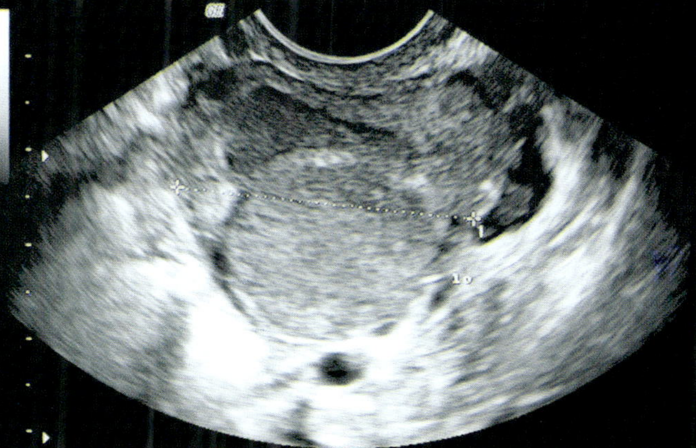

Fig. 7.14: A small endometrioma in a left ovary. The cyst is well-circumscribed with a hyperechoic center, often referred to as "ground glass" appearance.

be associated with malignancy in the form of an endometrioid carcinoma or clear cell carcinoma, this should be suspected in women of advanced age associated with increasing size of the cyst. Typically, the ovarian lesions will demonstrate vascularity in the papillary projection on its internal wall. This is further detailed in chapter 7.

CYSTIC TERATOMA

Usually found in younger women and the benign cystic teratoma or dermoid cyst originates from all three germ cell layers. Appearance of a dermoid cyst varies considerably to being cystic with weak echogenic (sebaceous) content to being multiloculated or solid. They demonstrate a hyperechoic center while the surrounding demonstrates low-level echoes (Fig. 7.15). They are known to contain structures from primitive germ cell lines such as teeth, hair, or nerve tissue. Doppler will reveal no blood flow and the cysts are bilateral in 15% of cases. They usually present as asymptomatic lesion on ultrasound examination but may present with pain or features of torsion. In cases of torsion, if not diagnosed early and treated, there is likelihood of loss of ovarian function.

MALIGNANT OVARIAN PATHOLOGIES

While it is very rare that we come across with ovarian malignancies in women of reproductive age group, it is important to rule out neoplastic lesions if there are large ovarian cysts. Ovarian cancer is one of the leading causes of death for gynecological malignancy and is still detected at very advance stages.

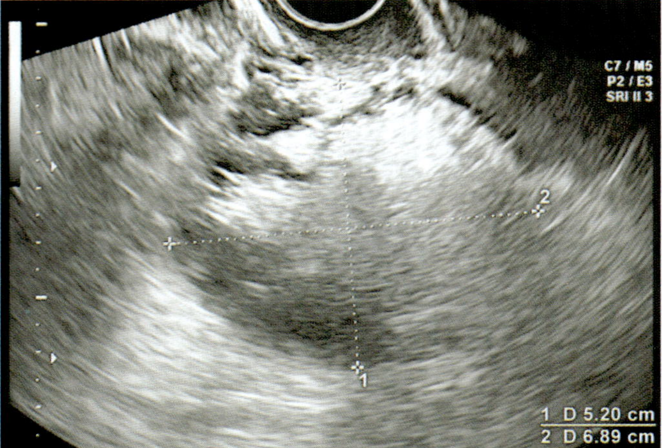

Fig. 7.15: A benign dermoid cyst. The outline of the cyst is difficult to delineate. This is because of the high sebaceous content of the cyst is similar to its pelvic surrounding.

Ultrasound characterization plays a key role in determining malignancies. Most malignancies will have central blood low and will demonstrate certain characteristics which are unique to cancers. In the United Kingdom, a risk of malignancy index (RMI) has been developed to help in the diagnosis and management of ovarian cancer.

Malignancy index combines three presurgical features: (1) serum CA125 (CA125), (2) menopausal status (M), and (3) ultrasound score (U). The RMI is a product of the ultrasound scan score, the menopausal status, and the serum CA125 level (IU/mL). Risk of malignancy index = $U \times M \times$ CA125. The ultrasound result is scored 1 point for each of the following characteristics: multilocular cysts, solid areas, metastases, ascites, and bilateral lesions. $U = 0$ (for an ultrasound score of 0), $U = 1$ (for an ultrasound score of 1), and $U = 3$ (for an ultrasound score of 2–5).

The menopausal status is scored as 1 = premenopausal and 3 = postmenopausal.

The classification of "postmenopausal" is a woman who has had no period for more than 1 year or a woman over 50 who has had a hysterectomy. Serum CA125 is measured in IU/mL and can vary between 0 and hundreds or even thousands of units.[27] However, even using the RMI model, the findings are not easily reproducible in all populations studied.[28]

More recently the International Ovarian Tumor Analysis (IOTA) group, set up in 1999, attempted to tackle this task.[29] The principal aim of the IOTA project has been to develop approaches to the evaluation of adnexal pathology using ultrasound that can be transferred to all examiners. Creating models that use simple, easily reproducible ultrasound characteristics is one approach.

The IOTA study phase 1 data led to the development of a set of simple rules based on the ultrasound features of a mass.[30] Five ultrasound features to predict malignancy (M-features) and five to predict a benign tumor (B-features) were identified on the basis of the highest positive predictive value (PPV) for malignancy for M-rules and the lowest PPV for malignancy for B-rules.[31] Using this approach, a mass is classified as malignant if one or more M-features apply in the absence of a B-feature. A mass is classified as benign if one or more B-features apply in the absence of an M-feature. A mass cannot be classified if either both M-features and B-features apply, or if no B-feature or M-feature is present. On temporal and external validation using the IOTA 2 dataset, the simple rules could be applied in 77% of masses.[30] The sensitivity and specificity for ovarian cancer were 92% and 96%, respectively, which was similar to the performance of subjective assessment by an experienced operator (91% and 96%, respectively).

The M-rules and B-rules are:

M-rules	B-rules
M1—Irregular solid tumor	B1—Unilocular
M2—Presence of ascites	B2—Presence of solid components where the largest solid component is less than 7 mm
M3—At least four papillary	B3—Presence of acoustic structures shadows
M4—Irregular multiloculated with largest solid component, with a diameter less than 100 mm	B4—Smooth multilocular solid tumor with largest diameter of more than 100 mm
M5—Very strong blood flow	B5—No blood flow (external iliac visualized next to ovary)

Serous Cystadenocarcinoma

The cyst is usually multiloculated with many septae; it will have mixed solid components (Fig. 7.16) with vascular papillary projections (Fig. 7.17), which will demonstrate low resistance to flow. The fluid component of the cyst is usually bloody. In 50% of cases, the tumor is bilateral.

Mucinous Cystadenocarcinoma

Twenty percent of mucinous cysts will be malignant, 10% being borderline, and the other half showing true malignancy potential. It is suspected when a cyst, which otherwise looks serous, produces low-level echoes. Ten percent of cysts are bilateral and the tumor can spread to the peritoneal cavity causing myxoma peritonei where ultrasound scan will demonstrate a multilocular mesh-like content filling (Figs. 7.18 and 7.19) and extending above the pelvis.

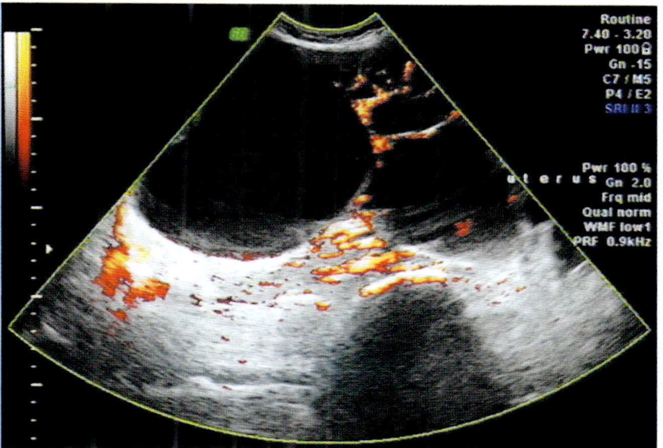

Fig. 7.17: Doppler examination reveals flow in the septae and the capsule.

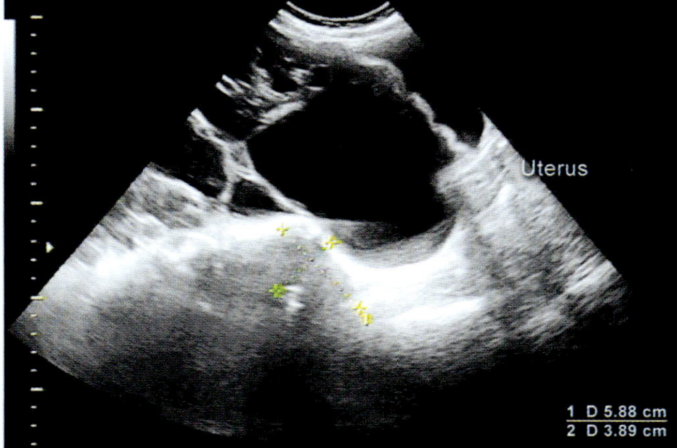

Fig. 7.16: A serous cystadenocarcinoma lying behind the uterus. The cyst has an irregular outline, the capsule appears thickened and it is multiloculated with some solid component.

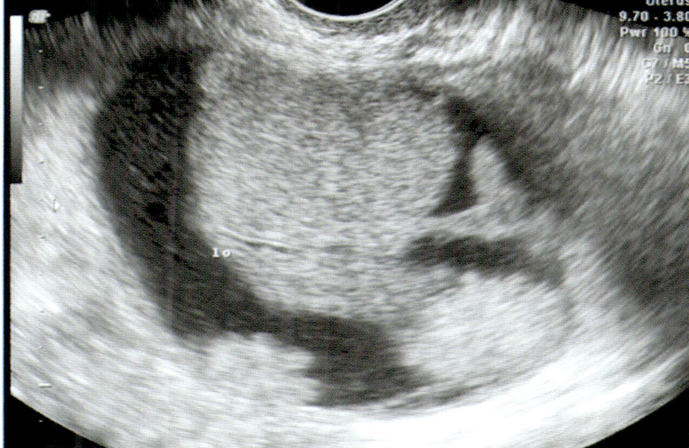

Fig. 7.18: A mucinous cystadenocarcinoma. Note the mixed echogenicity with thickened capsule, papillary projections, and solid component.

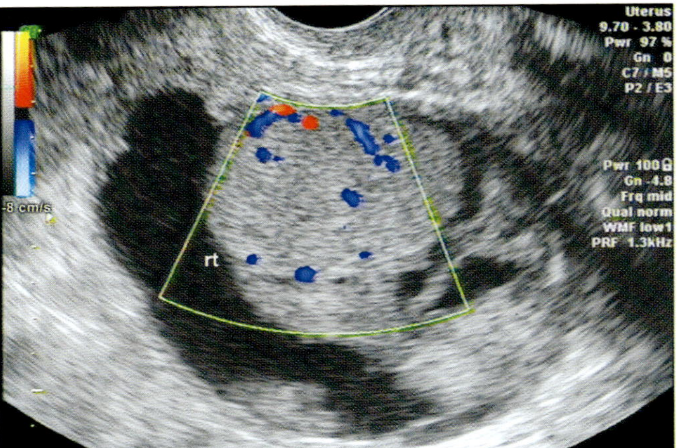

Fig. 7.19: Doppler examination reveals abnormal vasculature in the solid component.

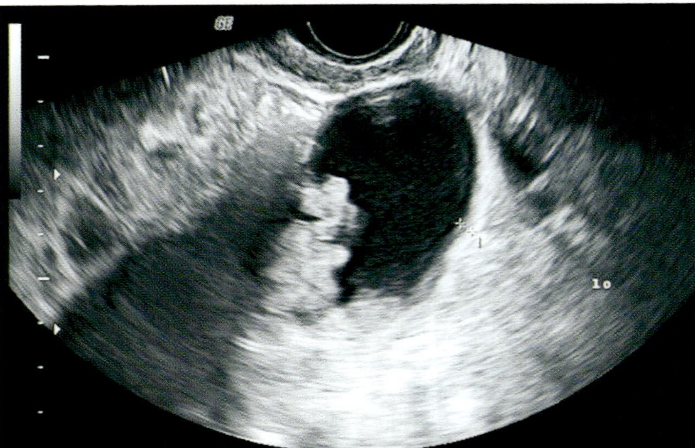

Fig. 7.20: A borderline serous cystadenoma with a thickened capsule and papillary projection.

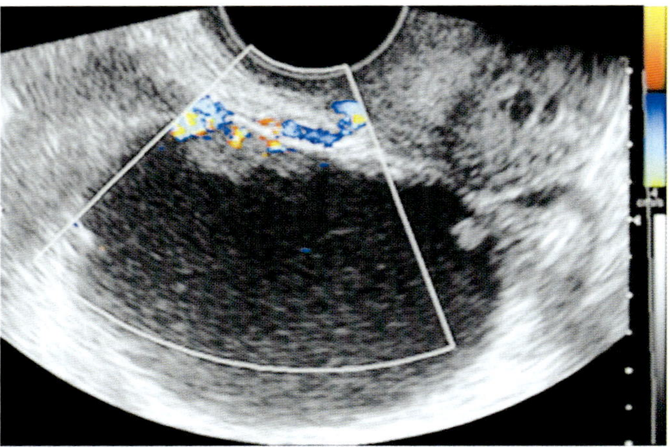

Fig. 7.21: Doppler examination reveals flow in the capsule.

Paraovarian cysts

Paraovarian cyst are remnants of Wolffian duct in mesosalpinx that do not arise from the ovary. They account for ~10-20% of adnexal masses. They typically occur in women around the ages of 20-40 years old. Most are asymptomatic, although patients with large lesions can present with pelvic pain. They usually occur around the broad ligament and arise from paramesonephric, mesothelial, or mesonephric remnants. They are usually simple cysts. A paraovarian cyst is easier to recognise if the ipsilateral ovary is demonstrated to be separate from it. Paraovarian cysts occasionally can be complicated by rupture, torsion, or hemorrhage. Large or symptomatic cysts may need to undergo surgical removal by laparoscopic cystectomy. Smaller asymptomatic ones are treated conservatively. For simple paraovarian cysts with no suspicious features on ultrasound, follow-up recommendations are the same as for ovarian cyst. Paraovarian cysts have sometimes been referred to as paratubal cysts or a hydatid cysts of Morgagni.

Ultrasound features are the following

- typically thin-walled and smooth margins
- most often appear as unilocular 'simple' cysts (in ~66%) and rarely as multilocular (~4%)
- Seen separate from the ovary

BORDERLINE OVARIAN TUMORS

They account for 15% of all epithelial ovarian tumors and are of low malignant potential. They are different histologically from invasive ovarian cancers, they tend to occur in younger patients and stage-by-stage, survival is better. Unfortunately, there are no reliable distinguishing markers and can only be suspected by their large size (Fig. 7.20) and atypical vascularity (Fig. 7.21).

CONCLUSION

Ultrasound assessment of ovaries is an integral part of pretreatment assessment of women seeking fertility treatment. The principal aims are to identify any ovarian pathology that may influence the fertility chances and risks associated with fertility treatment and to assess ovarian reserve. Polycystic ovarian syndrome is the most common ovarian pathology seen in subfertile population. Ovarian cysts seen in women of reproductive age group are usually benign and include endometrioma, hemorrhagic cysts, and dermoid cysts. It is rare to see any sinister ovarian pathology in women of reproductive age, but is important to rule out any malignant tumors. Ovarian cysts are readily diagnosed with TVS, which offers a sensitivity of 88–100% and specificity of 62–96% in the discrimination between benign and malignant adnexal masses.

KEY POINTS

- Ultrasound assessment of ovaries is an integral part of pretreatment assessment of women seeking fertility treatment
- While transabdominal ultrasound provides good information on the exact anatomical relationship of the pelvic organs, TVS with a high-frequency transducer is the tool of choice for imaging the female pelvis and for fine detailing of the ovary
- To image the ovary, the transvaginal probe is usually rotated anticlockwise and directed toward the side wall until the iliac vein comes into view and then the probe is slowly moved up until the ovaries are located just above
- The ovary is best imaged by TVS in the early follicular phase
- Polycystic ovarian syndrome and ovarian cysts are readily diagnosed with TVS as these pathologies have typical ultrasound features
- Ultrasound offers a high accuracy in the discrimination between benign and malignant ovarian pathologies

REFERENCES

1. Goswamy RK, Campbell S, Royston IP, et al. Ovarian size in post menopausal women. Br J Obstet Gynaecol. 1988;95:795-801.
2. Grandberg S, Wickland M. Comparison between endovaginal and transabdominal transducers for measuring ovarian volume. J Ultrasound Med. 1987;6:649-53.
3. Ilan E, Timor-Tritsch IE. Ultrasound in Gynaecology, 2nd edition. New York: Churchill-Livingstone (Elsevier); 2007. pp. 104-5.
4. Hamilton-Fairley D, Taylor A. Anovulation. BMJ. 2003;327:546-9.
5. Agrawal R, Conway G, Sladkevicius P, et al. Serum vascular endothelial growth factor and Doppler blood flow velocities in in vitro fertilization: relevance to ovarian hyperstimulation syndrome and polycystic ovaries. Fertil Steril. 1998;70:651-8.
6. Delvigne A, Rozenberg S. Epidemiology and prevention of ovarian hyperstimulation syndrome (OHSS): a review. Hum Reprod Update. 2002;8:559-77.
7. Hart R. PCOS and infertility. Panminerva Med. 2008;50: 305-14.
8. Legro RS. Polycystic ovary syndrome: the new millenium. Mol Cell Endocrinol. 2001;184:87-93.
9. Polson DW, Adams J, Wadsworth J, Franks S. Polycystic ovaries—a common finding in normal women. Lancet. 1988;1:870-2.
10. Balen A. Pathogenesis of polycystic ovary syndrome—the enigma unravels? Lancet. 1999;354:966-7.
11. Azziz R, Carmina E, Dewailly D, et al. Positions statement: criteria for defining polycystic ovary syndrome as a predominantly hyperandrogenic syndrome: an Androgen Excess Society guideline. J Clin Endocrinol Metab. 2006;91:4237-45.
12. Rotterdam ESHRE/ASRM-Sponsored PCOS Consensus Workshop Group. Revised 2003 consensus on diagnostic criteria and long-term health risks related to polycystic ovary syndrome (PCOS). Hum Reprod. 2004;19:41-7.
13. Adams J, Franks S, Polson DW, et al. Multifollicular ovaries: clinical and endocrine features and response to pulsatile gonadotropin releasing hormone. Lancet. 1985;2:1375-9.
14. Rotterdam ESHRE/ASRM-Sponsored PCOS Consensus Workshop Group. Revised 2003 consensus on diagnostic criteria and long-term health risks related to polycystic ovary syndrome. Fertil Steril. 2004;81:19-25.
15. Raine-Fenning NJ, Campbell BK, Clewes JS, Johnson IR. The interobserver reliability of ovarian volume measurement is improved with three-dimensional ultrasound, but dependent upon technique. Ultrasound Med Biol. 2003;29:1685-90.
16. Raine-Fenning NJ, Clewes JS, Kendall NR, Bunkheila AK, Campbell BK, Johnson IR. The interobserver reliability and validity of volume calculation from three-dimensional ultrasound datasets in the in vitro setting. Ultrasound Obstet Gynecol. 2003;21:283-91.
17. Lam PM, Johnson IR, Raine-Fenning NJ. Three-dimensional ultrasound features of the polycystic ovary and the effect of different phenotypic expressions on these parameters. Hum Reprod. 2007;22:3116-23.
18. Dewailly D. Diagnostic criteria for PCOS:Is there a need for rethink?:Best Practice & Research Clinical Obstetrics & Gynaecology. 2016;37:5-11.
19. Fulghesu AM, Angioni S, Frau E, et al. Ultrasound in polycystic ovary syndrome—the measuring of ovarian stroma and relationship with circulating androgens: results of a multicentric study. Hum Reprod. 2007;22:2501-8.
20. Buckett WM, Bouzayen R, Watkin KL, Tulandi T, Tan SL. Ovarian stromal echogenicity in women with normal and polycystic ovaries. Hum Reprod. 1999;14:618-21.
21. Ozkan S, Vural B, Caliskan E, Bodur H, Turkoz E, Vural F. Color Doppler sonographic analysis of uterine and ovarian artery blood flow in women with polycystic ovary syndrome. J Clin Ultrasound. 2007;35:305-13.
22. Tugrul S, Oral O, Guclu M, Kutlu T, Uslu H, Pekin O. Significance of Doppler ultrasonography in the diagnosis of polycystic ovary syndrome. Clin Exp Obstet Gynecol. 2006;33:154-8.
23. Raine-Fenning NJ, Campbell BK, Clewes JS, Kendall NR, Johnson IR. The interobserver reliability of three-dimensional

power Doppler data acquisition within the female pelvis. Ultrasound Obstet Gynecol. 2004;23:501-8.

24. Jarvela IY, Mason HD, Sladkevicius P, et al. Characterization of normal and polycystic ovaries using three-dimensional power Doppler ultrasonography. J Assist Reprod Genet. 2002;19:582-90.
25. Ng EH, Chan CC, Yeung WS, Ho PC. Comparison of ovarian stromal blood flow between fertile women with normal ovaries and infertile women with polycystic ovary syndrome. Hum Reprod. 2005;20:1881-6.
26. Geomini P, Kruitwagen R, Bremer GL, et al. The accuracy of risk scores in predicting ovarian malignancy—a systematic review. Obstet Gynecol. 2009;113:384-94.
27. Mashiach R, Melamed N, Gilad N, Ben-Shitrit G. and Meizner I, Sonographic Diagnosis of Ovarian Torsion. Journal of Ultrasound in Medicine, 2011;30:1205–10.
28. Mol BW, Boll D, De Kanter M, et al. Distinguishing the benign and malignant adnexal mass: an external validation of prognostic models. Gynecol Oncol. 2001;80:162-7.
29. Timmerman D, Van Calster B, Testa AC, et al. Ovarian cancer prediction in adnexal masses using ultrasound-based logistic regression models: a temporal and external validation study by the IOTA group. Ultrasound Obstet Gynecol. 2010;36:226-34.
30. Timmerman D, Testa AC, Bourne T, et al. Simple ultrasound-based rules for the diagnosis of ovarian cancer. Ultrasound Obstet Gynecol. 2008;31:681-90.
31. Timmerman D, Ameye L, Fischerova D, et al. Simple ultrasound rules to distinguish between benign and malignant adnexal masses before surgery: prospective validation by IOTA group. BMJ. 2010;341:c6839.

Chapter

8

Pelvic Endometriosis and Adnexal Pathologies

Narendra Malhotra, Jaideep Malhotra, Sonal Panchal

Chapter Outline

ENDOMETRIOSIS

Endometriosis is defined as presence of endometrial tissue at any other location than endometrial cavity. Though the precise etiology is still not known, it may be because of regurgitation of viable endometrial cells into the peritoneal tissues during menstruation followed by oestrogen stimulation. Though the genetic predisposition for the same cannot be excluded.[1]

It is a very debilitating, frustrating, and perplexing disease. The common presenting symptoms are pelvic pain of variable intensity, dysmenorrhea, dyspareunia, and infertility.[2] Patients with bladder or bowel endometriosis may also present with dysuria and dyschezia.[3] No predictable relationship has been established between the extent of the lesion and severity of symptoms. Though several imaging modalities have been tried to diagnose endometriosis, confirmation is possible only by laparoscopy and biopsy confirming the presence of endometrial glands and stroma in ectopic location.[4]

DIAGNOSTIC MODALITIES

While gold standard diagnostic modality for endometriosis is laparoscopy, this is invasive and is associated with operative risks. There are various noninvasive diagnostic modalities such as ultrasound (US), magnetic resonance imaging (MRI), and serum markers. Serum markers are rarely used, as its specificity is very low. Ultrasound is the commonly used diagnostic modality as it is widely available and cost-effective. Magnetic resonance imaging is used as an adjunctive noninvasive test for diagnosis of endometriosis with US and also for detection of endometriotic tissue in laparoscopically inaccessible areas. This chapter focuses primarily on application of US in diagnosing pelvic endometriosis.

ROLE OF ULTRASOUND

It is usually the most preferred modality for assessment of any gynecological pathology and transvaginal is the route of choice. High-resolution (6–12 MHz or 5–9 MHz) transvaginal probe is used for these scans. Ovarian and uterine lesions like chocolate cyst/endometriomas and adenomyosis are easy to diagnose by transvaginal US but diagnosis of superficial lesions, bowel lesions, or even bladder and ureteral lesions demands special skills.[5] Using harmonics imaging (HI), speckle reduction imaging (SRI), and cross-beam focusing (resolution) imaging (CRI) improves the quality of gray-scale imaging significantly to enable visualization of even subtle textural changes associated with early ovarian or extraovarian endometriosis. Certain modifications and maneuvers on transvaginal scans may improve the efficacy of these scans. Though endometriosis is likely to involve multiple organs and can be wide spread in pelvis. The approach to US assessment should therefore be flexible. Transabdominal and transrectal routes may be used as and when required. Moreover, different tools of US, like color and power Doppler (PD) and 3D US, should also be used and are helpful for diagnosis and assessment of patients with endometriosis.

Scanning Technique

Scanning should ideally begin with a survey of the whole abdomen with 3.5 MHz transabdominal sector or curvilinear probe. This should be followed up with a transvaginal scanning with slightly full bladder so that the bladder wall can be evaluated for chronic cystitis and or endometriosis.

In and out movement of the probe allows to assess the sliding of tissue planes over one another (sliding organ sign). It is used to rule out adhesions. Adhesions are common in patients with endometriosis. Therefore, eliciting "sliding organ sign" may give a clue to the presence of endometriosis. Negative sliding organ sign is an easy and practical method for prediction of the presence of deep infiltrating endometriosis involving the rectum. This could be a valuable "red flag sign" for triaging patients for detailed investigation.[6]

In addition, probe movements will also help to find out if there is any tenderness. Tenderness-guided approach is especially very useful to locate endometriotic patches.[7] Superficial or vaginal wall lesions can be better visualized by increasing the distance between the probe head and the lesion. This is done by placing more gel (12 mL) under the condom on the probe.

The efficacy of transvaginal sonography (TVS) for demonstration of rectovaginal lesions can be improved by providing better tissue interface. This is done by filling up the rectum with water, prior to transvaginal scan. Transvaginal sonography with water or contrast in rectum (RWC-TVS) is helpful to visualize rectovaginal nodules infiltrating rectal muscularis propria more accurately than TVS. This was described by Morotti et al.[8] A 6-mm flexible catheter is introduced in rectal lumen during transvaginal US. Water is slowly instilled into the rectum to permit intestinal distention. Colonic wall is evaluated by positioning the transvaginal probe against the length of the sigmoid colon. Obtain longitudinal or axial images. On this examination, rectosigmoid endometriotic nodules appear rounded or triangular hypoechoic masses, located anterior or lateral to bowel. It is the distance between these nodules and mucosal layer that permits to assess the infiltration of intestinal wall.[8]

Volume ultrasound (3D US) may be used to assess the multiorgan involvement and adhesions. It is also helpful to assess the ovarian reserve in diseased ovaries. A justified use of 3D US tools, like multiplanar imaging, tomographic ultrasound imaging (TUI), volume contrast imaging (VCI), and PD, may improve the accuracy of diagnosis significantly. Transrectal US may be used to demonstrate the lesions in the rectovaginal pouch.

What to check for in a case of endometriosis?

- Uterus mobility and adenomyosis
- Ovaries—endometrioma and mobility
- Mobility of anterior compartment
- Mobility of posterior compartment
- Bladder endometriosis
- Bowel endometriosis
- Hydronephrosis

TYPES OF ENDOMETRIOTIC LESIONS

Endometriosis can be seen at different locations (Fig. 8.1):

1. Superficial endometriosis
2. Ovarian endometriomas
3. Adenomyosis
4. Deep retroperitoneal endometriosis
5. Bladder endometriosis
6. Ureteral endometriosis leading to obstructive uropathy
7. Diaphragmatic endometriosis
8. Bowel endometriosis

Superficial Endometriosis and Adhesions

Transvaginal scan is unable to delineate or diagnose superficial peritoneal endometriosis and ovarian surface or ovarian fossa powder burn lesions or flimsy adhesions

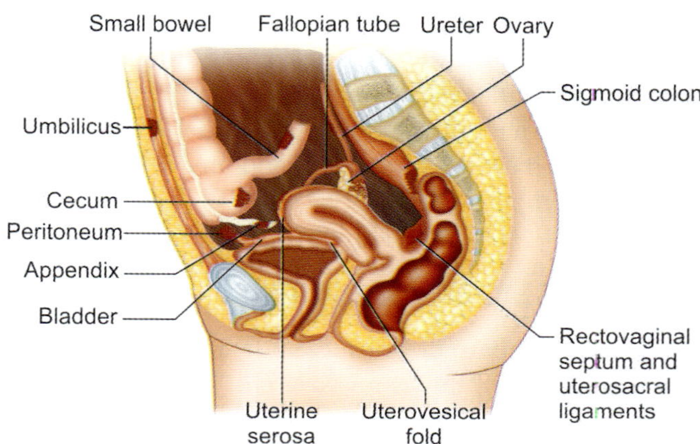

Fig. 8.1: Different possible locations of endometriosis.

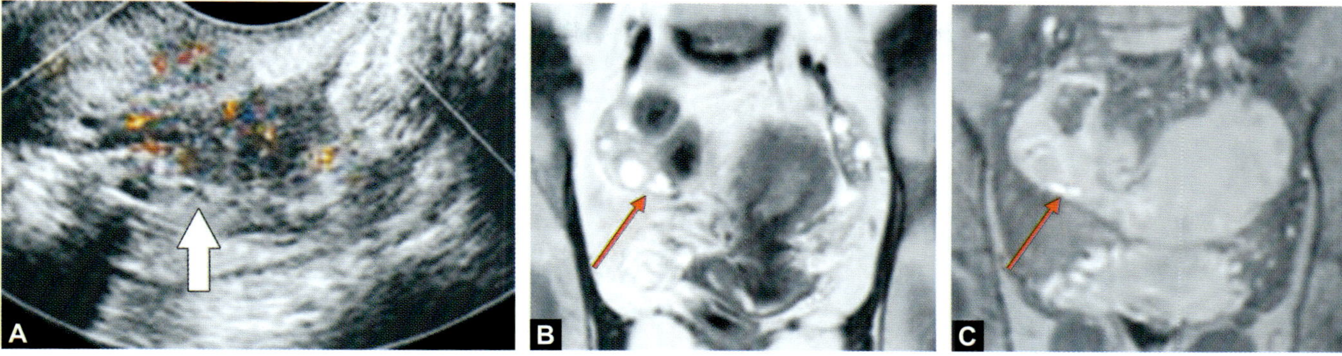

Figs. 8.2A to C: Superficial endometriosis on US and MRI: From "the radiology assistant."

confidently. Though some studies have described these lesions as hypoechoic ill-defined areas, these are very rare to be picked up on US. Even MRI cannot delineate subtle endometriosis (4% detection rate for lesions < 5 mm). Though fat-saturated MRI improves the detection rate of small hemorrhagic lesions to 50%[5] (Figs. 8.2A to C).

Ovarian Endometrioma

Whenever repeated retrograde menstruation occurs over the ovarian surface, endometrial tissue settles over the ovarian surface and repeatedly starts proliferating and shedding.[7] More than 90% of endometriomas are pseudocysts formed by invagination of the ovarian cortex, which is sealed off by adhesions. Inside of the cyst is characterized by fibrosis and retraction of cortex, the presence of islands of glandular endometrial tissue and organized blood clots. There is no evidence that endometriotic tissue invades ovarian stroma; however, it is common to see combined corpus luteum or lutein cysts with endometriomas. The chocolate-like content of the cyst represents old and chronic bleeding but it is not a specific feature for endometriomas and is seen in other hemorrhagic cysts of the ovary also. One-third to half of the ovarian endometriotic cysts are bilateral. These are commonly associated with adhesions of uterus and ovaries with each other or surrounding structures. Ovarian endometriomas on TAS may appear cystic that are entirely or predominantly anechoic.[9] They may appear as complex masses.[10] Transvaginal sonography has 82–89% sensitivity and 89–97% specificity for diagnosis of ovarian endometriomas.

Ultrasound Features

Small endometriotic ovarian lesions are usually uniform and slightly hyperechoic than ovarian stroma. These lesions usually do not change their echotexture during different phases of menstrual cycle. Even ovarian stroma shows areas of mildly increased echogenicity in very early disease. Endometriomas usually have thick, smooth, or shaggy wall and often have low-level internal echoes. In Kupfer's study by TVS, 82% of 32 surgically proven endometriomas showed the presence of a homogenous hyperechoic "carpet" of low-level echoes (ground glass appearance)[11] (Figs. 8.3A and B). These low-level echoes are because of thick fluid, and therefore when the probe is held steady after a single short swift probe movement on the lesion, it shows continuously "falling down" effect of these low-level echoes known as acoustic streaming sign. This was thought to be fairly typical of endometriomas. However, the recent studies have shown that acoustic streaming cannot discriminate reliably between endometriomas and other adnexal lesions.[12]

Echogenicity of the lesion can be objectively measured by mean gray value utilizing 3D US and associated software. It has been shown in a study by Alcazar et al. that mean gray value is significantly higher in ovarian endometrioma compared to all other kinds of ovarian cysts. Mean gray value, which is a quantitative measurement of grayness, with a cut-off of more than 15.56 has a sensitivity of 85% and specificity of 76.5% for diagnosis of endometrioma.[13]

Some endometriomas may have no internal echogenicity, and/or may show septae. Fluid level may be seen, which separates echogenic (thick) from nonechogenic (thin) fluid (Fig. 8.4). This fluid interface appears vertical on the screen when probe is oriented longitudinally. Echogenic fluid is seen on the posterior aspect of the lesion in endometriosis and consists of solid components of blood, debris, and fresh blood and the anechoic anterior layer consists of serum.[14] Atypically, endometriomas may contain solid areas (Fig. 8.5). These areas may be retracted blood clots and have concave margins in at least one plane

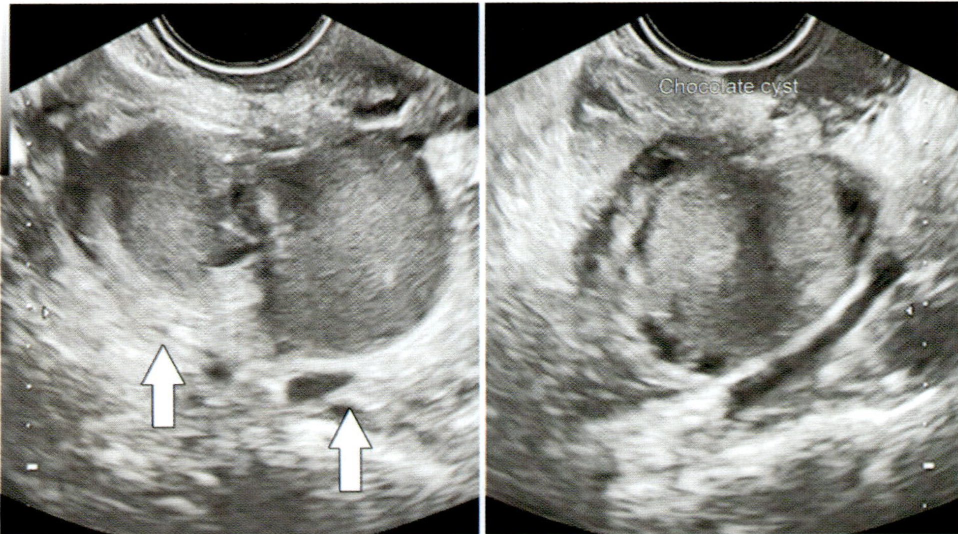

Fig. 8.3: Ground glass appearance of endometrioma.

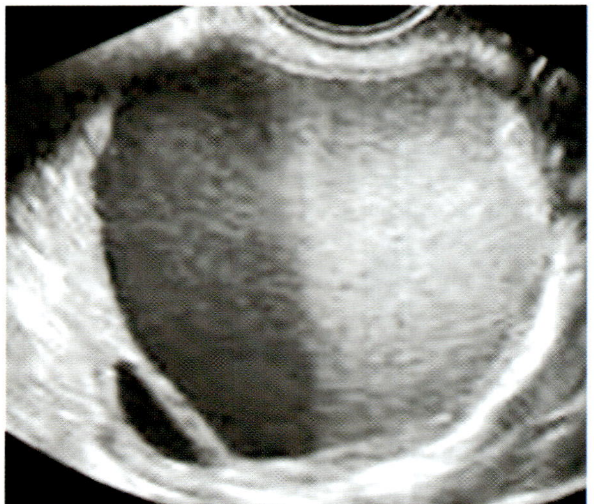

Fig. 8.4: Vertical fluid level in endometrioma.

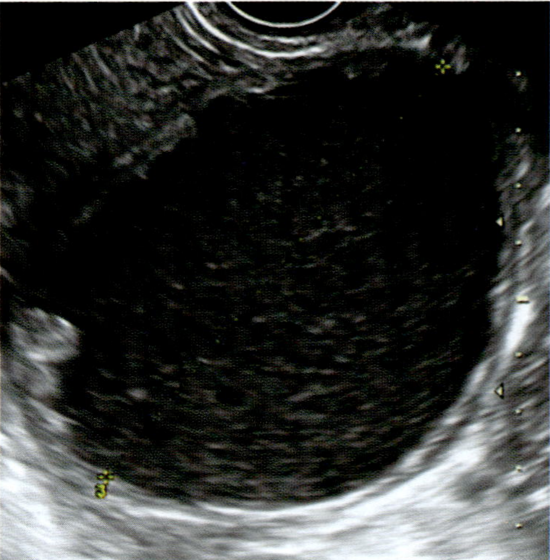

Fig. 8.5: Solid components in endometrioma.

when these are observed on probe rotation. Probe pressure will displace free clots/debris and move them away from the walls. It is because of these, that the endometriomas may be commonly mistaken for hemorrhagic cyst.

Other ovarian lesions like hemorrhagic cysts, dermoid cysts, and some epithelial tumors can show sonographic features similar to that of endometriomas.[15] Though punctate or linear, bright echogenicities in the wall favor the diagnosis of endometrioma. Moreover, it is interesting to know that textural changes are noted in endometriomas with the phase of menstrual cycle. These changes reflect the ovarian activity and exposure to exogenous hormonal influences. Endometriotic cysts usually increase in size following each menstrual period along with internal changes. These cyclical changes may help to differentiate endometriomas from other complex lesions of ovary. Therefore, serial scanning has a role for confirmation of diagnosis. Single postmenses follow-up study may considerably enhance diagnostic accuracy.

Unusually, endometriomas may show calcifications. Decidualization of solid projections may be rarely seen in endometriomas during pregnancy and then these appear hyperechoic and vascular.[16] These changes may mimic malignancy. About 0.3–0.8% of endometriomas

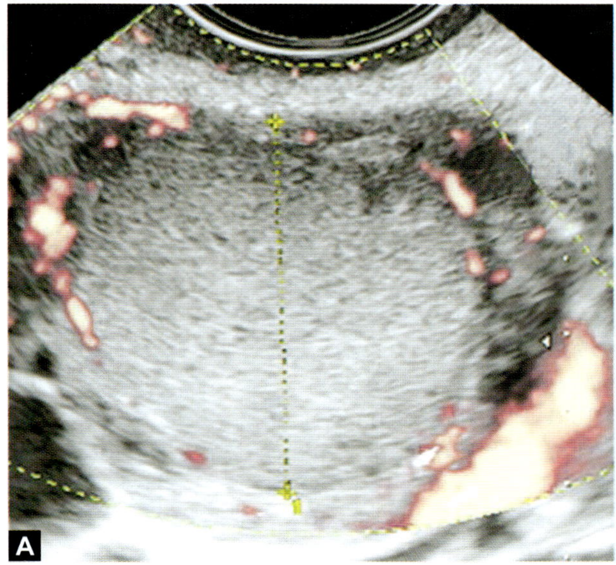

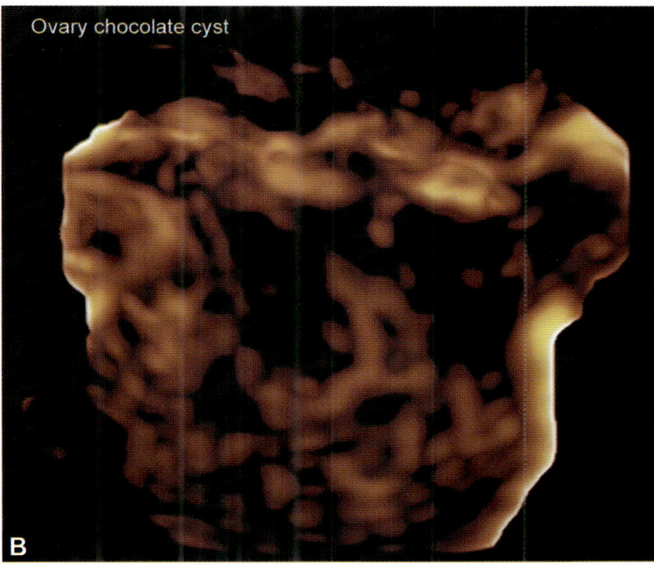

Figs. 8.6A and B: (A) Color Doppler showing scattered vascularity in endometrioma. (B) Three-dimensional power Doppler of endometrioma showing bird's nest appearance.

may contain malignant cells as has been described in one study, but this does not mean there is conversion to malignancy in these lesions. Moreover, this study looks at a very selected population and actual incidence is much lower than this. A systematic review by Moore et al.[17] has shown that US is an effective tool to both confirm and exclude the diagnosis of an endometrioma with moderate accuracy (+LR 7.6–29.8, –LR 0.1–0.4).

Addition of color Doppler studies (Fig. 8.6A) improve the diagnostic accuracy and this enables detection of vascularity within endometriomas and may help in ruling out malignancy.[18]

Kurjak and Kupesic were the first to report on the combined use of TV color Doppler and CA 125 levels in patients with ovarian endometriomas.[19] The scoring system proved to be very useful in distinguishing ovarian endometriosis from other benign and malignant ovarian lesions, with a sensitivity of 99.02% and a specificity of 99.64%, compared with morphological scoring system's sensitivity of 83.91% and specificity of 97.12%. Aleemet et al.,[20] however, concluded that scattered vascularity is typical of ovarian endometriomas and distinct from the dense vascularization associated with corpus luteum cysts and ovarian neoplasms. Guerriero et al.[21] believed that endometriomas had poor vascularization, whereas nonendometriomas were characterized by rich vascularization and presence of arterial flow in papillary projections and in solid echogenic areas. Moreover, endometriomas show low-resistance vascularity [resistance index (RI) 0.4] in menstrual period but is high (RI 0.4–0.56) in preovulatory and secretory period. Vascular lesions are more responsive to medical treatment as delivery of drugs is better in these patients.

Endometriomas have been shown to typically have short-coursed vessels. Three-dimensional-PD shows a well-perfused lesion with regularly placed vessels with a short course, with minimal variability in diameter. This gives a "bird's nest" appearance[22] (Fig. 8.6B).

Ultrasound characteristics of endometriomas may differ between premenopausal and postmenopausal patients. Masses with ground glass appearance in menopausal patients have high chances of malignancy.

Torsions of large endometriotic cysts, although rare, are of clinical concern. It may be suspected when there are changes in the outline of the lesion, differential internal bleeding outside of menstruation, and decrease in vascularity of course along with the typically acute clinical presentation of severe pain of sudden onset and vomiting.

Ultrasound features of endometrioma

- Thick, shaggy walls
- Low-level echogenecity—ground glass echogenecity
- Septae
- Echogenic flecks in walls
- Vertical fluid level
- Scattered hilar vascularity
- Short-coursed vessels
- Bird's nest appearance of vascularity

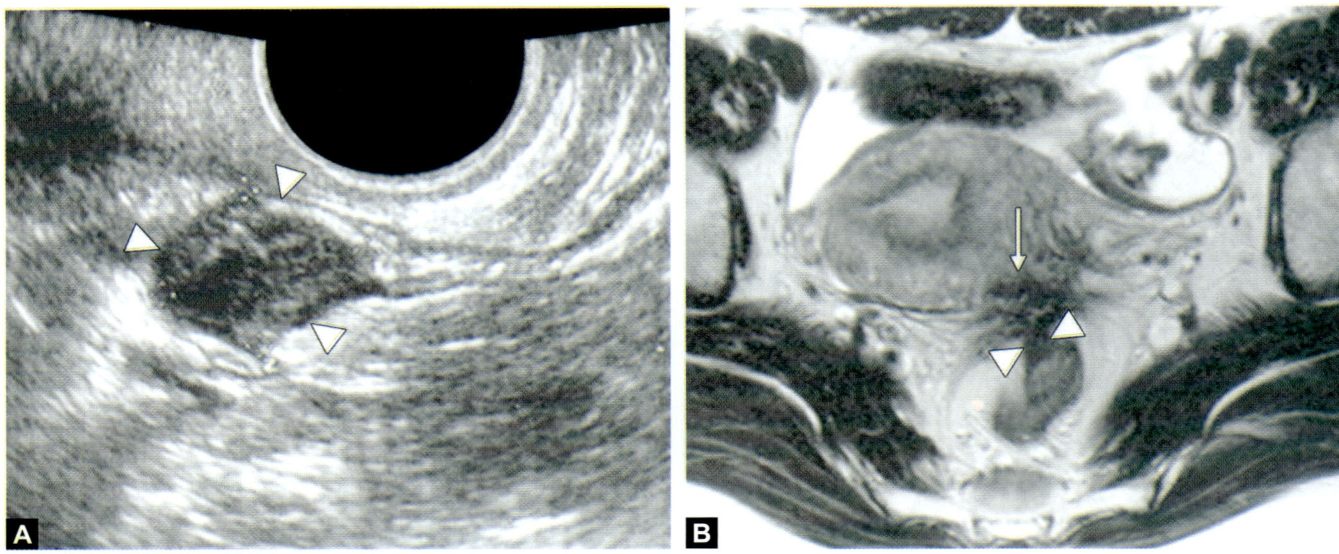

Figs. 8.7A and B: Deep endometriosis in US and MRI (arrows showing endometriotic nodule between upper vagina and rectum on US and MRI).

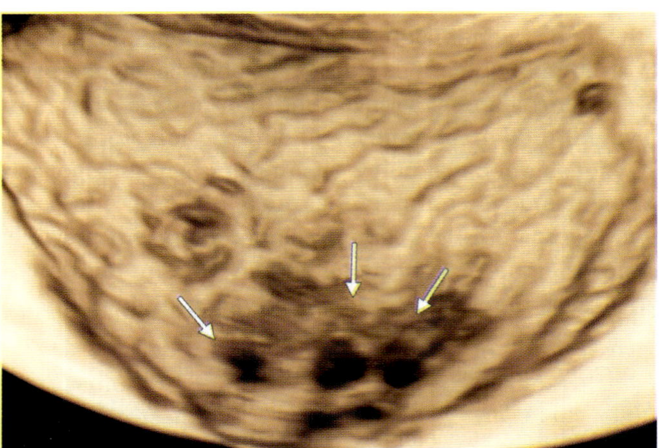

Fig. 8.8: Bladder endometriosis: Endometriotic patches and nodules seen in urinary bladder on 3D surface rendering of the bladder.

Rupture of the endometriotic cysts result in subcapsular hemorrhage within the ovary and collapse of the lesion.

Deep Retroperitoneal Endometriosis

Deep endometriosis is a nodular myeloproliferative lesion with very little glandular and stromal tissue. Deep retroperitoneal endometriosis occurs usually in the rectovaginal and vesicouterine spaces, uterosacral ligaments, bladder, and bowel. Bowel endometriosis can affect the rectosigmoid colon, appendix, and ileum.[23]

On US (TAS/TVS), these lesions appear as solid hypoechoic linear thickening or nodules with or without regular contour (Figs. 8.7A and B). They may vary in size from as small as 0.5 cm to more than 4 cm. These lesions will exhibit probe tenderness especially during menstruation. Rectal US (TRUS) can visualize uterosacral ligament thickness and also rectal infiltration.[24] Tenderness-guided US is an important technique to diagnose deep-seated endometriosis. Transvaginal sonography is more accurate than TRUS for prediction of deep infiltrating endometriosis in specific locations.[25,26]

Bladder Endometriosis

Bladder endometriosis may be suspected in patients with dysmenorrhea and urinary symptoms. Heamaturia with menstruation may be a helpful clue. Transvaginal sonography may reveal a solid nodule within the posterior bladder wall if the bladder is slightly filled (Fig. 8.8). Magnetic resonance imaging also helps in such cases.

Ureteral Endometriosis Leading to Obstructive Uropathy

This is a rare but serious complication of deep peritoneal endometriosis. Magnetic resonance imaging is most useful for diagnosing periuretric endometriomas.

Bowel Endometriosis

Endometriotic implants can also present on the small bowel and omentum. These are usually diagnosed by laparoscopy. However, with high-resolution US scanners, these lesions are seen as irregular hypoechoic areas typically described as "red Indian head sign"[7] (Fig. 8.9). For rectosigmoid endometriosis, TVS is an investigation of choice.

Bowel involvement was established when long, nodular, predominantly solid, and hypoechoic lesion adherent to the wall of the intestinal loop was detected.[27,28] The external hyperechoic margins are due to congested adipose tissue, submucosa and mucosa. Internal hyperechoic spots may be due to calcification.

However, TVS with water contrast in rectum (RWC-TVS) determines the presence of rectovaginal nodules infiltrating rectal muscularis propria more accurately than TVS. This technique is especially used when information achieved by TVS is incomplete and doubtful (Fig. 8.10). Diagnostic accuracy of RWS-TVS has been reported to be superior to TVS.[29]

To improve the near-field visualization for rectosigmoid endometriosis, 12 mL of gel under the probe cover can be tried instead of routine 4 mL. This increases the distance between the lesion and the probe head and allows better visualization. Posterior fornix is then evaluated accurately with up and down sliding movement of the probe. Tender areas were further checked more closely.[30]

Vaginosonography (Figs. 8.11A and B) may also be tried for rectovaginal endometriosis. This is TVS with acoustic

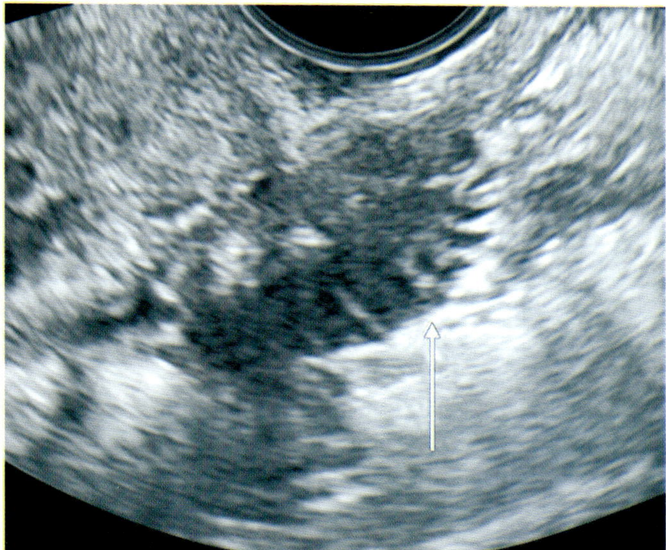

Fig. 8.9: Endometriotic nodule showing irregular hypoechoic area like red Indian head (Bowel endometriosis).

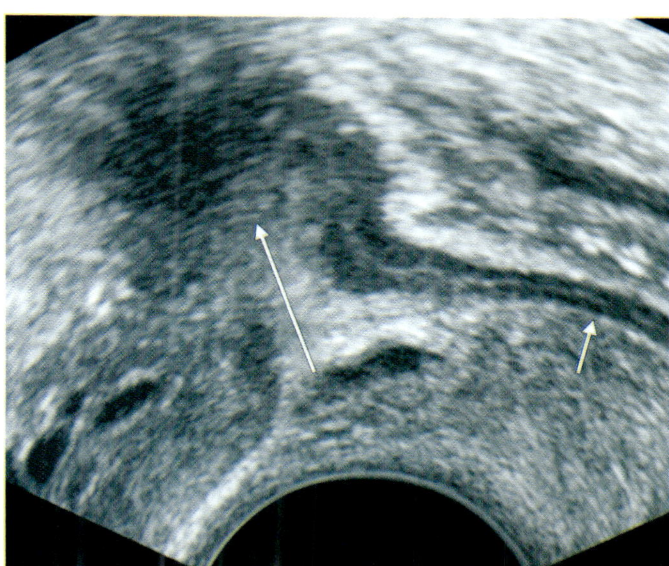

Fig. 8.10: Rectal endometriosis: Endometriotic nodule leading to thickened rectal wall.

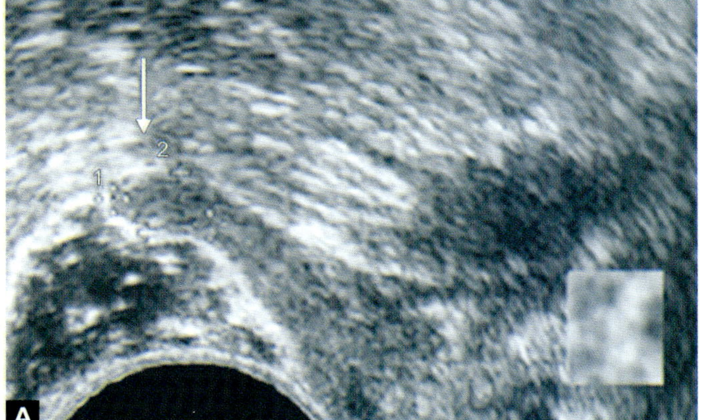

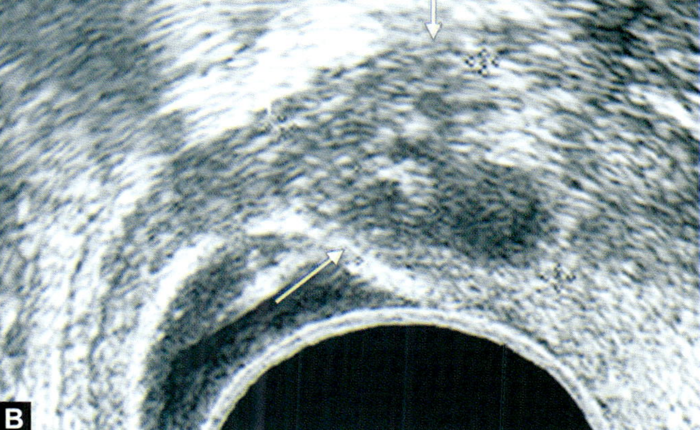

Figs. 8.11A and B: Vaginosonography demonstrating rectovaginal endometriosis.

window created in vagina by introduction of saline solution. This was more accurate than TVS for detection of rectovaginal septum endometriosis with sensitivity and specificity of 90.6% versus 43.7% and 85.7% versus 50%, respectively.[31]

As is known that saline can easily flow out of the vagina very quickly, Condous et al.[32] have tried US coupling gel for the same purpose with much better image quality and more informative assessment. For rectovaginal endometriosis, TRUS has a sensitivity of 97% and specificity of 96%,[23] and TVS: sensitivity of 99.3% and specificity of 87.2%.[33]

Uterosacral Ligament Endometriosis

On TRUS examination, thick uterosacral ligaments of more than 14 mm are suggestive of uterosacral ligament endometriosis.[34] Ligaments are seen as low echogenic thick and irregularly shaped arcs on both sides of cervix. Rectal US has 80% sensitivity and 97% specificity for detection of uterosacral ligament endometriosis. Transvaginal sonography has a sensitivity of 70.6% and specificity of 95.9% for detection of uterosacral ligament endometriosis.[33] Though on TVS these are difficult to locate if these are not floating in fluid.

Three-dimensional image rendering could allow a better analysis of a nodule because this 3D reconstruction might make the irregular shapes and borders more evident. Three-dimensional image rendering may show the particular shape of an endometriotic nodule with its irregular contour in a simpler way. The relationship between the nodule and the bowel could be evaluated in more detail.[32] The TUI display could be particularly useful for evaluating the extension of a nodule in the rectovaginal septum and also the depth of infiltration in the coronal plane and the relationship with the rectosigmoid junction.

ADNEXAL PATHOLOGIES

Adnexal pathologies consist of ovarian and tubal lesions. The ovarian pathologies other than endometriomas are discussed in Chapter 7. We shall therefore discuss the tubal pathologies here.

Anatomically, the tubes arise from the cornual end of the uterus and are 9–11 cm in length. Tubal lumen shows variations in its caliber but is very small and is nearly impossible to visualize on US, unless there is some fluid in the tubal lumen or outside the tube. The distal end of the tube is free and shows widening and finger-like processes called fimbriae. Tubes are loosely attached to broad ligament by mesosalpinx which is a peritoneal fold. Medial two-thirds of the tube is supplied by branches of uterine artery and lateral one-third by the branches of ovarian artery.

Commonest of the tubal pathologies is inflammation, which is often seen as a result of pelvic inflammatory disease (PID). PID, most commonly, is a result of ascending infection through vagina and cervix, but may rarely be seen as a result of hematogenous spread. Pelvic inflammatory disease often is asymptomatic or may have only minimal symptoms, but may also present sometimes as an acute pelvic pain with systemic signs of infection.

In the acute phase of infection, the tube becomes thick-walled and echogenic. It is also hyperperfused, but these features can be demonstrated only if the tube is identified by the fluid interface due to inflammatory free pelvic fluid or fluid in the tube.

Tube then appears like a dilated tubal structure in its long-axis-hydrosalpinx, but if scanned in its transverse axis, it may appear like a rounded cystic structure, similar to ovarian or paraovarian cyst. It is the sliding organ sign, which will enable us to confirm its extraovarian origin. As a rule, therefore any lesion in the pelvis must be scanned in two orthogonal planes and sliding organ sign must also be elicited to decide its organ of origin.

Though hydrosalpinges and tuboovarian mass may also be seen as a result of endometriosis. Details of hydrosalpinx and tuboovarian masses are described in detail in Chapter 5.

CONCLUSION

With current improved high-resolution scanning, it is now possible to diagnose most of the endometriotic lesions. Addition of color Doppler helps in scoring and detecting endometriosis and differentiating it from malignancies. However, current scoring systems are not yet very accurate as TVS still cannot diagnose and visualize superficial peritoneal implants, ovarian implants, bowel endometriosis, or extent of adhesions. Adenomyosis and adnexal pathologies like hydrosalpinx can be easily diagnosed by conventional US with confidence.

KEY POINTS

- Endometriosis is the leading cause of pelvic pain and disability in reproductive age group of women and results in almost 10–15% as a cause of infertility

- Scanning should ideally begin with a survey of the whole abdomen, followed up with a transvaginal scanning with slightly full bladder so that the bladder wall can be evaluated for chronic cystitis or endometriosis
- In and out movement of the probe allows to assess the sliding of tissue planes over one another (sliding organ sign)
- The efficacy of transvaginal sonography for demonstration of rectovaginal lesions can be improved by providing better tissue interface
- Volume US (3D US) may be used to assess the multiorgan involvement and adhesions
- Currently available resolution on transvaginal scans is unable to delineate or diagnose superficial peritoneal endometriosis and ovarian surface or ovarian fossa powder burn lesions or flimsy adhesions
- Small endometriotic ovarian lesions are usually uniform and slightly hyperechoic than stroma
- Atypically, endometriomas may contain solid areas and calcifications
- Doppler studies do not improve diagnostic accuracy, but this may help in ruling out malignancy
- Deep endometriotic lesions appear as solid hypoechoic linear thickening or nodules with or without regular contour
- Three-dimensional image rendering may allow better visualization of uterosacral endometriotic nodule because 3D reconstruction might make the irregular shapes and borders more evident

REFERENCES

1. Simpton JL, Elias S, Malinak LR, et al. Heritable aspects of endometriosis. I: genetic studies. Am J Obstet Gynecol. 1980;137:327-31.
2. Eskenazi B, Warner ML. Epidemiology of endometriosis. Obstet Gynecol Clin North Am. 1977;4:235-58.
3. Ballweg ML. Overcoming Endometriosis: New Help from the Endometriosis Association. New York: Congdon and Weed; 1987.
4. Anaf V, Simon P, Fayat I, et al. Smooth muscles one frequent components of endometriotic lesions. Hum Reprod. 2000;15:767-71.
5. Takahashi K, Okada M, Okada S, et al. Studies on the detection of small endometrial implants by magnetic resonance imaging using a fat saturation technique. Gynecol Obstet Invest. 1996;41:203-6.
6. Hudelist G, Fritzer N, Staettner S, et al. Uterine sliding sign: a simple sonographic predictor for presence of deep infiltrating endometriosis of rectum. Ultrasound Obstet Gynecol. 2013; 41:692-5.
7. Guerriero S, Ajossa S, Gerada M, et al. Tenderness-guided transvaginal ultrasonography: a new method for the detection of deep endometriosis in patients with chronic pelvic pain. Fertil Steril. 2007;88:1293-7.
8. Morotti M, Ferrero S, Boqliolo S, et al. Transvaginal ultrasonography with water contrast in the rectum in the diagnosis Dinecol. 2010;62(3):179-85.
9. Athey PA, Diment DD. The spectrum of sonographic findings in endometriosis. J Ultrasound Med. 1989;8(9):487-91.
10. Goldman SM, Minkin SI. Diagnosing endometriosis with ultrasound: accuracy and specificity. J Reprod Med. 1980;25:4-8.
11. Kupfer MC, Schwimer RS, Lebovic J. Transvaginal sonographic appearance of endometriomata: spectrum of findings. J Ultrasound Med. 1992;11:129-32.
12. Van Holsbeke C, Zhang J, Van Belle V, et al. Acoustic streaming cannot discriminate reliably between endometriomas and other types of adnexal lesion: a multicenter study of 633 adnexal masses. Ultrasound Obstet Gynecol. 2010;35:349-53.
13. Alcazar JL, Leon M, Galvan R, et al. Assessment of cyst content using mean gray value for discriminating endometrioma from other unilocular cysts in premenopausal women. Ultrasound Obstet Gynecol. 2010;35:228-32.
14. Asch E, Levine D. Variations in appearance of endometriomas. J Ultrasound Med. 2007;26(8):993-1002.
15. Patel MD, Feldstein VA, Chen DC, et al. Endometriomas: diagnostic performance of US. Radiology. 1999;210:739-45.
16. Fruscella E, Testa AC, Ferrandina G, et al. Sonographic features of decidualize endometriosis suspicious for malignancy. Ultrasound Obstet Gynecol. 2004;24(5):578-80.
17. Moore J, Copley S, Morris J, et al. A systematic review of the accuracy of ultrasound in the diagnosis of endometriosis. Ultrasound Obstet Gynecol. 2002;20(6):630-4.
18. Kurjak A, Schulman H, Socic A, et al. Transvaginal ultrasound, color flow and Doppler waveform analysis of the postmenopausal adnexal mass. Obstet Gynecol. 1992;80:917-21.
19. Kurjak A, Kupesic S. Scoring system for prediction of ovarian endometriosis. Fertil Steril. 1994;62:81-8.
20. Aleem F, Pennisi J, Zeitoum K, et al. The role of color Doppler in diagnosis of endometriomas. Ultrasound Obstet Gynecol. 1995;5:51-4.
21. Guerriero S, Ajossa S, Mais V, et al. The diagnosis of endometriomas using color Doppler energy imaging. Hum Reprod. 1998;13:1691-5.
22. Raine-Fenning N, Jayaprakasan K, Deb S. Three-dimensional ultrasonographic characteristics of endometriomata. Ultrasound Obstet Gynecol. 2008;31:718-24.
23. Brosens IA. New principles in the management of endometriosis. Acta Obstet Gynaecol Scand Suppl. 1994;159:18-21.
24. Fedele L, Bianchi S, Portuese A, et al. Transrectal ultrasonography in the assessment of rectovaginal endometriosis Obstet Gynaecol. 1998;91:444-8.

25. Bazot M, Thomassin I, Hourani R, et al. Accuracy of transvaginal sonography and rectal endoscopic sonography in the diagnosis of deep infiltrating endometriosis. Ultrasound Obstet Gynecol. 2007;30:994-1001.
26. Posnaik HV, Keshavarzian A, Jabamoni R. Diaphragmatic endometriosis; CT and MR findings. Gastrointest Radiol. 1990;15:349-51.
27. Abrao MS, Goncalves MO, Dias JA, Jr., Podgaec S, Chamie LP, Blasbalg R. Comparison between clinical examination, transvaginal sonography and magnetic resonance imaging for the diagnosis of deep endometriosis. Hum Reprod. 2007;22:3092-7.
28. Bazot M, Thomassin I, Hourani R, Cortez A, Darai E. Diagnostic accuracy of transvaginal sonography for deep pelvic endometriosis. Ultrasound Obstet Gynecol. 2004;24:180-5.
29. Valezano Menada M, Remorgida V, Abbamonte LH, et al. Does transvaginal ultrasonography combined with water-contrast in the rectum aid in the diagnosis of rectovaginal endometriosis infiltrating the bowel? Hum Reprod. 2008;23:1069-75.
30. Guerriero S, Ajossa S, Gerada M, et al. Diagnostic value of transvaginal tenderness-guided ultrasonography for the prediction of location of deep endometriosis. Hum Reprod. 2008;23:2452-7.
31. Dessole S, Farina M, Rubattu G, et al. Sonovaginography is a new technique for assessing rectovaginal endometriosis. Fertil Steril. 2003;79:1023-7.
32. Condous G, Bignardi T, Alhamdan D, Lu C. Sonovaginography: defining the normal rectovaginal septum. UOG. 2008;32(3):249.
33. Bazot M. Thomassin I, Hourani R, et al. Diagnostic accuracy of transvaginal sonography for deep pelvic endometriosis. Ultrasound Obstet Gynecol. 2004;24:180-5.
34. Ohba T, Mizutani H, Maeda T, et al. Evaluation of endometriosis in uterosacral ligaments by transrectal ultrasonography. Hum Reprod. 1996;11:2014-7.35.

Chapter

9

Ultrasound Monitoring of Natural and Stimulated Cycles

Sonal Panchal

Chapter Outline

- Introduction
- Monitoring a Natural Cycle
- Monitoring of Stimulated Cycles
- Conclusion
- Key Points

INTRODUCTION

Continuous complex hormonal changes occurring during the menstrual cycle result into cyclical morphological changes and vascular changes in ovaries and uterus, and these are the basis of reproductive function in human. Transvaginal ultrasound (TVS) is the modality of choice to study these changes. The accuracy of diagnosis and monitoring of infertility treatments, such as ovulation induction, has greatly increased because of the availability of sophisticated ultrasound (US) technology and equipment.[1]

The cyclical changes in uterus and ovaries that are seen in the natural cycle can be a basis for treatment planning and management of infertile patients. Therefore, this chapter has been discussed chiefly under two headings:

1. Monitoring a natural cycle
2. Monitoring a stimulated cycle

MONITORING A NATURAL CYCLE

Ovarian Follicle Tracking

Follicular tracking describes the serial ultrasonographic study of the ovary during the menstrual cycle. The aim is to estimate follicular maturity, so that the time of ovulation can be predicted and to follow the corpus luteum to assess the secretory phase. During follicular tracking, the mean diameter of each of the follicles is measured and their growth is followed. Ultrasound is often used in conjunction with serum measures of estradiol, luteinizing hormone (LH), and progesterone to improve accuracy.

Monitoring of a menstrual cycle should start in early proliferative phase, preferably days 2–3 of the cycle. At this time estrogen, progesterone, follicle-stimulating hormone (FSH), and LH are at baseline levels. Secondary antral follicles (1–2 mm) are the first follicular structures that may be visualized on US. A cohort of small antral follicles develops during the luteal phase of previous menstrual cycles independently of gonadotropin stimulation. Follicles up to 2 mm diameter grow independent of gonadotropins (FSH).[2] Further development of the follicle is only possible in the presence of appropriate levels of gonadotropin, subsequently the most mature follicle is selected and the others become atretic. Before day 5 of the cycle, selection of the dominant follicle occurs. Between days 5 and 7, dominance of the follicle becomes apparent on US. Follicle that is 10–12 mm in size is known as a dominant follicle and it is this follicle that is most likely to grow to become a mature follicle. It is interesting to know that often first largest follicle on baseline scan may not always be the dominant follicle. A normal growth rate of a healthy follicle is approximately 2 mm/day and reaches a size of 18–24 mm (Fig. 9.1A) by the time of ovulation.[3]

In response to LH surge, resulting preovulatory changes in follicle are seen as appearance of a sonolucent halo surrounding the follicle and appearance of cumulus (a small solid projection from the follicle wall) within 24 hours before ovulation. Ovulation is characterized by blurring

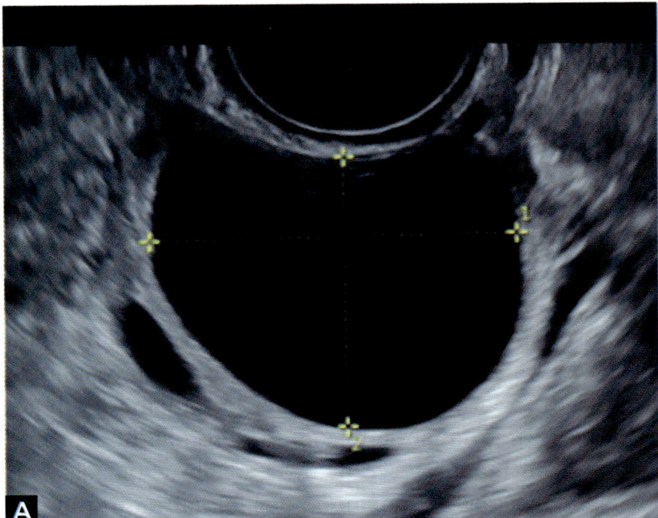

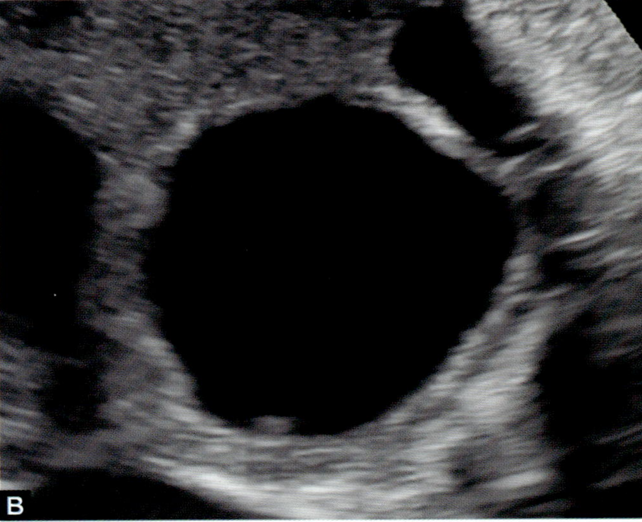

Figs. 9.1A and B: Preovulatory follicle on B-mode (A) and a few hours before rupture (B).

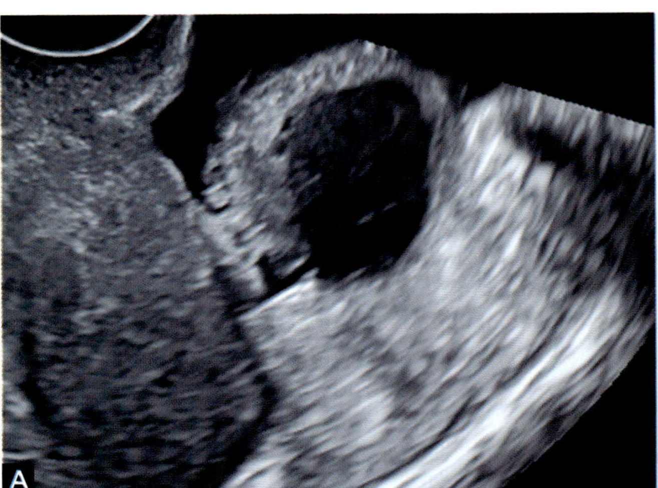

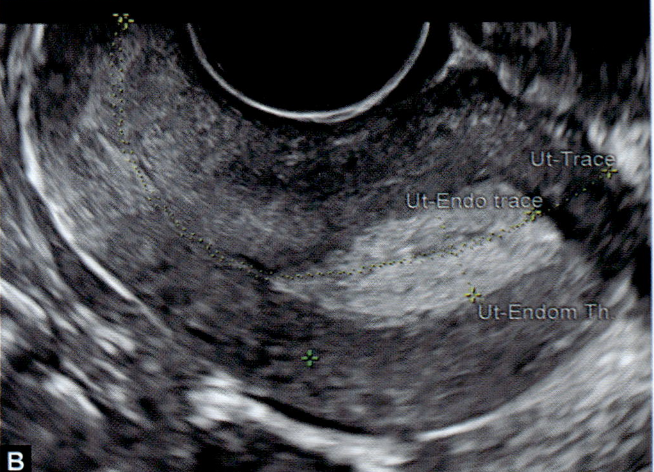

Figs. 9.2A and B: (A) Corpus luteum and (B) secretory endometrium.

of the follicular margins, the appearance of intrafollicular echoes (Fig. 9.1B), and the appearance of free fluid in the pouch of Douglas. Ovulation results in collapse of the follicle with irregular contour followed by filling of its cavity with echogenic fluid, now called corpus luteum. Corpus luteum typically has variable appearances with ground glass echogenicity in lumen or lace-like echogenicities (Fig. 9.2A) and has circumferential blood flow referred to as a "ring of fire" (Fig. 9.3). Secretory changes are seen in the endometrium in the form of echogenicity of the endometrium which starts from outside, proceeding to the central line making a ring sign of the endometrium[4] (Fig. 9.2B).

The corpus luteum has a limited life expectancy and resolves if pregnancy does not occur at the end of the luteal phase. Rarely, ovulation fails to occur leading to a luteinized, unruptured follicle in which, despite the absence of follicular rupture and release of the oocyte, the unruptured follicle undergoes luteinization under the action of LH. Ultrasound, but not the mid-luteal progesterone levels, aids in diagnosing this condition as there is normal production of progesterone.

Blood flows close to the follicle can be seen by Doppler when follicle reaches 10 mm in diameter and this may be used as a hemodynamic parameter of its growth,

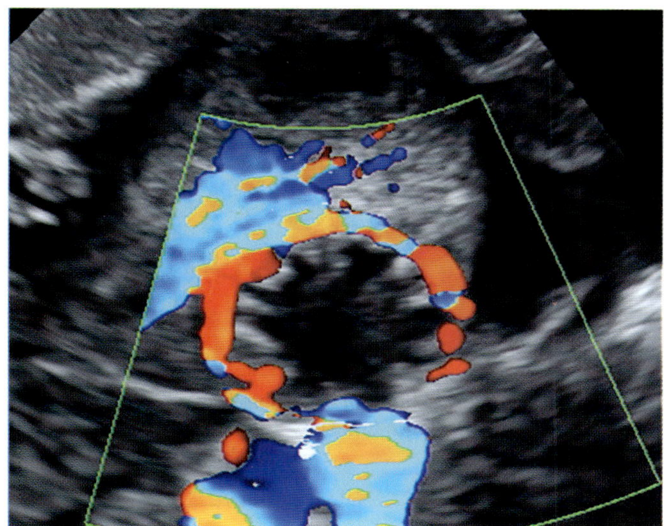

Fig. 9.3: A typical corpus luteum with vascularity around it.

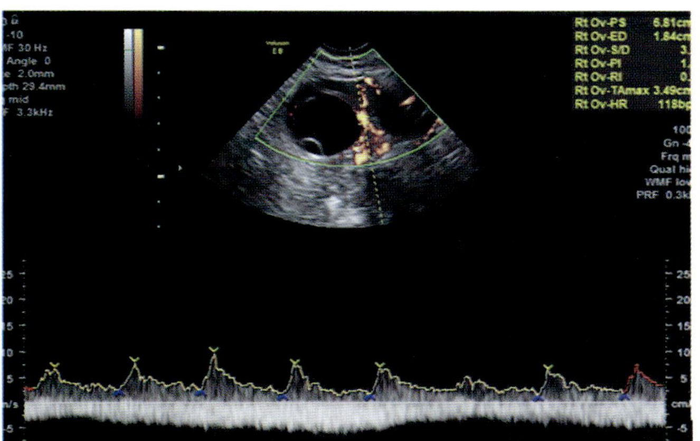

Fig. 9.5: High-resistance flow in luteinized unruptured follicle.

maturation, and ovulation. Resistance index (RI) of these vessels is reported as 0.54 ± 0.04. Resistance index starts falling 2 days prior to ovulation and reaches its nadir of 0.44 ± 0.04 at ovulation.[5] Just prior to rupture, the vascularity surrounding the follicle increases along with the increase in its flow velocity.[6] The mean changes in peak systolic velocity (PSV), follows the mean rise in LH by approximately 12 hours. Peak systolic velocity increases 29 hours before the time of follicular rupture and continues for at least 72 hours after corpus luteum is formed.[7] Three to seven times increase in the blood flow is noted in the dominant ovary (ovary from which ovulation occurs) during the luteal phase.[8] The flow is highest in the mid-luteal phase, which declines till menstruation in absence of conception.

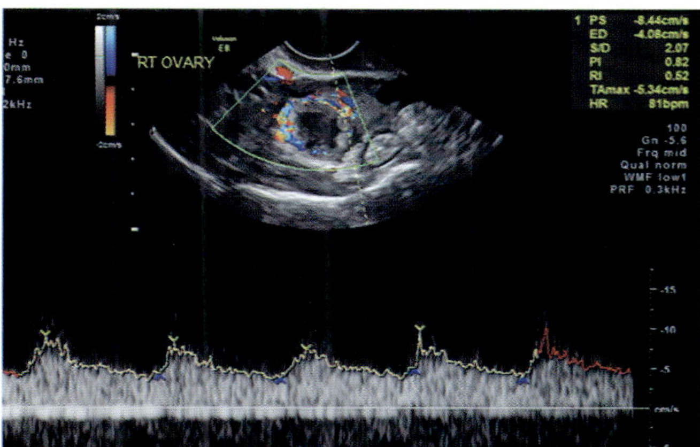

Fig. 9.4: Doppler wave form analysis of vascularity around a corpus luteum.

Resistance index of the corpus luteum has been suggested as an adjunct to plasma progesterone assay as an index of luteal function.[9] A healthy corpus luteum will show a vascular ring surrounding itself on color Doppler and on power Doppler, and these vessels show RI 0.35–0.50, pulsatility index (PI) 0.70–0.80, and PSV 10–15 cm/s[10,11] (Fig. 9.4). This resistance starts increasing on day 23 of the cycle in a nonconception cycle to RI 0.5–0.55. Based on these values, abnormal parameters indicate luteal phase problems like luteinized unruptured follicle (Fig. 9.5) or luteal phase defect (Figs. 9.6A and B).[10]

Uterine Monitoring

Ultrasound appearance of endometrium is a result of dynamic, histological, and physiological changes. These changes are reflection of the changes in the reproductive steroids—estrogen and progesterone. These changes are seen in the form of changes in echogenicity and reflectivity.

Endometrial thickness is less than 5 mm in early follicular phase and slightly more echogenic than the myometrium. It grows at a rate of 1–2 mm/day. Endometrium starts becoming triple line from 6 days before LH surge. Endometrial thickness can be correlated with the rise in estradiol.[12] It grows to a thickness of 10–12 mm at ovulation and becomes multilayered or trilaminar,[13] though relationship of endometrial thickness to histological dating is controversial. Endometrial wave-like activity can be seen on US throughout the menstrual cycle and is highest in the periovulatory period and in 30–40% of spontaneous

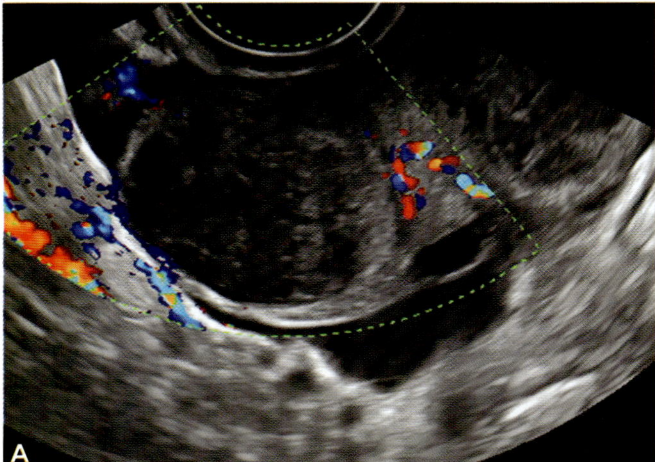

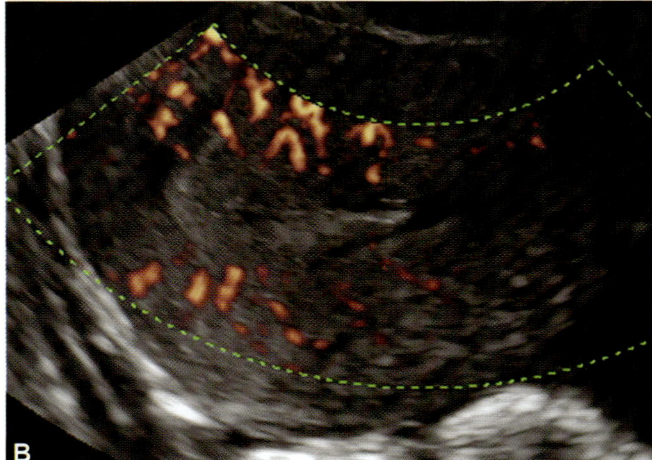

Figs. 9.6A and B: Possible luteal phase defect: Decreased corpus luteal and endometrial vascularity.

cycles its rate is 3–4/minute.[14] During the secretory phase, the endometrium starts becoming echogenic from the periphery, echogenicity progresses toward the central line and is described as "endometrial ring sign."[4] Its thickness decreases by 0.5 mm on the day of LH surge and then increases by 2 mm in the luteal phase.[15]

Endometrial and subendometrial vascular flow increases to its maximum 3 days prior to ovulation and then decreases until fifth postovulatory day (due to probably vasodilatation of subepithelial capillary plexus leading to stromal edema) and then again increases for the rest of the luteal phase.[16] The proliferative phase flow is thought to be due to vasodilatory effect of estrogen and the secretory phase vascularity can be attributed to serum progesterone levels. Blood flow in the uterine vascular bed can be correlated to the estrogen/progesterone ratio.[17]

Uterine artery usually shows a moderate- to high-resistance flow and shows variations in resistance according to phase of the cycle, but is also affected by age. The RI of the uterine artery flow is 0.88 ± 0.04 till day 13 of the 28-day menstrual cycle.[18] It is due to postovulatory drop in serum estradiol concentration that leads to increased resistance in uterine artery, 3 days after LH peak with highest resistance on day 16.[19,20] The uterine artery resistance then falls and reaches its lowest during the peak luteal function. Persistently, low RI of uterine artery is maintained in the luteal phase till menstruation.

Though in anovulatory cycles, this fall is not seen and there is persistent rise in the uterine artery RI.[18] Blood flow to the endometrium, which is by spiral arteries, follows the similar pattern as the uterine arteries but shows a lower resistance and lower velocity than the uterine arteries.[21]

MONITORING OF STIMULATED CYCLES

The purpose of monitoring in stimulated cycles:

- To evaluate ovarian response to stimulation in terms of the number and size of ovarian follicles:
  - To identify exaggerated response
  - To identify poor response
- To decide the correct time of ovulation trigger and intrauterine insemination (IUI) or ovum pick up.
- To evaluate the luteal phase to look back and analyze if the proliferative phase was managed optimally or not

The aforementioned aims for monitoring the stimulated cycle can only be achieved in the light of the changes occurring in the natural cycle.

Early Proliferative Scan

The ovarian response can be assessed by a baseline or an early proliferative scan. Ovary is quiescent at this stage and so only antral follicles are visualized on this scan in the ovaries. It should be done on days 2–4 of the cycle. Number of antral follicles (antral follicle count: AFC) in the ovary on this scan decides the ovarian reserve and may therefore help to plan the stimulation protocol.

Number of antral follicles, measuring 2–10 mm in diameter, correlates well with the female's age, ovarian reserve, and ovarian response to gonadotropin stimulation.[22] Normal AFC in one ovary ranges from 5 to 10.

Antral follicle count less than 6 correlates well with reduced ovarian reserve and poor response to ovarian stimulation, with positive predictive value of 75%. Total AFC more than 21 could lead to the decision to adjust the gonadotropin dose in trying to prevent a hyper-response leading to ovarian hyperstimulation syndrome (OHSS).[23]

Ovarian volume is a poor predictor of number of oocytes obtained in an in vitro fertilization (IVF) cycle.[23] The mean ovarian diameter significantly correlated with age, day 3 FSH, day 3 LH, and day 3 estradiol.[24]

Commonly used morphological US markers for deciding the stimulation protocol are:[25]

- Antral follicle count
- Ovarian volume
- Mean ovarian diameter and size
- Ovarian stromal blood flow

Details of the assessment of ovarian reserve by AFC and ovarian volume have already been mentioned in Chapter 6.

Measurement of ovarian stromal flow in early follicular phase is related to subsequent ovarian response in IVF treatment.[26] Ovarian stromal PSV after pituitary suppression may be predictive of ovarian responsiveness and outcome of IVF treatment.[27] Even the three-dimensional (3D) power Doppler studies have shown correlation between the ovarian stromal blood flow and the ovarian response. Merce et al. have demonstrated that vascularization index (VI), flow index (FI), and vascularization flow index (VFI) of the ovary were significantly related to ovarian response to stimulation.[28] Vascularization index, FI, and VFI are 3D power Doppler indices used for quantitative assessment of 3D vascularity. (1) The VI, which represents the ratio of power Doppler information within the total dataset relative to both color and gray information; (2) the FI, which is proportional to the power Doppler signal intensity; and (3) the VFI, which reflects a combination of the two.

Therefore, Doppler of ovaries on baseline scan can be helpful to decide stimulation protocol. Undetectable basal ovarian stromal blood flow in at least one ovary is related to low ovarian response in infertile women undergoing IVF-embryo transfer (ET).[29] Ovarian stromal PSV was the most important single independent predictor of ovarian response in patients with normal basal serum FSH level. Patients with PSV more than or equal to 10 cm/s had significantly higher median number of mature oocytes and higher clinical pregnancy rates. Ovarian stromal blood flow velocity after 2–3 weeks of pituitary suppression is a true representative of baseline ovarian blood flow and predictive of ovarian responsiveness and outcome of IVF treatment.[27]

Preovulatory Scan

Maturation of follicle and endometrium, ovulation and luteinization is a process of multiple biochemical, morphological, and vascular changes. Vascular changes may therefore reflect the hormonal changes and combining Doppler to B-mode scans may help to understand the hormonal changes occurring during the menstrual cycle in response to stimulation. Three-dimensional US has an advantage of providing follicular and endometrial volume readily, than two-dimensional (2D) US and 3D power Doppler give quantitative idea of global vascularity rather than just information on velocity flow of an individual vessel.

B-Mode Features of a Mature Follicle

The follicular diameter is measured when the follicle is seen as a rounded structure on US image. Single diameter measurement in this case may be considered adequate for practical purposes. However, for optimal assessment of the size of the follicle, it is scanned to find the longest diameter and this image is stored as one of the dual frame images. Probe is then rotated 90° to achieve the transverse section of the follicle. On the long section, the longest diameter is measured. The second measurement taken is the largest diameter perpendicular to the longest diameter and the third measurement is taken on the transverse image as side-to-side or transverse diameter. The mean of these three is the mean diameter of the follicle (Figs. 9.7A to C). The follicle shape may become ellipsoid, if pressure is applied by the transvaginal probe on the follicle, and therefore scans should be done with only optimum pressure applied by the probe. When there is multifollicular development, shape of follicles changes from round to polygonal, due to pressure effect from adjacent follicles. In such follicles, the follicular volume assessment may be more reliable instead of a single diameter. Follicle volume can be calculated from the three diameters that have been measured earlier, but assessment of the ovarian volume by 3D US and Virtual Organ Computer-Aided Analysis (VOCAL) software is more accurate.

A mature follicle is 17–18 mm (Fig. 9.1A). A follicular size of 17–18 mm is for gonadotropin stimulated cycle, whereas for clomiphene citrate (CC) stimulated cycles minimum size of 18–20 mm is considered to be the size for

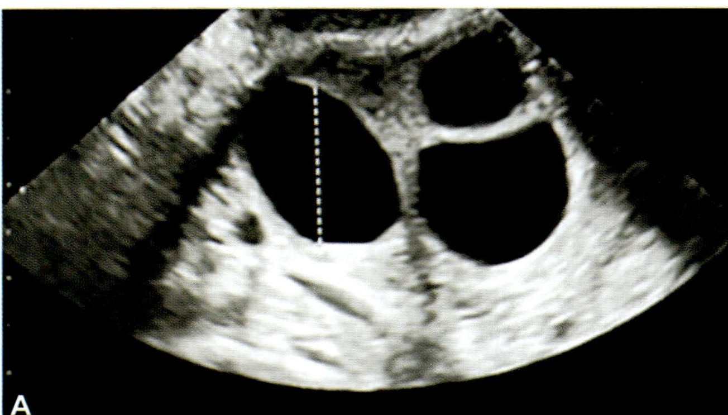

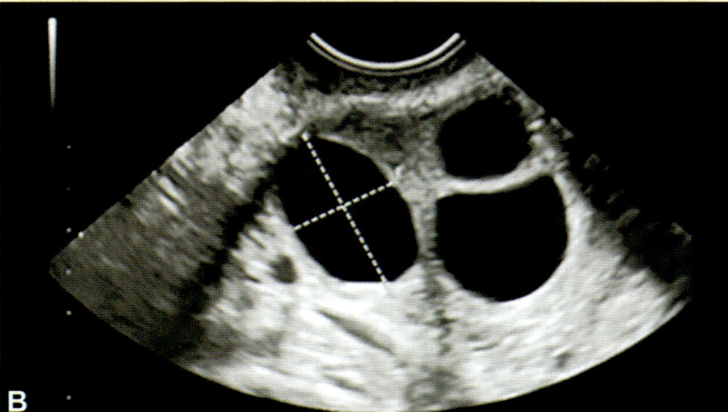

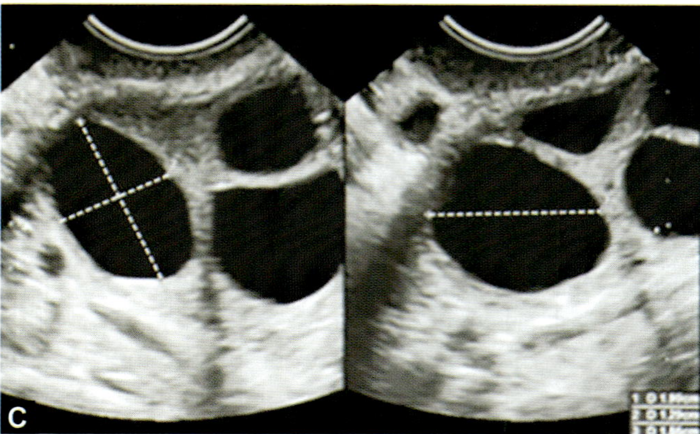

Figs. 9.7A to C: Measurement of a preovulatory follicle: (A) Single oblique diameter; (B) two diameters, (B) longitudinal and transverse, and (C) three diameters, longitudinal, two transverse diameters.

a mature follicle.[29] Though at times in CC cycles the follicle may reach physiological maturity till the diameter of 24 mm. A good-quality follicle has thin walls, regular round shape, and no echogenicity in the lumen. A thin hypoechoic halo surrounding the follicle and cumulus-like shadow (a tiny solid projection from the follicular wall) in the follicle appears approximately 36 hours before rupture. A flimsy irregular line is seen inside the follicle parallel to the wall about 6–10 hours before rupture (Fig. 9.1B).[30]

Doppler Features of a Mature Pre-hCG Follicle

Perifollicular vascularity of dominant follicle starts developing as early as eighth day of the cycle. Fall in perifollicular RI starts 2 days before ovulation, reaches nadir at ovulation, remains low for 4 days, and then with gradual rise reaches a peak in mid-luteal phase.[5] When mature, on color Doppler, the follicle shows blood vessels covering at least three-fourth of the follicular circumference (Fig. 9.8). Chui et al. graded the follicular flow on the day of oocyte collection as grade 1–4 when in a single cross area slice the flow covered less than 25%, 25–50%, 50–75%, and more than 75% of follicular circumference, respectively. The conception was related to grade 3–4 vascularity.[31]

On pulse Doppler, these blood vessels show an RI of 0.4–0.48[5] and PSV of more than 10 cm/s (Fig. 9.9). Vascular changes at the time of impending ovulation include increased vascularity of the inner wall of the follicle and a coincident surge in blood velocity just prior to erruption. A marked increase in the PSV around the follicle, in the presence of a relatively constant PI, could be a sign of follicle maturity and impending ovulation.[32,33]

Implications of Flow Parameters on Ovum Quality

Perifollicular vascularity correlates well with oocyte recovery rates and hence may be useful in determining the most appropriate time to administer human chorionic gonadotropin (hCG) to optimize recovery rate. Oocytes from

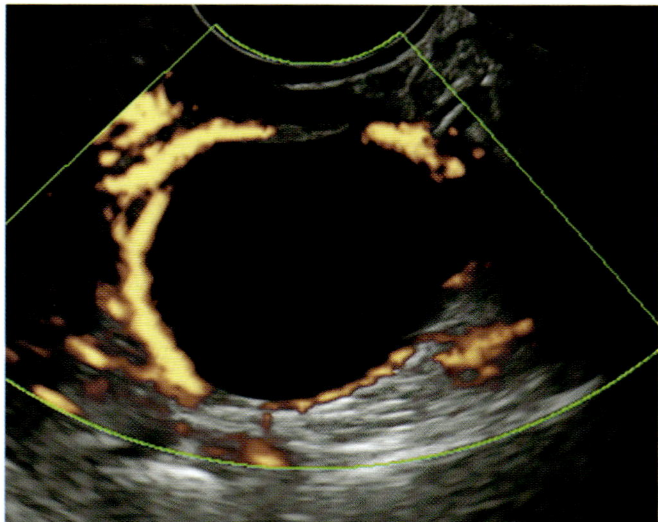

Fig. 9.8: Preovulatory follicle with vascular ring surrounding the follicle.

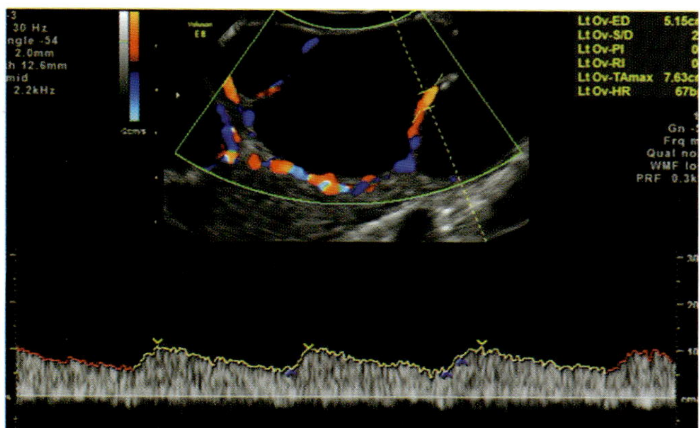

Fig. 9.9: Preovulatory follicle with pulse Doppler showing low-resistance flow.

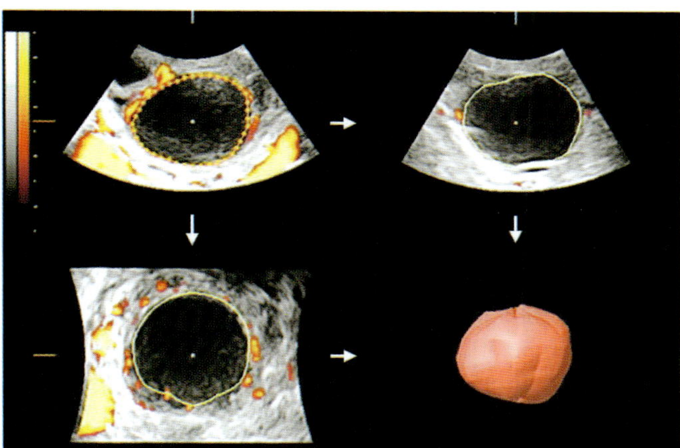

Fig. 9.11: Three-dimensional model of a follicle generated using VOCAL software, which is utilized for manual delineation of ovarian follicle at different desired angle to 180° and this gives follicular volume.

severely hypoxic follicles are associated with high frequency of abnormalities of organization of chromosomes on metaphase spindle and may lead to segregation disorders and catastrophic mosaics in embryo.[34]

Higher RI indicates higher resistance flow to the follicle meaning lower flow during diastolic phase and so reduced phasic oxygen supply to the ovum. Lower PSV again indicates lower blood supply and hence ovum hypoxia. It has been quoted in a study by Nargund et al.[35,36] that embryos produced by fertilization of the ova obtained from the follicles, which had a perifollicular PSV of less than 10 cm/s, are less likely to be grade 1 embryos and also have higher chance of chromosomal malformations. In the same study, it has been shown that the probability of developing a grade 1 or 2 embryo is 75% if PSV was more than 10 cm/s,

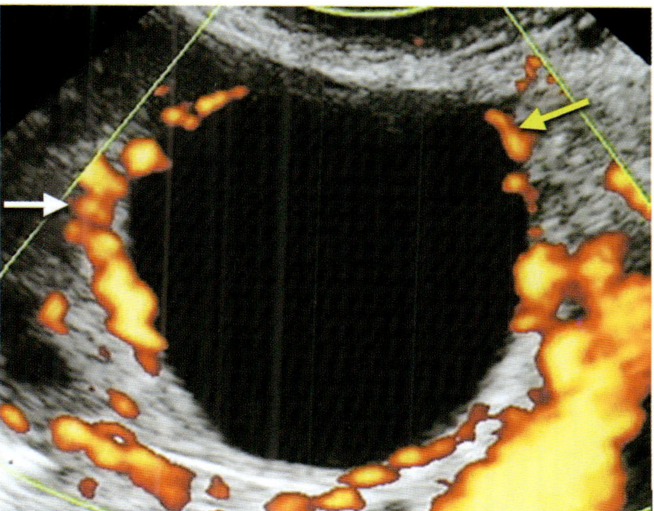

Fig. 9.10: True perifollicular vessel (yellow arrow), not a perifollicular vessel (white arrow).

40% if PSV was less than 10 cm/s, and 24% if there was no perifollicular flow.

Our unpublished data of more than 3,000 IUI cycles has shown that when the perifollicular RI more than 0.53 and PSV less than 9 cm/s, 12 hours before hCG injection, the conception rates were only 8.3% and 10%, respectively, as compared to 32.8% and 28.2%, respectively, and individually when perifollicular RI less than 0.50 and PSV more than 11 cm/s. We have therefore always preferred to wait with no extra medication when patient is on CC stimulation or continue with the same dose of gonadotropin till we get desired perifollicular RI and PSV, though sometimes the follicular size may reach up to 22 mm. Almost 90% of the time, the desired RI and PSV are reached by the time follicular size is 22 mm maximum.

When evaluating perifollicular vascularity, the pulse repetition frequency (PRF) settings for color Doppler are set at 0.3 and wall filter at the lowest (30 MHz). The perifollicular vessels are only those that obscure the follicular wall with color. If the follicular wall is seen and the vessel is seen just beside it, it is probably not considered a perifollicular vessel (Fig. 9.10).

Volume Ultrasound Parameters of Mature Pre-hCG Follicle

On 3D, the follicular volume of 3–7.5 cc has been found to be optimum for a mature follicle[37] (Fig. 9.11). It has been shown that in IVF-ET cycles, follicles with mean follicular

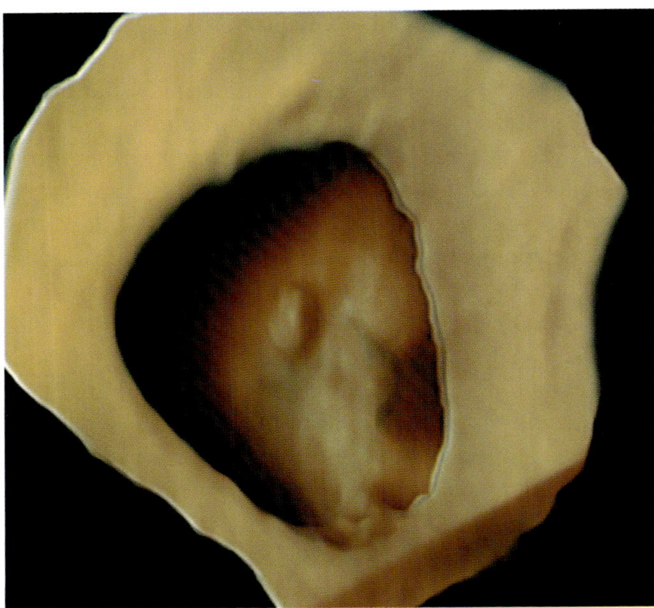

Fig. 9.12: Cumulus oophorus in preovulatory follicle on a 3D model of a preovulatory follicle.

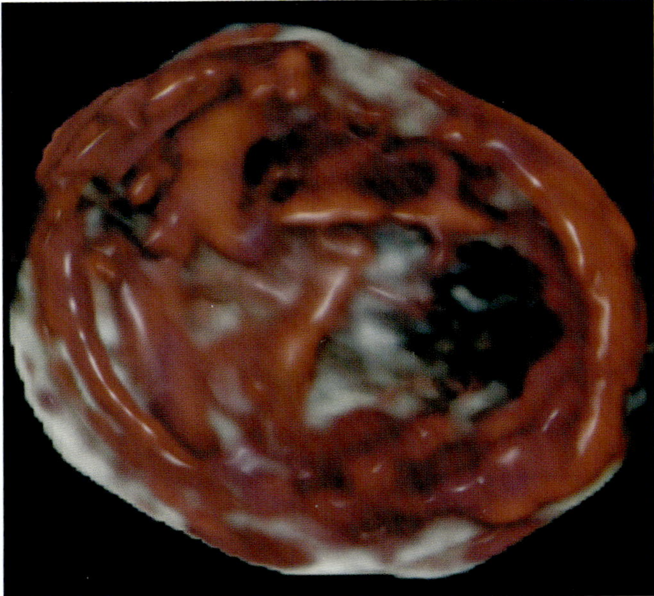

Fig. 9.13: Power Doppler angiography of a preovulatory follicle demonstrating a uniform and distinctive perifollicular vascularity.

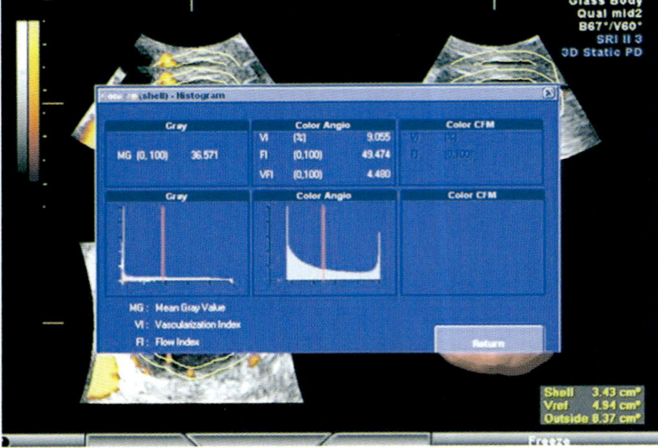

Fig. 9.14: Histogram for perifollicular flow giving values of 3D vascular indices, vascular index (VI), flow index (FI), and vascular flow index (VFI).

diameter of 12–24 mm is associated with optimal rates of oocyte recovery, fertilization, and cleavage.[36] This corresponds to the follicular volumes of between 1 and 7 mL. The accuracy of 3D US measurement of follicular volume was better when compared to the standard 2D techniques by comparing the volume of aspirates from individual follicles with the limits of agreement between aspirates and calculated volume was +3.47 to –2.42 for 2D measurements as compared to +0.96 to –0.43 when calculated by 3D US using VOCAL.[38] However, the follicles of less than 10 mm in diameter cannot be assessed accurately by 3D US as the limits of agreement are too wide in this range.

Feichtinger et al. in their study have shown presence of cumulus in follicles more than 15 mm by 3D US.[39] Follicles without visualization of cumulus in all three planes are not likely to contain mature oocytes. Appearance of the intrafollicular cumulus-like structures by 3D US (Fig. 9.12) was correlated with the recovery rate of the mature oocytes.[40] A significant correlation was found between the number of detected cumuli and the number of retrieved oocytes ($P < 0.0001$), mature oocytes ($P < 0.0001$), and number of fertilized oocytes ($P < 0.0001$). We, in our unpublished data of 500 IUI cycles, have been able to identify the cumulus in 94.6% of cases in conception cycles and in 53% of nonconception cycles. It has been shown that follicular fluid concentration of leptin, a follicular angiogenesis-related factor is inversely related to the stromal blood FI.[41] It has also been suggested that the follicles containing oocytes capable to produce a pregnancy have a perifollicular vascular network more uniform and distinctive[42] (Fig. 9.13).

Quantification of power Doppler information within a 3D model of an ovarian follicle (Fig. 9.11) can be performed using the “histogram facility” (Fig. 9.14).

In our study,[37] we have found perifollicular VI of between 6 and 20 and perifollicular FI more than 35 as most optimum. Around 68.4% of patients conceived when the VI was between 6 and 18 and 50% when it was between

18 and 20. However, the pregnancy rates were less than 25% when VI was less than 6 and only 7.4% when VI was more than 20. Only 7.4% of patients with FI less than 27 conceived whereas with FI beyond 27, the conception rates rose consistently. It was 50% with FI between 27 and 35, 70% when FI was between 35 and 43, and almost all patients had conceived when FI was more than.[42] A study by Kupesic and Kurjak reported that when the ratio of follicular volume to blood flow index (FV/FI) were 0.4, 0.4–0.6, and 0.6, the pregnancy rates were 21%, 39%, and 52%, respectively.[43]

The above data from different studies indicate that even when the follicle appeared mature according to the 2D US and color and pulse Doppler parameters, the pregnancy rates were significantly better, when the follicular volume was between 3 and 7.5 cc, cumulus was present and the perifollicular VI and FI values were optimum as mentioned earlier. Although it is possible to assess the follicular flow as expressed by the PSV and perifollicular color map,[44] 3D power Doppler provides a more detailed quantitative information about the ovarian vascularization and perifollicular blood flow.[45]

Another 3D US-based software, SonoAVC (Automatic Volume Calculation; GE Medical Systems), has been used to provide automated measurements of follicle size from the stored 3D datasets (Fig. 9.15). SonoAVC is a software program designed to provide automatic volume calculations of fluid-filled areas. It is either incorporated into the US machine or installed on a personal computer for offline analysis of the datasets acquired by any US machine of the same manufacturer. SonoAVC identifies and quantifies anechoic areas within a 3D dataset and provides automatic estimation of their absolute dimensions, mean diameter, and volume. While this technique has been proven to be more reproducible and valid in measuring follicular diameter and volume than conventional 2D US method and may have implications for improving the work flow within an IVF center,[46] timing final follicle maturation and oocyte retrieval on the basis of such automated measures do not appear to improve the clinical outcome of assisted reproductive technology (ART).[47]

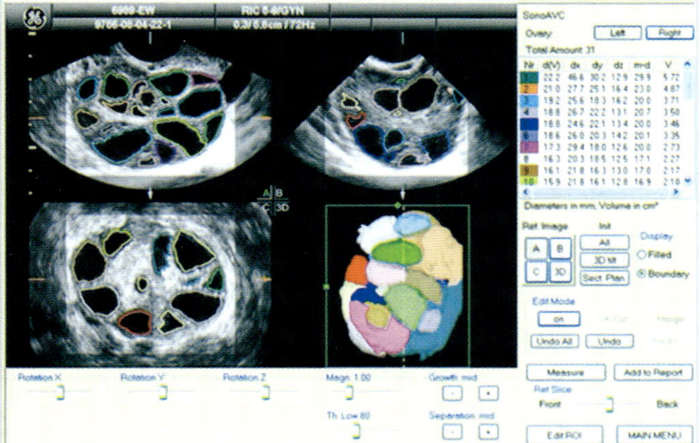

Fig. 9.15: Three-dimensional ultrasound imaging using SonoAVC software within a stimulated ovary during IVF treatment. The color-coded follicles are visible. The number of follicles and their individual measurements are seen on the output box seen on the right-hand side.

Endometrial Evaluation

Implantation has been the weakest link in the success of infertility treatment. Endometrium is a receptor organ for majority of the hormones involved in fertility and therefore study of its morphology and vascularity is thought to explain the mysteries of implantation failure. Ultrasound assessment of the endometrium is important in the analysis of factors that affect embryo implantation.

B-Mode Features of Endometrium with Good Receptivity

Endometrial growth does not differ significantly in stimulated and nonstimulated cycles. However, in CC stimulated cycle, the endometrial thickness may be less in the days immediately after CC is taken because of its antiestrogenic effect. However, during late proliferative phase, endometrial thickness increases at a faster rate than in spontaneous cycles as it escapes from the antiestrogenic effect and effect of increased estrogen due to multifollicular growth. However in gonadotropin-stimulated cycles the endometrial thickness is greater than in spontaneous cycles.[48] On TVS, an endometrial thickness of 6 mm is considered minimum that is required on the day of ovulation or on the day of hCG trigger for a successful outcome, although 8 mm is generally considered optimum.[49] Even when pregnancy occurs with endometrial thickness of 6–8 mm on the day of hCG, the rates of preclinical miscarriage (biochemical pregnancy) and clinical miscarriage were 21.9% and 15.6%, respectively, as compared to 0% and 12.9%, respectively, when endometrial thickness was more than 8 mm.[50] Endometrial thickness has more negative predictive value for implantation.[51] In healthy endometrium, the endometrial-myometrial interface is always seen as a clear hypoechoic halo surrounding the whole endometrium (Figs. 9.16A and B). Breach or irregularity of

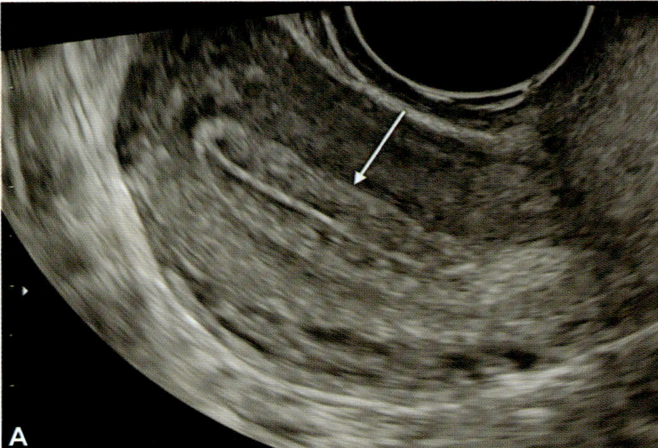

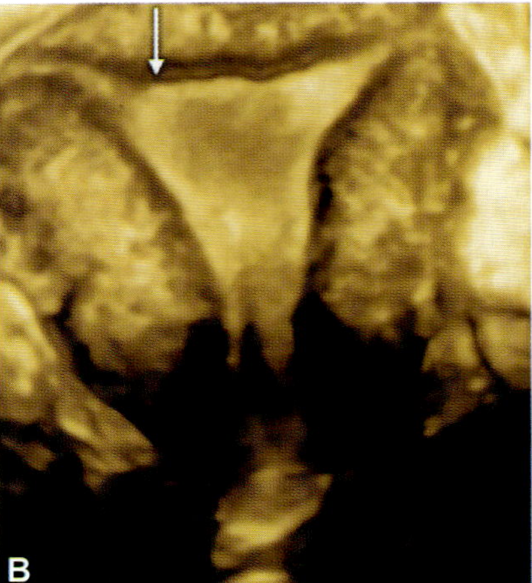

Figs. 9.16A and B: Endometrial-myometrial junction on B mode and 3D US.

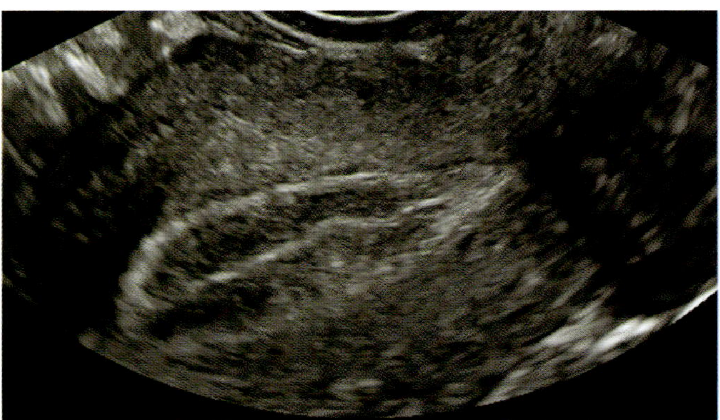

Fig. 9.17: Grade A multilayered endometrium with echogenicity of intervening area is similar to that of myometrium.

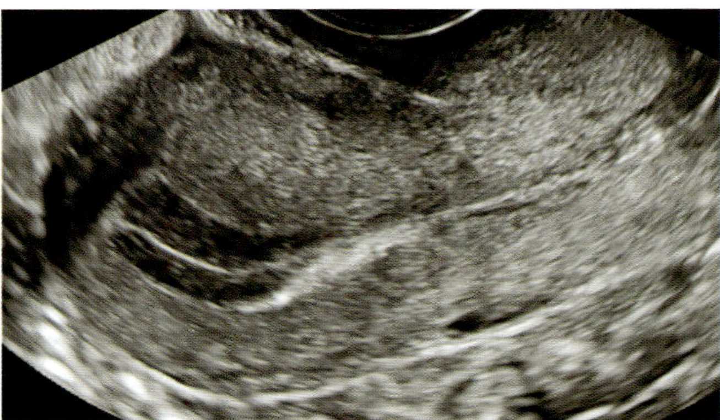

Fig. 9.18: Multilayered endometrium grade B—intermediate.

endometrial-myometrial junction may be an indication of unhealthy endometrium and therefore poor receptivity.

Morphology of the endometrium is as important as thickness of the endometrium. Popularly, multilayered endometrium is considered a desired endometrial pattern. Morphologically, the endometrium is graded as the best, grade A, when it is a triple-line endometrium with the intervening area as hypoechoic as the anterior myometrium. The echogenicity is attributed to the development of multiple vessels penetrating in the endometrium producing multiple tissue interfaces and due to glycogen storage in the endometrial columnar epithelium (Fig. 9.17). It may also be because of secretions in endometrial glands and scarce stromal edema.[52]

The endometrium is graded as intermediate or grade B (Fig. 9.18), when it is multilayered or triple line with anechoic intervening area. In grade C, the endometrium would be a homogenous isoechoic (to myometrium) endometrium[53] (Fig. 9.19). Actually as the estradiol level starts increasing, the single-line endometrium becomes multilayered and develops into grade B endometrium, with further increase in the estradiol levels it converts into grade A and with supraphysiological levels of estradiol it becomes grade C. Grade C endometrium therefore is commonly seen in patients with polycystic ovarian syndrome (PCOS) or with multifollicular development.

Doppler Features of Receptive Endometrium

There are several reports by different groups[54] that agree on the fact that implantation rates can be more correlated to the vascularity of the endometrium than the thickness and morphology of the endometrium. Segmental uterine artery perfusion demonstrates significant correlation with

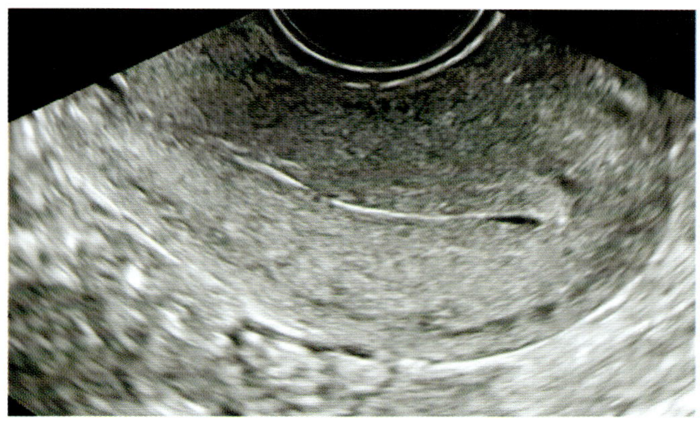

Fig. 9.19: Isoechoic homogenous grade C—endometrium.

hormonal and histological markers of uterine receptivity, reaching the highest sensitivity for subendometrial blood flow.[43] But the endometrial neoangiogenesis differ in natural and stimulated cycles. There may be 35% decrease in endometrial and subendometrial vascularity in stimulated cycles as compared to natural cycles.[55] However, it is important to mention here that in spite of this fact, in stimulated cycles, the stimulation needs to be designed and continued till the endometrium shows sufficient vascularity.

On color Doppler, the endometrium that has vascularity in zones 3 and 4 or in subendometrial and endometrial layers (Fig. 9.20) has been reported to have a high degree of endometrial receptivity. Endometrial vascularity has been divided into four zones for the convenience of description and semiquantitative assessment by Applebaum.[56] These are described as follows:

- Zone 1: When the vascularity on power Doppler is seen only at endometrial-myometrial junction
- Zone 2: When vessels penetrate up to the hyperechogenic endometrial edge
- Zone 3: When vessels reach the intervening hypoechogenic zone
- Zone 4: When vessels reach the endometrial cavity—the central line

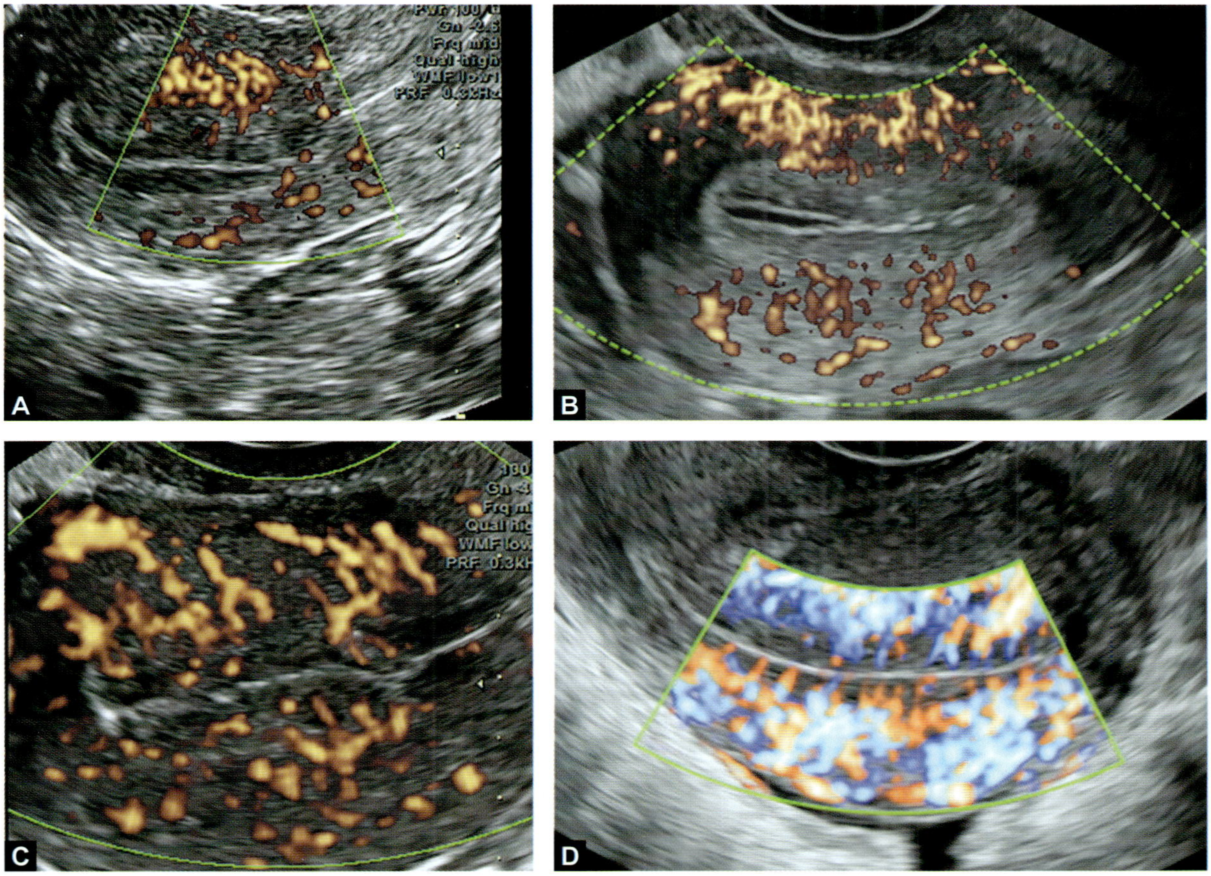

Figs. 9.20A to D: Endometrial vascularity zones (zones 1–4).

The pregnancy rates related to the zones of vascular penetration during IVF were 26.7% for zone 1, 36.4% for zone 2, and 37.9% for zone 3.[56] Another comparative study has also shown similar results[57] with pregnancy rates for zone 1, zone 2, zone 3, and zone 4 were 5.2%, 28.7%, 52%, and 74%, respectively.

Zaidi et al. found that absence of flow in the endometrial and subendometrial zones on day of hCG indicates minimal chance for a successful implantation.[54] In our study, we have found only 19% pregnancy rates for zone 1 and 21.87% for zone 2 vascularity. The conception rates with zones 3 and 4, the pregnancy rates were comparable and were 39.77% and 70.14%, respectively. A very interesting finding in this study was also that the abortion rates also were 50% and 23.8%, respectively with vascularity in zone 1 and zone 2, but were as low as 5.6% and 1.5% when the vascularity was present in zone 3 and zone 4, respectively.[58]

While the reported correlation between vascularity in the endometrium and subendometrium and pregnancy rates is controversial, it has been concluded in two studies that no difference was found in patients with good prognosis for cycle outcome, but in patients with poor embryo quality, better endometrial vascularity seemed to improve the cycle outcome.[59,60] The vessels that reach the endometrium covering at least 5 mm^2 area of the endometrium are reported to be good prognostic factors.[61] The pulse Doppler of these arteries indicating RI of less than 0.6 and PI of between 1.1 and 2.3 has also been reported to be good prognostic factor[62] (Fig. 9.21).

Uterine Artery Doppler

Pulse Doppler analysis of the uterine artery waveform is also reported to be predictive of endometrial receptivity with its PI less than 3.2 being desirable (Fig. 9.22). Several authors have shown that the optimum uterine receptivity was obtained when average PI of the uterine artery was between 2 and 3 on the day of hCG.[63,64] Coulam et al. and Cacciatore et al. have also reported that no pregnancy was achieved after ET when uterine artery PI was above 3.3 in an IVF program.[65,66] Tsai and colleagues[67] evaluated the prognostic value of uterine perfusion on day of hCG for IUI cycles and showed that no pregnancy occurred when the PI of ascending branch of uterine artery was more than 3. Fecundity rate was 18% when PI was less than 2 and 19.8% when PI was between 2 and 3. In our study, we have found no conceptions when uterine artery PI more than 3.5 on the day of hCG.[68]

The hypothesis is that the high-resistance blood flow in the uterine artery may lead to higher-resistance flow in endometrial vessels and inadequate endometrial oxygenation and causes low implantation rates.

3D and 3D Power Doppler Features of Food Endometrial Receptivity

The correlation of IVF outcome with 3D US volume of the endometrium (Fig. 9. 23) has been reported to be better than with endometrial thickness.[37] It has been reported that pregnancy and implantation rates were significantly lower when endometrial volume was 1–2 mL.[62,69] In a study of IVF population by our group, no pregnancy was observed in the group with endometrial volume of less than 2 on the day of hCG ovulation trigger.[37] The pregnancy rates were 16.7%, 47%, and 62%, respectively when the endometrial volume was 2–3, 3–5, and 5–7 cc, respectively.

While there is no consensus regarding the role of 3D power Doppler indices (Figs. 9.24 and 9.25) in predicting

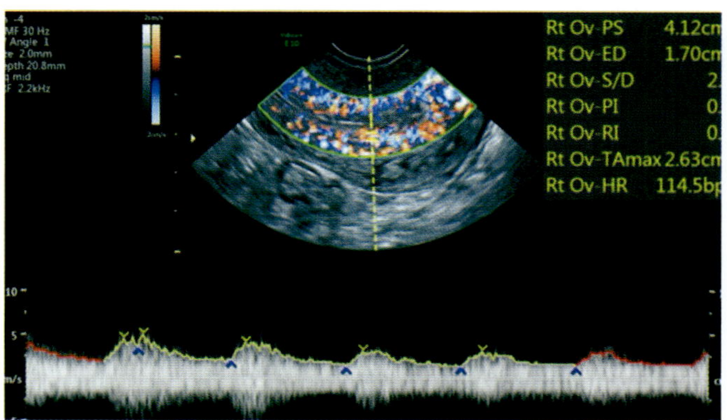

Fig. 9.21: Pulse Doppler of endometrial vascularity.

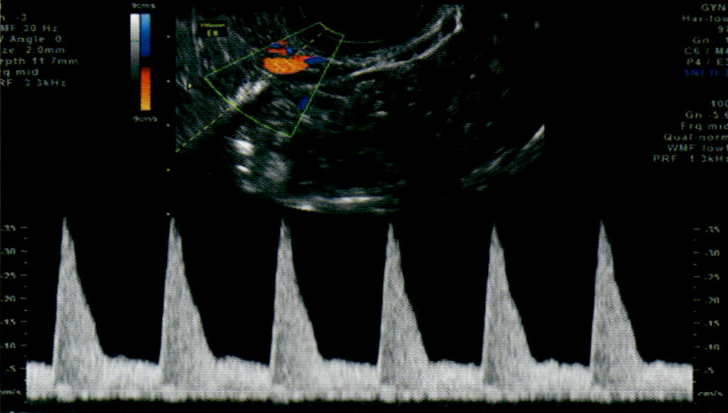

Fig. 9.22: Preovulatory uterine artery waveform.

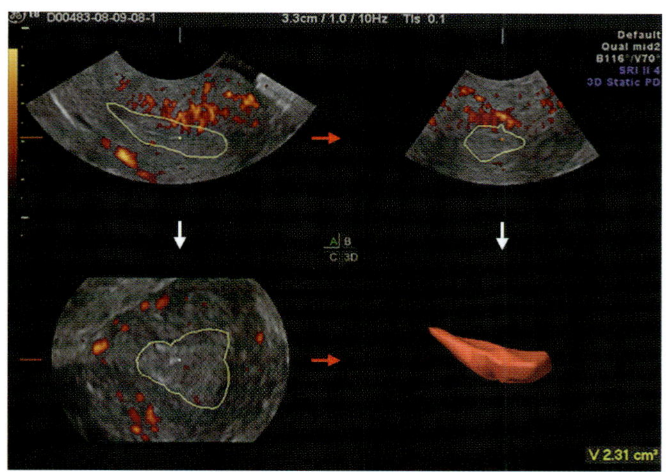

Fig. 9.23: Calculating endometrial volume by VOCAL software.

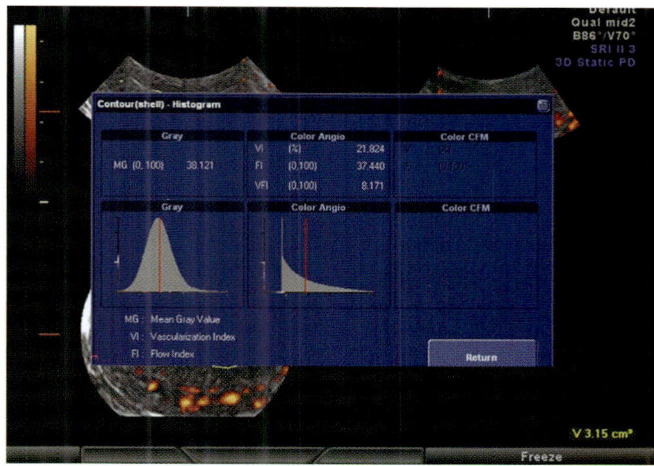

Fig. 9.24: Histogram of endometrium showing VI, FI, and VFI values.

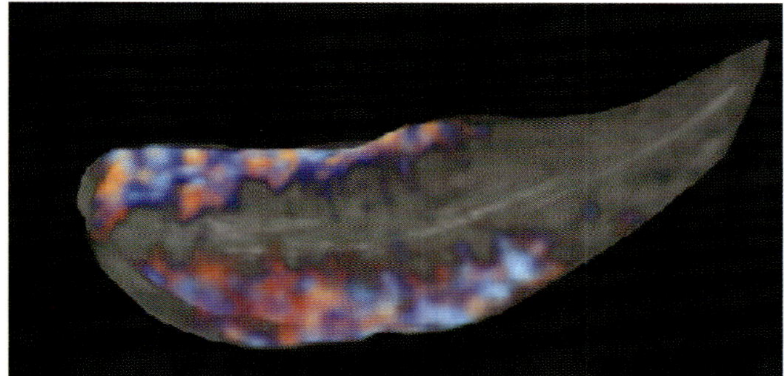

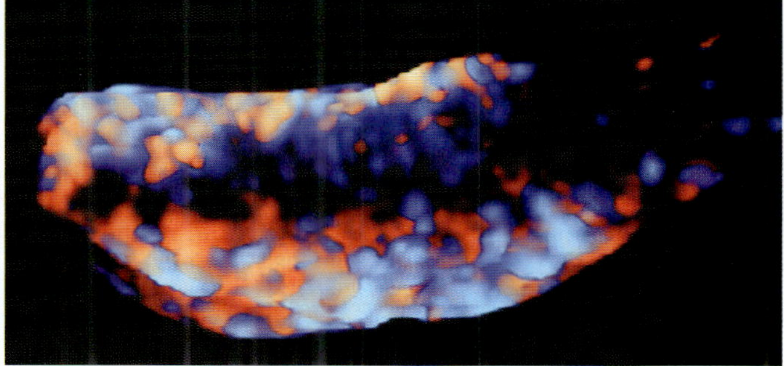

Fig. 9.25: Glass body mode of endometrial 3D power Doppler vascularity.

endometrial receptivity, a study by Kupesic et al.,[62] reported a subendometrial FI of less than 11 on the day of ET as a cut-off level for predicting poor implantation. No pregnancies occurred when FI was less than 11 and the conception group showed FI of 13.2 ± 2.2. Contrary to this, Ng et al.[70] reported a low endometrial VI and VFI in pregnant group on the day of oocyte retrieval and also a nonsignificant trend of higher implantation and pregnancy rates in patients with absent subendometrial and endometrial flow. This probably can be explained on the basis that hCG administration or LH peak causes increased uterine artery resistance and hence decrease in endometrial perfusion also on the day of oocyte retrieval. This also correlates with the observation made by Ng et al., which says that subendometrial vascularization flow indices are significantly lower in patients with uterine artery RI of 0.95 or more.[71] They concluded that number of embryos replaced and endometrial VFI were the only two predictive factors for pregnancy. Wu et al.[72] reported that endometrial VFI was more reliable than VI and FI, and best prediction rate was achieved by VFI cut-off value of more than 0.24. As there are conflicting reports, the routine application of 3D power Doppler indices for predicting endometrial receptivity in women undergoing ART currently is limited.

Three-dimensional or four-dimensional (4D) US allows visualization of coronal plane of uterus and has been recommended by some researchers to identify the point of maximum implantation potential (MIP) within the endometrium while performing ET.[73] Embryo transfers at the MIP were reported to be associated with good implantation and pregnancy rates. The MIP point is an intersection of two lines that are drawn parallel to both cornua on a mid-coronal section of uterus (Fig. 9.26). This was hypothesized as the MIP point, as this point of

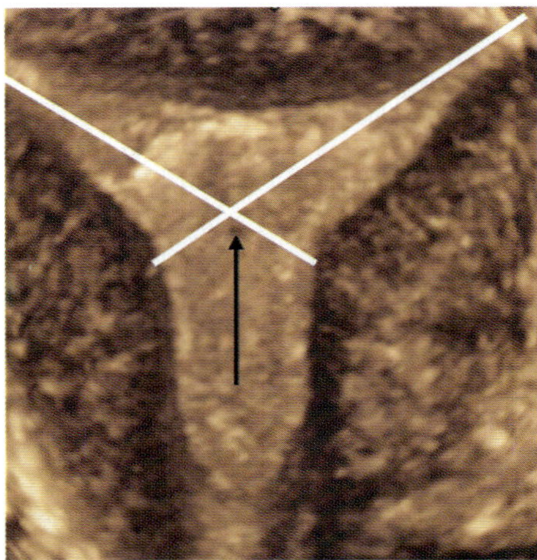

Fig. 9.26: Maximum implantation potential (MIP) point.

endometrium is in the trajectory line when the embryo falls into the uterus during the process of natural conception and is thought to be the thickest and having the greatest blood flow. Considering lack of universal availability of 3D US machine and limited evidence base on its advantage, 3D/4D US-guided ET cannot be recommended for routine use.

Uterine Contractions

The uterus demonstrates periodic contractile activity that varies throughout the menstrual cycle. The contractions increase in frequency throughout the follicular phase to peak at four to five contractions per minute in the late follicular phase before reducing in frequency during the transition to luteal phase when the uterus essentially becomes quiescent. This pattern of contraction frequency has been suggested as being sex steroid dependent in that it parallels the rise in serum estradiol and the subsequent postovulatory increase in progesterone. Initial studies used intrauterine pressure transducers but due to the invasiveness of this approach and its potential to induce myometrial activity assessment have largely been superseded by the digital storage and subsequent fast-forward, play-back of video recordings of transvaginal US examinations.

The exact physiological benefit of such uterine activity is unknown but the propagation of contractions from the cervix toward the fundus during the periovulatory period may favor the passage of spermatozoa through the uterus to the Fallopian tubes. The relative quiescence during the luteal phase is more readily understandable and has been shown to occur during ART 7 days following the administration of hCG at the time of blastocyst transfer.[74] A contraction frequency of more than five per minute on the day of ET is associated with a very low implantation rate in comparison to one of three or less per minute (4% vs 21%, respectively). Further studies have confirmed this negative association of symmetrical contractions with the chances of pregnancy following assisted reproduction.[75] Early administration of vaginal progesterone decreases the contraction frequency at the time of embryo transfer but this has yet to be shown to significantly increase the conception rates[76-78] and may result in premature luteinization if given too early.

CONCLUSION

Ultrasound is an excellent tool for cycle monitoring. Doppler helps to understand the hormonal changes occurring during the cycle. Volume assessments both for follicle and the endometrium are much more reliable parameter than follicular diameter or endometrial thickness. The presence of cumulus, can be confirmed by 3D US, increases the surety of the presence of a mature ovum in the follicle. The 3D power Doppler gives idea about the global vascularity of follicle and endometrium. Though larger studies and standardization of US parameters and settings are required to establish more precise values for follicular and endometrial VI, FI, and VFI, the results are fairly promising. We can hope to understand the follicular and endometrial physiological status better with these parameters and achieve better pregnancy rates with ART procedures and reduce the span of unexplained infertility.

KEY POINTS

- Follicular tracking describes the serial ultrasonographic study of the ovary during the follicular phase of the menstrual cycle
- Monitoring of a menstrual cycle should ideally start in early proliferative phase
- A normal growth rate of a healthy follicle is approximately 2 mm/day and reaches a size of 18–24 mm by the time of ovulation
- Corpus luteum typically has variable appearances with ground glass echogenicity in lumen or lace-like echogenicities and has circumferential blood flow referred to as a "ring of fire"

- Follicular tracking is important during controlled ovarian stimulation as it is used as part of IVF treatment when multifollicular recruitment is desired
- SonoAVC has been used to provide automated measures of follicle size and may have implications for the work flow within IVF centers
- Commonly used markers of endometrial receptivity include endometrial thickness and endometrial pattern
- Conception is unlikely in association with an endometrial thickness of 5 mm or less, although most centers would prefer to see it measure 8 mm or more prior to ET
- While a trilaminar pattern is more frequently associated with conception, a homogenous, hyperechogenic endometrium lacking an echogenic central line has been shown to be associated with nonconception both in natural and ART cycles
- The 3D power Doppler gives idea about the global vascularity of follicle and endometrium

REFERENCES

1. Kyei-Mensah A, Zaidi J, Pittrof R, et al. Transvaginal three dimensional ultrasound: accuracy of follicular volume measurements. Fertil Steril. 1996;65:371-6.
2. Hackeloer BJ, Sallam HN. Ultrasound scanning of ovarian follicles. Clin Obstet Gynecol. 1983;10:603-20.
3. Hackelöer BJ, Fleming R, Robinson HP, et al. Correlation of ultrasonic and endocrinological assessment of human follicular development. Am J Obstet Gynecol. 1979;135(1):122-8.
4. Bald R, Hackeloer BJ. Ultraschall-darstellung verschiendener. endometriumformen. In: Otto R, Jan FX (Eds). Ultraschalldiagnostik 1982. Stuttgart: Thieme; 1983. p. 187.
5. Kurjak A, Kupesic-Urek S. Infertility. In: Kurjak A (Ed). Transvaginal Color Doppler. Carnforth, UK: Parthenon Publishing; 1991. pp. 33-8.
6. Bourne T, Jurkovic D, Waterstone J, et al. Intrafollicular blood flow during human ovulation. Ultrasound Obstet Gynecol. 1991;1(1):53-9.
7. Bourne TH, Athanasiou S, Bauer B. Ovulation and the periovulatory follicle. In: Bourne TH, Jauniaux E, Jurkovic D (Eds). Transvaginal Colour Doppler. Berlin: Springer-Verlag; 1995. pp. 119-30.
8. Niswender GD, Moore RT, Akbar AM, et al. Flow of blood to the ovaries of ewes throughout the oestrous cycle. Biol Reprod. 1975;13:381-8.
9. Glock JL, Brumsted JR. Colour flow pulsed Doppler ultrasound in diagnosing luteal phase defect. Fertil Steril. 1995;64:500-4.
10. Kupesic S, Kurjak A. The assessment of normal and abnormal luteal function by transvaginal colour Doppler sonography. Eur J Obstet Gynecol. 1997;72:83-7.
11. Salim A, Kurjak A, Zalud I. Ovarian luteal flow in normal and abnormal early pregnancies. J Matern Fetal Invest. 1992;2:119-24.
12. Bakos O, Lundkvist O, Bergh T. Transvaginal sonographic evaluation of endometrial growth and texture in spontaneous ovulatory cycles—a descriptive study. Hum Reprod. 1993;8:799-806.
13. Kupesic S. The first three weeks assessed by transvaginal colour Doppler. J Perinat Med. 1996;24:301-17.
14. Ijland MM, Evers JLH, Dunselman GAJ, et al. Endometrial wavelike movements during menstrual cycle. Fertil Steril. 1996;65:746-9.
15. Randall JM, Fisk MM, McTavish A, et al. Transvaginal ultrasonic assessment of endometrial growth in spontaneous and hyperstimulated menstrual cycles. Br J Obstet Gynecol. 1989;96:954-9.
16. Rainne-Fenning NJ, Campbell BK, Kendall NR, et al. Quantifying the changes in endometrial vascularity throughout the normal menstrual cycle with three dimensional power Doppler angiography. Hum Reprod. 2004;19:330-8.
17. Killam AP, Rosenfeld C, Battaglia FC, et al. Effect of oestrogens on the uterine blood flow in oophorectomized ewes. Am J Obstet Gynecol. 1973:115;1045-50.
18. Kurjak A, Kupesic-Urek S, Schulman H, et al. Transvaginal colour Doppler in the assessment of ovarian and uterine blood flow in infertile women. Fertil Steril. 1991;56(5): 870-3.
19. Goswamy RK, Steptoe PC. Doppler ultrasound studies of the uterine artery in spontaneous ovarian cycles. Hum Reprod. 1988;3:721-5.
20. Sholtes MCW, Wladimiroff JW, van Rijen HJM, et al. Uterine and ovarian flow velocity waveforms in the normal menstrual cycle: a transvaginal study. Fertil Steril. 1989;52:981-5.
21. Andreotti RF, Thompson GH, Janowitz W, et al. Endovaginal and transabdominal sonography of ovarian follicle. J Ultrasound Med. 1989;8(10):555-60.
22. Scheffer GJ, Broekmans FJM, Looman CWN, et al. The number of antral follicles in normal women with proven fertility is best reflection of reproductive age. Hum Reprod. 2003;18:700-6.
23. Kwee J, Elting ME, Schats R, et al. Ovarian volume and antral follicle count for the prediction of low and hyper responders with in vitro fertilization. Reprod Biol Endocrinol. 2007;5:9.
24. Fratelli JL, Levi AJ, Miller BT. A prospective novel method of determining ovarian size during in vitro fertilization cycles. J Assist Reprod Genet. 2002;19(1):39-41.
25. Soldevila PN, Carreras O, Tur R, et al. Sonographic assessment of ovarian reserve. Its correlation with outcome of in vitro fertilization cycles. Gynecol Endocrinol. 2007;23(4):206-12.

26. Zaidi J, Barber J, Kyei-Mensah A, et al. Relationship of ovarian stromal blood flow at baseline ultrasound to subsequent follicular response in an in vitro fertilization program. Obstet Gynecol. 1996;88:779-84.
27. Engmann L, Sladkevicius P, Agrawal R, et al. Value of ovarian stromal blood flow velocity measurement after pituitary suppression in the prediction of ovarian responsiveness and outcome of in vitro fertilization treatment. Fertil Steril. 1999;71(1):22-9.
28. Merce LT, Barco MJ, Bau S, Troyano JM. Prediction of ovarian response and IVF/ICSI outcome by three-dimensional ultrasonography and power Doppler angiography. Eur J Obstet Gynecol Reprod Biol. 2007;132:93-100.
29. Younis JS, Haddad S, Matilsky M, Radin O, Ben-Ami M. Undetectable basal ovarian stromal blood flow in infertile women is related to low ovarian reserve. Gynecol Endocrinol 2007 May 23(5):284-9.
30. Hackeloer BJ, Fleming R, Robinson HP. Correlation of ultrasonic and endocrinological assessment of human follicular development. Am J Obstet Gynecol. 1979;135(1):122-8.
31. Kupesic S, Kurjak A. Uterine and ovarian perfusion during the periovulatory period assessed by transvaginal colour Doppler. Fertil Steril. 1993;3:439-43.
32. Van Blerkom J, Antezak M, Schrader R. The developmental potential of human oocyte is related to the dissolved oxygen content of follicular fluid: association with vascular endothelial growth factor levels and perifollicular blood flow characteristics. Hum Reprod. 1997;12(5):1047-55.
33. Lunenfeld E, Schwartz I, Meizner I, et al. Intra-ovarian blood flow during spontaneous and stimulated cycles. Hum Reprod. 1996;11(11):2481-3.
34. Nargund G, Doyle PE, Bourne TH, et al. Ultrasound-deviced indices of follicular blood flow before HCG administration and prediction of oocyte recovery and preimplantation embryo quality. Hum Reprod. 1996;11:2512-7.
35. Nargund G, Bourne TH, Doyle PE, et al. Association between ultrasound indices of follicular blood flow, oocyte recovery and preimplantation embryo quality. Hum Reprod. 1996;11:109-13.
36. Wittmack FM, Kreger DO, Blasco L, et al. Effect of follicular size on oocyte retrieval, fertilization, cleavage and embryo quality in in vitro fertilization cycles: a 6 year data collection. Fertil Steril. 1994;62:1205-10.
37. Panchal SY, Nagori CB. Can 3D PD be a better tool for assessing the pre HCG follicle and endometrium? A randomized study of 500 cases. Presented at 16th World Congress on Ultrasound in Obstetrics and Gynecology, 2006, London. J Ultrasound Obstet Gynecol. 2006;28(4):504.
38. Kyei-Mensah A, Zaidi J, Pittrof R, et al. Transvaginal three dimensional ultrasound reproducibility of ovarian and endometrial volume measurements. Fertil Steril. 1996;66:718-22.
39. Feichtinger W. Transvaginal three dimensional imaging for evaluation and treatment of infertility. In: Merz E (Ed). 3D Ultrasound in Obstetrics and Gyneacology. Philadelphia: Lipincott Williams & Wilkins; 1998. pp. 37-43.
40. Poehl M, Hohlagschwandtner M, Doerner V, et al. Cumulus assessment by three dimensional ultrasound for in vitro fertilization. Ultrasound Obstet Gynecol. 2000;16:251-3.
41. Wu MH, Tsai SJ, Pan HA, et al. Three dimensional power Doppler imaging of ovarian stromal blood flow in women with endometriosis undergoing in vitro fertilization. Ultrasound Obstet Gynecol. 2003;21:480-5.
42. Vlaisavljevic V, Reljic M, Gavric Lovrec V, et al. Measurement of perifollicular blood flow of the dominant preovulatory follicle using three dimensional power Doppler. Ultrasound Obstet Gynecol. 2003;22:520-6.
43. Kupesic S, Kurjak A. Prediction of IVF outcome by three dimensional ultrasound. Hum Reprod. 2002;17:950-5.
44. Merce LT. Ultrasound markers of implantation. Ultrasound Rev Obstet Gynecol. 2002;2:110-23.
45. Merce LT, Barco MJ, Kupesic S, et al. 2D and 3D power Doppler ultrasound from ovulation to implantation. In: Kurjak A, Chervenak F (Eds). Textbook of Perinatal Medicine. London: Parthenon Publishing; 2005.
46. Raine-Fenning N, Jayaprakasan K, Clewes J. Automated follicle tracking facilitates standardization and may improve work flow. Ultrasound Obstet Gynecol. 2007;30:1015-8.
47. Raine-Fenning N, Deb S, Jayaprakasan K, et al. Timing of oocyte maturation and egg collection during controlled ovarian stimulation: a randomized controlled trial evaluating manual and automated measurements of follicle diameter. Fertil Steril. 2009;94(1):184-8.
48. Yagel S, Ben-Chetrit A, Anteby E, et al. The effect of ethinyl oestradiol on endometrial thickness and uterine volume during ovulation induction by clomiphene citrate. Fertil Steril. 1992;57:33-6.
49. Dickey RP, Olar TT, Taylor SN, et al. Relationship of biochemical pregnancy to preovulatory endometrial thickness and pattern in patients undergoing ovulation induction. Hum Reprod. 1993;8;327-30.
50. Boue J, Boue A, Lazar P. Retrospective and prospective epidemiological studies of 1500 karyotyped spontaneous human abortions. Tetrology. 1973;12:11-26.
51. Weissman A, Gotlieb I, Casper RF. The detrimental effect of increased endometrial thickness on implantation and pregnancy rates and outcome in an in vitro fertilization program. Fertil Steril. 1999;71:147-9.
52. Fleischer AC, Keppe DM. Benign conditions of the uterus, cervix and endometrium. In Nyberg Am Hill LM, Bohm-Velez M, Mendelson EB eds. Transvaginal Ultrasound. St. Louis: Mosby Year Book 1992:21-43.
53. Smith B, Porter R, Ahuja K, et al. Ultrasonic assessment of endometrial changes in stimulated cycles in an in vitro fertilization and embryo transfer program. J In Vitro Fertil Embryo Transf. 1984;1(4):233-8.
54. Zaidi J, Campbell S, Pittrof R, et al. Endometrial thickness, morphology, vascular penetration and velocimetry in predicting implantation in an in vitro fertilization program. Ultrasound Obstet Gynecol. 1995;6:191-8.
55. Ng EH, Chan CC, Tang OS, et al. Comparison of endometrial and subendometrial blood flow measured by three dimensional power Doppler ultrasound between

stimulated and natural cycles in the same patients. Hum Reprod. 2004;19:2385-90.
56. Applebaum M. The 'steel' or 'teflon' endometrium—ultrasound visualization of endometrial vascularity in IVF patients and outcome. Presented at the Third World Congress of Ultrasound in Obstetrics and Gyneacolgy. Ultrasound Obstet Gynecol. 1993;3(Suppl 2):10.
57. Chein LW, Au HK, Chen PL, et al, Assessment of uterine receptivity by the endometrial-subendometrial blood flow distribution pattern in women undergoing IVF-ET. Fertil Steril. 2002;78:245-51.
58. Nagori C, Panchal S. Endometrial vascularity: its relation to implantation rates. IJIFM. 2012;3(2):48-50.
59. Merce LT, Barco MJ, Bau S, et al. Prediction of ovarian response and IVF/ICSI outcome by three dimensional ultrasonography and power Doppler angiography. Eur J Obstet Gynecol Reprod Biol. 2007;132:93-100.
60. Merce LT, Barco MJ, Bau S, et al. Are endometrial parameters by three-dimensional ultrasound and power Doppler angiography related to in vitro fertilization/embryo transfer outcome? Fertil Steril. 2008;89(1):111-7.
61. Yang JH, Wu MY, Chen CD, et al. Association of endometrial blood flow as determined by modified colour Doppler technique with subsequent outcome of in vitro fertilization. Hum Reprod. 1999;14:1606-10.
62. Kupesic S, Bekavac I, Bjelos D, et al. Assessment of endometrial receptivity by transvaginal colour Doppler and three dimensional power Doppler ultrasonography in patients undergoing in vitro fertilization procedures. J Ultrasound Med. 2001;20(2):125-34.
63. Steer CV, Campbell S, Tan SL, et al. The use of transvaginal colour flow imaging after in vitro fertilization to identify optimum uterine conditions before embryo transfer. Fertil Steril. 1992;57:372-6.
64. Zaidi J, Pittrof R, Shaker A, et al. Assessment of uterine artery blood flow on the day of human chorionic gonadotrophin administration by transvaginal colour Doppler ultrasound in an in vitro fertilization program. Fertil Steril. 1996;65:377-81.
65. Coulam CB, Stern JJ, Soenksen DM, et al. Comparison of pulsatility indexes on the day of oocyte retrieval and embryo transfer. Hum Reprod. 1995;10:82-4.
66. Cacciatore B, Simberg N, Fusaro P, et al. Transvaginal Doppler study of uterine artery blood flow in in vitro fertilization embryo transfer cycles. Fertil Steril. 1996;66:130-4.
67. Tsai YC, Chang JC, Tai MJ, et al. Relationship of uterine perfusion to outcome of intrauterine insemination. J Ultrasound Med. 1996;15:633-6.
68. Panchal SY, Nagori CB. Role of 3D and 3D power Doppler to access endometrial receptivity in IUI cycles. IJIFM. 2010;1(1):19-24.
69. Raga F, Bonilla-Musoles F, Casan EM, et al. Assessment of endometrial volume by three dimensional ultrasound prior to embryo transfer: clues to endometrial receptivity. Hum Reprod. 1999;14:2851-4.
70. Ng EH, Chan CC, Tang OS, et al. The role of endometrial and subendometrial blood flows measured by three dimensional power Doppler ultrasound in prediction of pregnancy during IVF treatment. Hum Reprod. 2006;21(1):164-70.
71. Ng EH, Chan CC, Tang OS, et al. Relationship between uterine blood flow and endometrial and subendometrial blood flows during stimulated and natural cycles. Fertil Steril. 2006;85(3):721-7.
72. Wu HM, Chiang CH, Huang HY, et al. Detection of subendometrial vascularization flow index by three dimensional ultrasound may be useful for predicting pregnancy rate for patients undergoing in vitro fertilization-embryo transfer. Fertil Steril. 2003;79(3):507-11.
73. Gergely RZ, DeUgarte CM, Danzer H, et al. Three dimensional/four dimensional ultrasound guided embryo transfer using the maximal implantation potential point. Fertil Steril. 2005;84(2):500-3.
74. Fanchin R, Ringhini C, Olivennes F, Taylor S, de Ziegler D, Frydman R. Uterine contractions at the time of embryo transfer alter pregnancy rates after in-vitro fertilization. Hum Reprod. 1998;13(7):1968-74.
75. Lesny P, Killick SR, Tetlow RL, et al. Uterine junctional zone contractions during assisted reproduction cycles. Hum Reprod Update. 1998;4:440-5.
76. Fanchin R, Righini C, de Ziegler D, et al. Effects of vaginal progesterone administration on uterine contractility at the time of embryo transfer. Fertil Steril. 2001:75;1136-40.
77. Kupesic S, Kurjak A, Vujisic S, et al. Luteal phase defect: comparison between Doppler velocimetry, histological and hormonal markers. Ultrasound Obstet Gynecol. 1997;9:105-12.
78. Steer CV, Tan SL, Mason BA, et al. Midluteal phase vaginal colour Doppler assessment of uterine artery impedance in a subfertile population. Fertil Steril. 1994;61(1):53-8.

Chapter

10

Ultrasound-Guided Procedures in Assisted Reproduction

Chaitanya Nagori

Chapter Outline

INTRODUCTION

Ultrasound has proved to be a unique noninvasive modality for diagnosis and management of subfertility and also as an aid to therapeutic procedures. Moreover, ultrasound has been found to be safe for its use in peri-implantation period and early pregnancy.

The procedures in which ultrasound is being used as a guiding aid in subfertile patients are as follows.

- Oocyte retrieval
- Embryo transfer (ET)
- Cyst aspiration
- Hydrosalpinx aspiration
- Aspiration of ascitic fluid in ovarian hyperstimulation syndrome (OHSS)
- Multifetal pregnancy reduction (MFPR)

OOCYTE RETRIEVAL

Oocyte retrieval was done by laparoscopy for first decade after the development of in vitro fertilization (IVF).[1] Being highly invasive it limited the use of the technology to very few patients. Lenz and colleagues first described percutaneous transabdominal or transvesical aspiration of follicles under ultrasound guidance in 1981.[2] Transvaginal ovum retrieval with transvaginal ultrasound guidance with mechanical transvaginal sector scanner was first described by Kemeter and Feichtinger in late 1980s.[3] This was a major breakthrough in IVF treatment and was soon universally accepted. Transvaginal oocyte retrieval is a very simple and well-accepted method with very low complication rate. The ease of the procedure was one of the important reasons for easy acceptability of the clinicians and the patients for the procedure.

Method

Preprocedure

Patient is asked to remain nil by mouth for at least 6–8 hours as a preanesthesia requirement. While there is no evidence that routine antibiotics reduce the risk of infection, the administration of an intravenous bolus of antibiotics is generally recommended to women with history of severe pelvic inflammatory disease or if an endometrioma is punctured. However, in certain units, antibiotics are routinely administered. The procedure is planned 34–35 hours after the trigger for ovulation induction is given.

Premedication and Anesthesia

It is important to provide effective anesthesia and analgesia for transvaginal oocyte retrieval as the procedure is painful. But it is also known that no technique of anesthesia, analgesia, or sedation is free from side effects. Especially because, anesthetic agents have been found in the follicular fluid, and these drugs may have adverse effects on oocyte fertilization and embryonic development. Prolonged period of exposure with general anesthesia (GA) can lead to lower pregnancy and delivery rates.[4]

It has been reported that due to stress there is 50-fold transient increase in serum prolactin levels during oocyte retrieval under GA which may affect IVF outcome.[4]

Conscious sedation should be offered to all women having the procedure as it is safe and acceptable method of providing analgesia. Intravenous fentanyl, propofol, and midazolam are the commonly used medications. Short-acting opioids, principally fentanyl and remifentanil, do not alter IVF success rates.[5] Rosen et al. did not find the deleterious effect of nitrous oxide (N_2O) on the rates of fertilization or pregnancy when used during an isoflurane-based general anesthetic technique.[6]

Though according to another study by Gonen et al. showed significantly lower clinical pregnancy rates in N_2O group (14.5%) compared with epidural group (23.7%; P = 0.018) or sedation group (25.8%; P = 0.0074). Nitrous oxide deactivates methionine synthetase thereby reducing the amount of thymidine available for DNA synthesis in dividing cells.[7]

Rafter and Sherry[8] in their study on 80 women found that total intravenous anesthesia (TIVA) with propofol and alfentanil is superior to inhalational anesthesia with N_2O and enflurane in view of less nausea and vomiting (64% in inhalational group and 39% in TIVA group), less requirement for antiemetic medication (62% in inhalational group and 32% TIVA group), and a lower probability of unplanned admission to hospital (21% in inhalational group and 5% in TIVA group) after day-care IVF procedures.[8]

Whatever technique is used, recognized standards of practice should be adhered to and all IVF professionals should follow the safe practice of administering sedative drugs. Pharmacological exposure to the anesthetic agents should be for the least possible duration with minimal penetration to follicular fluid. Assessment of specific anesthetic drugs must be interpreted with the method of administration, dose of anesthetic agents, combination with other drugs, timing of administration, and duration of exposure. Local anesthesia is rarely used as this does not provide effective analgesia. Though paracervical block (PCB) or preovarian block (POB) has been tried. In PCB, a local anesthetic is injected into two to six sites at a depth of 3–7 mm alongside the vaginal portion of the cervix in the vaginal fornices. In POB, the local anesthetic is infiltrated in the vaginal wall under ultrasound guidance between the vaginal wall and peritoneal surface near the ovary.[9]

Some workers have also tried spinal or epidural anesthesia, but the long recovery time and therefore a longer hospitalization that is required is the disadvantage.

Technique

All sterile precautions are taken with washing hands and wearing a sterile gown. Perfume-free washing and cleansing agents are preferred. It is best to use powder-free sterile gloves. The trolley for the procedure is prepared with all sterile precautions. Vagina can be cleaned thoroughly with normal saline. Some units use culture medium to cleanse the vagina, but this is not essential. Antiseptic agents must not be used. Ultrasound transducer is covered with a sterile plastic sleeve and then covered with a sterile condom with no spermicidal gel. Though to allow transmission of sound waves ultrasound gel or saline may be used between the transducer head and the condom. When cleansing the vagina with saline, as the last step, it is douched with normal saline, which acts as a coupling agent for the ultrasound at the time of ovum pick up. Prior to insertion into the vagina and after the procedure the transducer should be thoroughly cleaned with the probe cleansing agents and techniques recommended by the manufacturer. It is covered by sterile sleeve and condom. The biopsy guide on the probe is fixed (Fig. 10.1).

Place the probe in the vagina to assess the endometrial thickness, position and accessibility of the ovaries, and the number of follicles to be aspirated. Switch on the biopsy guide on the screen. The guide helps to identify the position of the needle and the path it will take when advanced through the vaginal fornix into the ovary.

Transducer is manipulated to position the follicles in the needle path (biopsy guideline) (Fig. 10.2).

The transducer should be positioned in such a way that the ovaries are placed closest possible to the needle tip. Needle path is usually at 2 o'clock position for puncturing

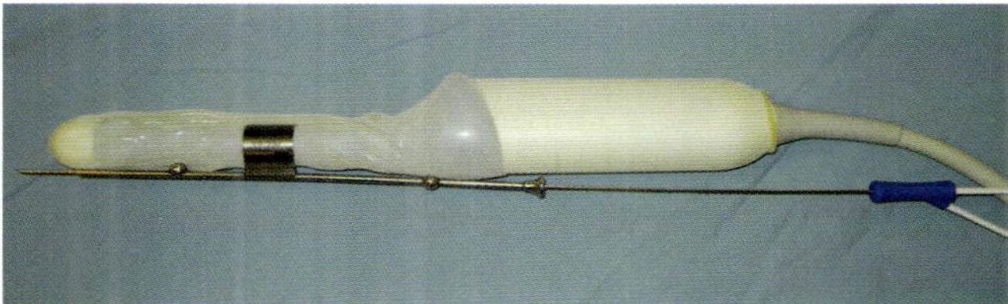

Fig. 10.1: Transvaginal probe, prepared for ovum pick up with biopsy guide fixed on it.

the left ovary and 10 o'clock position for right ovary in the vagina, lateral to the cervix. But when ovaries are fixed or positioned high up in the pelvis, the path may have to be changed. If possible, the follicle should be punctured from the side of the ovary, then entering each follicle systematically with an aim to induce minimal damage to the ovary. As far as possible, only single vaginal puncture with one or two ovarian punctures maximum should be done on each side. This approach reduces the risk of bleeding. Entering the ovary may be difficult with an ovary with a very few follicles. If ovaries are very mobile and then pressure on the abdomen may be required to fix the ovaries. Find the nearest leading follicle and then needle must be advanced.

Several designs of aspiration needles are available. They may have a single or double lumen to enable aspiration and flushing through different routes. The needle is usually 18–20 gauges and must have a very sharp tip to enable easy puncture of mobile ovaries and its distal 2 cm should be roughened to enhance ultrasound visualization (Fig. 10.3).

The needle is connected to a test tube, prewarmed at 37°C in hot blocks, by tubing and suction is applied either from a foot-operated pump (Fig. 10.4) or manually. Before

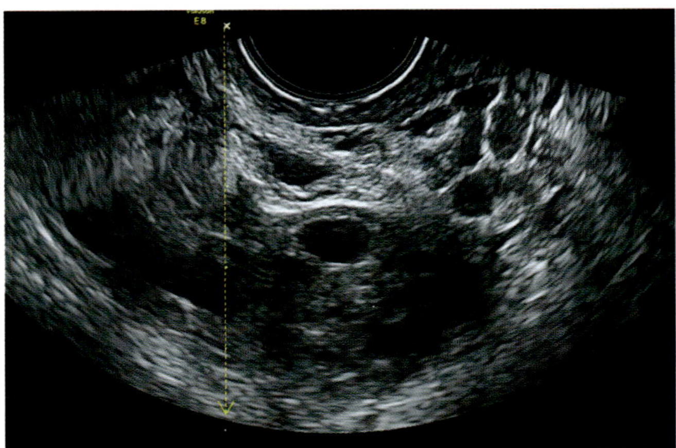

Fig. 10.2: Transvaginal ultrasound image with dotted line—biopsy guideline.

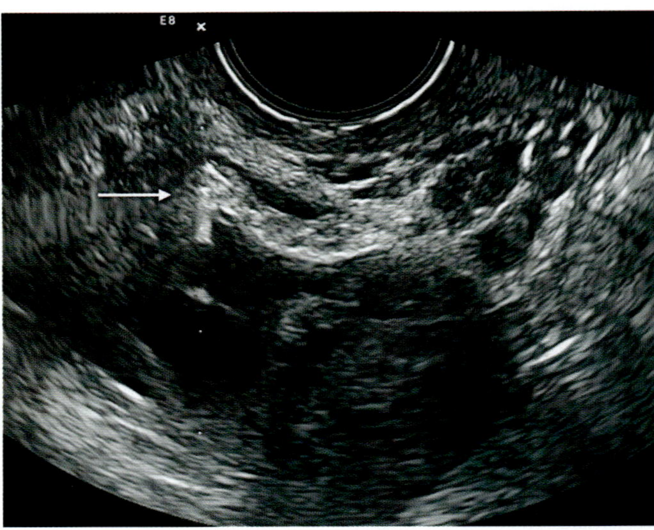

Fig. 10.3: Tranasvaginal ultrasound scan image with biopsy guideline and needle seen overlapping the biopsy guideline.

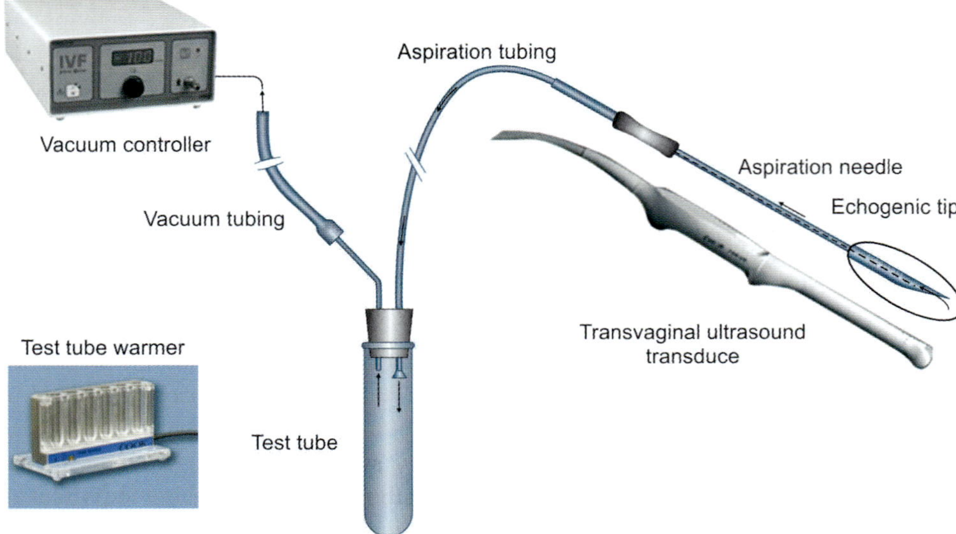

Fig. 10.4: Follicle aspiration equipment: An assembled follicle aspiration single lumen needle connected to a test tube. The test tube is in turn connected to a suction pump.

aspiration, the needle and the tubing are flushed with flushing medium. Several media are available. One with heparin is used for this purpose. This prevents clotting of blood in the tubing that may be aspirated along with the follicular fluid. Needle is advanced from the vagina into the ovary under vision.

The needle is attached to the transvaginal ultrasound transducer through needle guide and bracket firmly and quickly into the follicle. The negative pressure is applied at the same time when the needle punctures the follicle and should be released as soon as the follicle is completely aspirated. Pressure must not be continued while advancing to a new follicle. Negative pressure of 110–120 mmHg is required. Always confirm that you are puncturing the follicle and not the vessel by manipulating the probe to view the follicle in sagittal and transverse plane and if in doubt, use Doppler.

Gentle rotation of the needle helps to suck ovum from any part of the follicle. Contents are aspirated till the follicle is empty. The next follicle is entered without withdrawing the needle out of the ovary. Keep needle in the ovary and aspirate several follicles one after another with careful gentle manipulation. The order of aspiration of different follicles should be such that the needle manipulation is the least. All follicles of more than 10–12 mm size are aspirated as at times even a 10-mm-diameter follicle may contain a fertilizable ovum. Aspirating all these follicles also decreases the risk of OHSS.

After aspirating all the follicles from one ovary, the probe is still in the vagina, but the needle is withdrawn and flushed with media, before reintroducing it to puncture the second ovary. After finishing aspiration of all the follicles, remove the probe. Put the speculum and check for the bleeding from the puncture site. If required, apply pressure with a sterilized gauze for a few minutes to stop bleeding (Box 10.1).

Box 10.1: Oocyte retrieval technique

- Light general anesthesia or conscious sedation
- Consider antibiotic cover
- Aseptic technique
- Lithotomy position of patient, clean and drape
- Cleanse transvaginal probe and cover with sterile cover and condom with or without gel
- Set biopsy guideline on scanner and fix the biopsy guide on the probe
- Introduce the probe to image the ovary in alignment with the biopsy line
- Introduce the pick-up needle through fornix
- Apply suction as the follicle is punctured
- Aspirate all follicles one after the other and repeat the same on the other ovary
- Remove probe and check for bleeding

Difficulties and Controversies

Follicular flushing has been traditionally employed in the belief that it may improve the oocyte yield, although this may not improve the number of oocytes retrieved but increases the duration of retrieval and postoperative pain.[10,11] If the first aspirate does not contain an oocyte, the follicle is flushed few times until one is seen in the aspirate or the observer moves on to the next follicle. Flushing is recommended only if there are only very few follicles.

Some workers do recommend twisting of the needle in the follicular lumen, while aspirating. The explanation given is it may help the ovum to be sucked into the needle from any wall of the follicle. Though the advantage of the same has not been proved.

Bowels in the path of the needle can be displaced by rotating and pushing movements of the probe. At times the ovaries may not be accessible and rarely one may have to go through the uterus, but in such cases, one needs to ensure that vessels and endometrium are avoided. It is best not to puncture hydrosalpinx or endometriomas, if present, while doing oocyte retrieval. However, if a hydrosalpinx or an endometrioma is punctured inadvertently, prophylactic antibiotic should be administered. Transabdominal route may be needed rarely for oocyte retrieval, when ovary is not approachable from vaginal route, if it is placed high up in the pelvis, as in patients with absent uterus or if patient has had vaginoplasty. Though expert operators can still manage with the vaginal route.

Complications

Generally, very few complications are encountered during vaginal egg collections. The main risks of transvaginal oocyte recovery are pelvic infection (0.6%) and bleeding (>100 mL in 0.8% cases), which may be serious, sometimes even fatal. Appropriate preoperative vaginal preparation and minimizing the number of repeated vaginal penetrations may serve to lower the risk of infection. While there is no evidence that routine antibiotics reduce the risk of infection, the administration of an intravenous bolus of antibiotics is generally recommended to women with history of severe pelvic inflammatory disease or if an endometrioma or hydrosalpinx is punctured. Intestinal, vascular, uterine, and tubal injuries with the aspiration

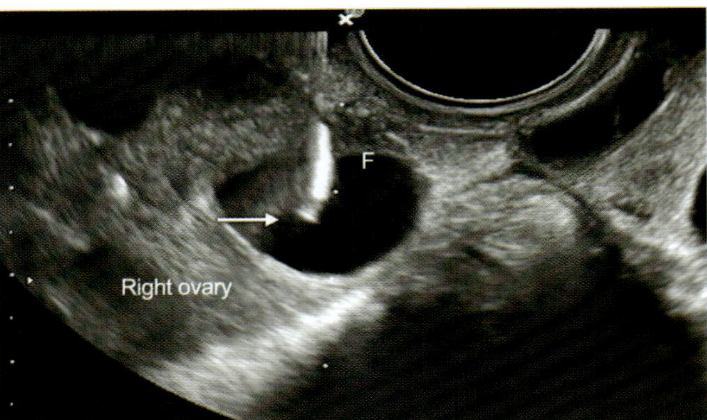

Fig. 10.5: Ultrasound image during vaginal egg recovery. The tip of the needle (arrow) is seen within the follicle (F).

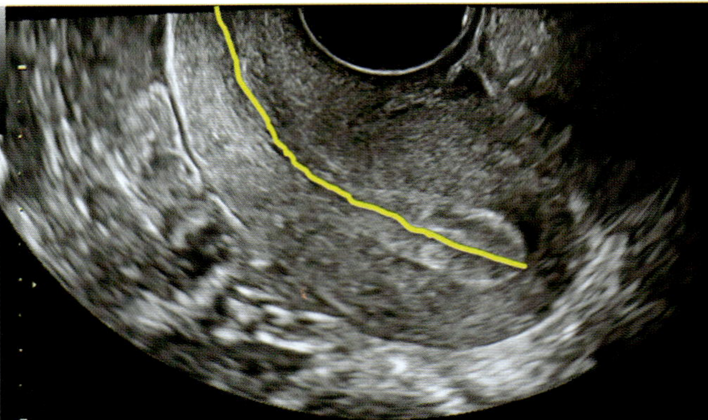

Fig. 10.6: Measuring the functional uterocervical length for embryo transfer.

needle have also been reported. Though bleeding and infections may be serious, sometimes even fatal.

Ovaries are located close to the iliac vessels and therefore iliac vessels are vulnerable to injury during ovum pick up in inexperienced hands. While bleeding from major vessel is a very rare occurrence in experienced hands, care must always be taken when aspirating the follicles that are close to major vessels. Another possible site of bleeding is from the vaginal wall. This is especially common when there is congestion of the vaginal wall. This bleeding is never severe, though may be frightening for the patient. It stops by manual pressure on the bleeding site for a few minutes or by tamponing. The third possible site from where the bleeding would occur is uterine vessels. This happens when the ovary is adherent to the uterus and placed high up in the pelvis. This can be prevented by carefully managing the needle path (Fig. 10.5).

EMBRYO TRANSFER

Embryo transfer is a critical step in determining the final outcome of IVF treatment. Though evidently simple, this procedure demands a lot of perfection and precision. It is a true blend of science and art. Optimizing the technique of ET would provide the best chance of pregnancy (Box 10.2).

Technique

Pretransfer ultrasound is done to check uterocervical curvature and uterocervical length. The length of the uterus is measured from the fundal end of the endometrium to external os (Fig. 10.6).

Box 10.2: Embryo transfer technique

Embryo transfer can be optimized by:

- Pretransfer assessment of uterine cavity and cervical canal
- Thorough and gentle removal of cervical mucus
- Avoid touching the uterine fundus to:
    - Avoid endometrial damage
    - Avoid initiation of uterine contractions
- Confirm proper delivery of embryos inside the uterine cavity; this can be done by:
    - Confirming the location of catheter tip
    - Visualize the easy passage of drop of media containing embryos followed by air bubble in the endometrial cavity

Asepsis is very essential. Patient lies in lithotomy position. Vagina is cleaned with warm normal saline. Gauze soaked in normal saline is used to wipe off all the vaginal secretions. Cusco's speculum is commonly used to visualize the cervix with minimal manipulation to cervix and uterus. Some units use Sim's speculum and Allis forceps or tenaculum to visualize the cervix and straighten the uterocervical canal to make the ET easier. However, it has been reported that this may lead to uterine contractions and may expel out the embryos and compromise the treatment outcome. But it is important to remember, on the other hand, that if the transfer is difficult, chance of implantation may be compromised. Embryo-loaded catheter is brought to the transfer room only when everything is set. Keep the theater lights dimmed when ET catheter is brought to the operation theater. It is also essential to maintain the room temperature at 27–29°C. Introduce the transfer catheter into the cervix, under transabdominal ultrasound guidance. If uterocervical canal on pretransfer ultrasound is not straight, one may electively use a stiff outer sheath or a cervical cannula for introduction of the transfer catheter through it. In any case, the embryo is not retained in the catheter for more than 2 minutes. If it takes longer, the embryos are replaced back into the culture dish and reloaded later. Double-sheathed ET catheter is to be used in such cases. After introducing the outer sheath, which is firm in consistency, its position is confirmed beyond the internal os. The inner cannula is introduced through this sheath later on. Cannula tip is placed 1–1.5 cm away from the fundus of the uterus or at 5–6 cm from the external os. Transfer is done in 15–25 µmol/L of medium. Volumes of 50 µmol/L or larger lead to lower-pregnancy rates, as this fluid may either flow out of the uterus or may fill up the tubes. Once the cannula is introduced to the desired level in the uterus, the piston of the syringe is pushed to introduce the desired amount of fluid containing embryos into the uterus. The ET cannula is seen as an echogenic line and can be traced from the internal os into the endometrial cavity and when the tip is placed at least 1 cm proximal to the fundal end of the endometrium. The passage of embryos with the air bubble is seen as a release of echogenic spot into the endometrial cavity and is also known as "bullet sign" (Figs. 10.7A to C). Then the cannula is steadily held in position for a few seconds. After that, it is gently pulled out with the piston pressed not to cause a suction action. Fluid remaining in the cannula is checked under the microscope to confirm that embryos are not remaining in the cannula. Uterine contractions, expulsion of embryos, blood or mucus on the catheter tip, bacterial contamination of catheter, and retained embryos have all been associated with difficult ETs.

Patient may be gently shifted into the bed and allowed to rest for 20–30 minutes. Success rates are similar regardless of the time for which the patient is kept motionless.

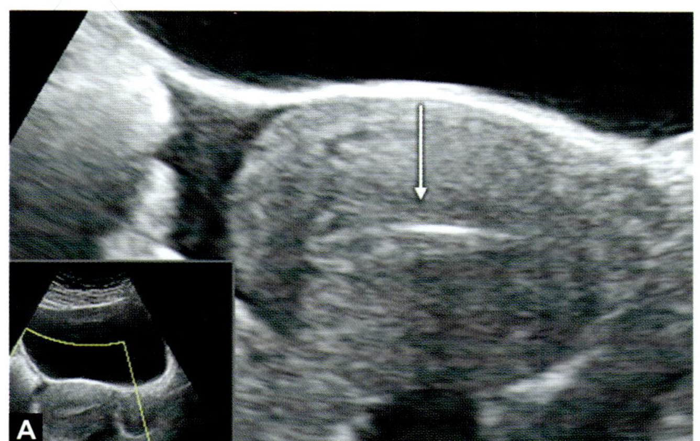

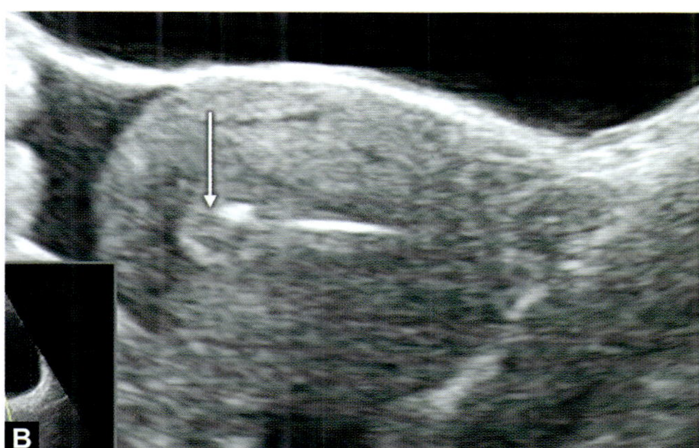

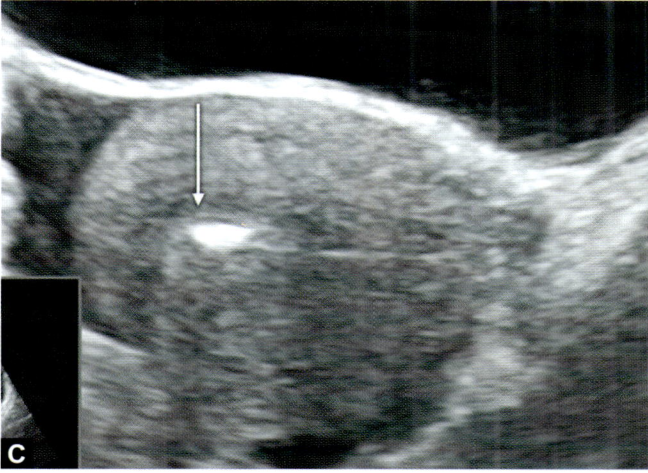

Figs. 10.7A to C: Embryo transfer: (A) Advancing the cannula in the uterus (arrows); (B) releasing the embryo bubble in the uterus (arrows); and (C) retained embryo bubble in uterine cavity after removal of cannula (arrow).

Variables affecting implantation rates and success of ET are:

- Ease of transfer and technique of transfer to avoiding uterine contractions and prevent blood or mucous on transfer catheter:
- Uterine depth and precise depth of ET in uterine cavity
- Type of catheter used
- Catheter loading
- Physician's experience: physician's perception of transfer difficulty was the most important variable

Variations in Embryo Transfer Technique

Ultrasound-Guided Instead of Clinical Touch Method

Ultrasound guidance in this procedure has shown advantage over clinical touch or blind ET by significantly increasing the chance of embryo implantation, ongoing pregnancy, and live birth due to the ease of transfer.[12,13] Transabdominal ultrasonographic guidance is used to determine the precise depth of embryo placement within the uterus. The tip of the catheter is placed approximately 1–1.5 cm from the uterine fundus so that the embryo/s are expelled gently into the mid-cavity of the uterus. Apart from the depth of the uterine cavity, the curvature of uterine cavity, angle between cervix and endometrial cavity may also be appreciated, and the angle of ET cannula may be accordingly adjusted to make the transfer easy. When the cervical canal appears curved or there is acute angle between cervix and uterus, double-sheathed catheter or a catheter with stilette is recommended. Use of stilette under ultrasound guidance to negotiate difficult cervical passage makes ET easy and less traumatic.[14]

In an exhaustive Cochrane Database Systematic Review that included 13/15 randomized controlled trials, Brown et al.[12] reported significantly higher live birth/ongoing pregnancies per woman randomized associated with ultrasound-guided ET (452/1,376 compared with 353/1,338) for clinical touch, odds ratio (OR) 1.40, 95% confidence interval (CI) 1.18–1.66, ($P < 0.001$) in six studies. This suggested that a population of women with 25% chance of pregnancy using clinical touch, would be increased to 32% (28–46%) using ultrasound-guided ET. Ultrasound guidance for ET is therefore recommended.

Studies have shown that no significant changes in results have been observed whether transabdominal or transvaginal ultrasound is used for guidance.[15] However, transabdominal ultrasound is preferred as it does not interfere with the transvaginal or transcervical procedure of ET.

Ultrasound-guided ET enables the visualization of:[15]

- Guiding cannula and transfer catheter placement in relation to the endometrial surface and uterine fundus during ET
- The position and movement of a transfer-associated air bubble
- The impact of subendometrial-myometrial contractions leading to endometrial movement

Advantages of ultrasound-guided ET:

- Helps placement of soft catheters
- Confirms that the catheter is beyond the internal os in cases of an elongated cervical canal
- Allows to guide the direction of the catheter along the contour of the endometrial cavity especially in uteri with acute curves
- Prevents damage to endometrium and plugging of catheter
- Full bladder that is required for transabdominal ultrasound and that straightens the uterocervical angle and helps catheter passage
- Helps to negotiate the catheter through difficult cervical canal
- Helps to correct position of catheter tip for embryo deposition (point of maximum implantation potential (MIP))

A total of eight prospective controlled trials were identified for a meta-analysis.[16] Of these studies, four were nonrandomized or quasirandomized and four were genuinely randomized. Meta-analysis demonstrated a significantly increased chance of clinical pregnancy following ultrasound-guided ET in all studies and in the genuinely randomized subgroup. The embryo implantation rate was also significantly increased following ultrasound-guided ET.[17]

Transfer at the Point of Maximum Implantation Potential

A large observational retrospective study by Gergely et al. has shown that if MIP is individually found in each patient by the help of three-dimensional (3D) ultrasound and embryos are deposited at this point can improve the implantation rates.[18] Point of MIP can be calculated by 3D ultrasound. On coronal section of the uterus, two lines are drawn, one on each side parallel to the cornu. The point at which these lines intersect is the point of MIP (Fig. 10.8).

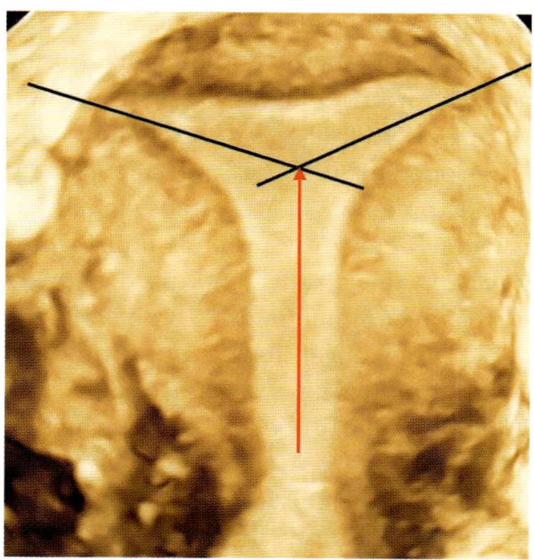

Fig. 10.8: Intersection of the lines drawn through and parallel to the uterine cornu, indicates the point of maximum implantation potential.

Transvaginal ultrasound-guided ET was performed on 121 consecutive patients. Observation was made of guiding cannula and transfer catheter placement in relation to the endometrial surface and uterine fundus during ET. The position and movement of a transfer-associated air bubble and the impact of subendometrial myometrial contraction leading to endometrial movement was observed. Results indicate that tactile assessment of ET catheter placement is unreliable: in 17.4% of transfers the outer guiding catheter inadvertently abutted the fundal endometrium. The outer guiding cannula indented the endometrium in 24.8% and the transfer catheter embedded in the endometrium in 33.1%.[15]

The use of ultrasound-guided transfer avoided tubal transfer in 7.4% of transfers. In a randomized trial, the use of transabdominal ultrasound guidance during ET improved the pregnancy rate from 33.7 to 50%[19] (Coroleu et al., 2000). In another retrospective study[20] (Wood et al., 2000), the pregnancy rate improved from 25 to 38% by using ultrasound during ET. However, three other prospective trials failed to show such a significant improvement.[15]

Catheter Types

Soft catheters are preferred over rigid ones as they are less likely to traumatize the cervix and endometrium and to invoke any uterine contractions. The commonly used soft catheters (Wallace) have a softer inner cannula and a stiffer outer sheath.[21] Occasionally, resistance to pass the soft inner cannula into the uterus usually at the level of internal os is encountered and in these cases the stiffer outer sheath is advanced in the cervical canal to negotiate the resistance with the inner cannula can now be advanced into the uterine cavity.

A firmer malleable catheter with a stilette and an outer sheath is another option in difficult cases, where the catheter is advanced up to the level of the internal os. The inner stilette is then removed and the softer cannula with embryos loaded in, is fed through the outer sheath to advance into the uterine cavity for transfer. The outer sheath or the malleable catheter should never be advanced beyond the internal os.

Bleeding at the time of the transfer may adversely affect the embryos. In difficult transcervical transfers, either transfer under anesthesia or a surgical transfer transfundally under ultrasound and laparoscopic guidance may be done.

Catheters with echogenic tips are better appreciated on ultrasound guidance and therefore reduce the time taken from loading the catheter to depositing the embryos in endometrial cavity. Coaxial catheter system has been preferred by some and has been claimed to be of help in difficult transfers. But in a prospective randomized study of 251 patients, no significant change was found in implantation rate, clinical pregnancy rate, or ongoing pregnancy rate between the two catheters.[22] Another group compared soft catheters and catheters with echogenic tip and concluded that catheters with echogenic tip simplify the ET and also improve implantation rates.

The pump-regulated ET (PRET) device generates a significantly smaller variance of the positioning of the embryo(s) into the uterine cavity. This resulted in an ongoing pregnancy rate of 21% in the PRET versus 17% in the manual (P = 0.22) transfer group; frozen-thawed ETs resulted in 17.5% versus 10.9% (P = 0.097), respectively.[23]

Mock Transfer

The role of mock transfers in reducing the frequency of unexpected difficult ETs has been controversial. Mock transfer is done to rehearse the transfer process so as to anticipate the difficulties and modify the selection of the catheter or speculum. Mock transfer can be done at the time of start of ovarian stimulation or at oocytes retrieval or at the time of actual transfer. In the initial studies by Mansour et al.,[24] trial transfers have been shown to reduce the incidence of difficult transfers. However in a study by Henne et al.,[25] it has been shown that uterine length and position changes with ovarian stimulation challenging the role of trial transfer.

Day of Embryo Transfer

The convention was to replace embryos on the second or third day postinsemination, when the embryos are usually two- to eight-cell stage of cleavage. With improvements in culture media and laboratory conditions, there is an increasing tendency for delaying ET till day 5 with an aim to improve the implantation rates. Delaying ET from day 2 or day 3, transfer of embryos at blastocyst stage (day 5/6) has shown significant increase in live birth rate (OR 1.35, 95% CI 1.05–1.74) when compared with day 2 or day 3 transfers.[26] It is a more physiological approach, allowing synchronization of the embryo with the endometrium and the selection of viable embryos for transfer will be more efficient.

However, the rates of embryos freezing are lower and the treatment cancellation rates are higher with blastocyst transfer. However in selected group of couples, the practice of blastocyst transfer has the potential to favor single ET without compromising the overall success rates, but can significantly reduce the occurrence of multiple pregnancies. The most favored groups for blastocyst transfer are those having high numbers of eight-cell embryos on day 3, in whom the cycle cancellation is not increased.

CYST ASPIRATIONS

Cysts in the ovary before starting stimulation are not desired and may delay the start of stimulation. Follicular or simple cysts of the ovaries can be aspirated transvaginally under ultrasound guidance. Transvaginal cyst aspiration has many advantages including short hospital stay, rapid recovery, excellent patient tolerance, and a low rate of procedure-related complications (Box 10.3).

Procedure

A thorough ultrasound evaluation and diagnosis must be done before planning the procedure. The procedure is best done in the operation theater. Proper asepsis is to be maintained. Patient is positioned in lithotomy-like position or the same position in which transvaginal scans are done. Short GA with propofol or local PCB with sedation may be used depending on operator's comfort and patient's cooperation.

We usually prefer a 5–9 MHz transvaginal probe with the biopsy attachment. The probe is thoroughly cleaned and disinfected. The disinfectants used depend on the manufacturer's recommendations. Probe is then covered with a sterile probe cover. Jelly is put on the probe and the probe is covered with a sterile condom. The biopsy guide is attached to the probe. A 17- to 20-gauge-long needle with Teflon tubing is used. The tubing is attached to the aspiration (suction) pump. When all the fluid is aspirated and the cyst is empty, the needle is removed. Scan is done to rule out any bleed or fluid collection in pelvis. Perioperative antibiotics are generally given. Usually postoperative pain is very little but if required analgesics may be given. Though refilling and recurrence risk is high after aspiration (Figs. 10.9A and B).

Box 10.3: Cyst aspiration technique

- Lithotomy position for patient with empty bladder
- Cleanse and drape parts including vagina with antiseptic solution
- Transvaginal probe is cleansed and covered with a sterile probe cover
- Biopsy guide attached and 17- to 20-gauge-long needle attached with Teflon tubing to suction pump is introduced into the cyst
- Aspiration is done till the cyst is empty
- Remove needle and check for bleeding

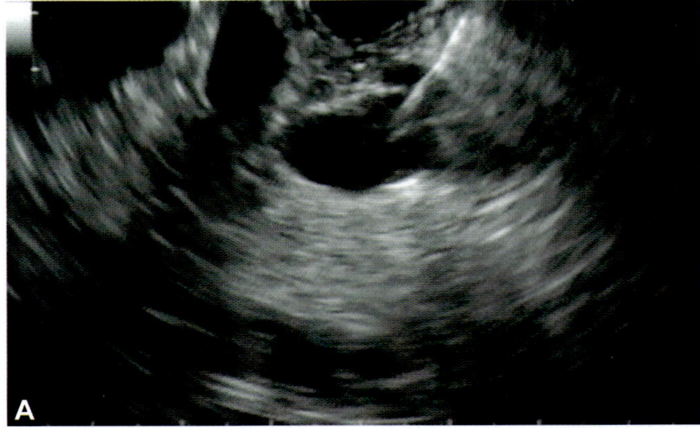

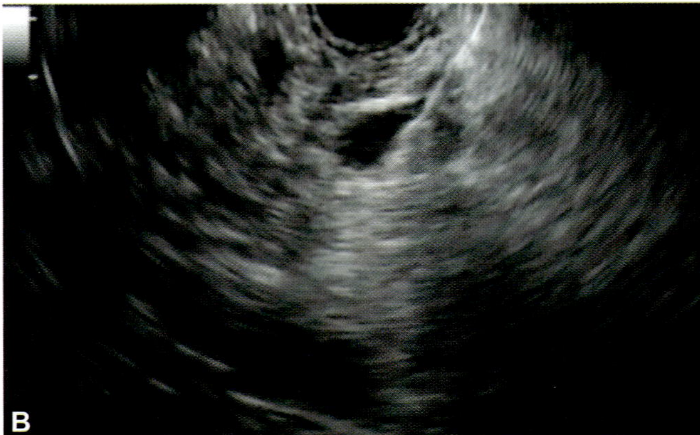

Figs. 10.9A and B: Pre- and postaspiration B mode ultrasound image of the cyst with aspiration needle in position.

The controversies in the cyst aspiration procedure are the size and the type of the cyst. According to most studies, the cysts that do not come in the way of pick up and are smaller than 5 cm in diameter. Simple cysts can be safely aspirated but the cysts with internal echogenecities are best avoided. This also includes the endometriotic cysts, as the risk of dissemination and infection is high.

There are studies that use sclerosants after the aspiration of the cyst to stimulate fibrosis in between the walls, which prevent refilling. Workers have tried using antibiotic solutions and askerol. Ultrasonography-guided transabdominal aspiration of cyst fluid and subsequent methotrexate injection appears to be an alternative treatment for both simple and endometriotic ovarian cysts in selected cases.[27]

ASPIRATION OF HYDROSALPINX

It has been proved beyond doubts in several studies that hydrosalpinx has a negative impact on IVF outcome.[28] This is due to the toxic effect of infected tubal fluid on the implanting embryo. This is why hydrosalpinx needs to be managed before ET. Salpingectomy or tubal ligation/clipping has been used as surgical therapy for hydrosalpinx in patients with subfertility. Ultrasound-guided transvaginal aspiration has also been recommended as a treatment option to remove hydrosalpingeal fluid. Fluid would reaccumulate if the procedure is done before starting stimulation. Because of fast refilling tendency, hydrosalpinx aspiration is not a therapy of choice, generally, instead clipping or surgical resection of the hydrosalpinx is preferred. However, many times, hydrosalpinx may be diagnosed on ultrasound scan while undergoing ovarian stimulation, and in these cases, hydrosalpinx aspiration can be offered and performed immediately after oocyte retrieval. Clinical pregnancy rates for aspiration versus control groups were 31.3% and 17.6%, respectively in a small study.[29] The procedure is same as that for cyst aspiration.

ASPIRATION OF ASCITIC FLUID IN OHSS

Ovarian hyperstimulation syndrome is one of the most dreaded complications of subfertility treatment. Various protocols have been devised to prevent it, but it still occurs, and the incidence is higher in IVF cycles than in patients on ovulation induction. Fluid collection in the third space (peritoneal, pleural, and pericardial) is one of the consequences. Pleural and pericardial fluid aspiration must be done by subspecialists, but the aspiration of peritoneal fluid is generally done by experienced radiologists and gynecologists. This procedure reduces the patient's weight, leg edema and abdominal circumference, and improves the derangements of renal function.[30] Aspiration may be done repeatedly at intervals, or an indwelling catheter may be placed. Whatever the technique is ultrasound guidance for the placement of the needle and the catheter is absolutely essential. Al-Ramahi et al. have described placing an indwelling catheter (closed system Dawson-Mueller catheter with "simp-loc" locking design) for continuous drainage.[31] Abuzeid and coworkers used a pigtail catheter for the same purpose.[32] Albumin supplementation may be required and a watch on serum protein balance as both these procedures lead to a significant protein loss. Koike et al. developed a continuous autotransfusion system of ascites (CATSA). This eliminated the need of protein supplementation because the ascitic fluid itself was again transfused. It was done for 5 hours every day at a rate of 100–200 mL/h.[33] Transvaginal approach is thought to be better than transabdominal approach. This approach is very convenient for those who are conversant with transvaginal ultrasound.[34] Ultrasound guidance helps to prevent ovarian injury, which is otherwise also large in OHSS.

FETAL REDUCTION

Twin and higher-order pregnancies are increasing with the increased use of fertility-inducing drugs and assisted reproductive techniques.[35] Prematurity and associated neurological sequelae can occur as complications of multiple pregnancies and these complications become worse with rising order of pregnancy (Table 10.1).[36] The risk of cerebral palsy is high in these patients. Its incidence in 1,000 survivors is 2.3 in singletons, 12.6 in twins, and 44.8 in triplets. More than 20% of babies with birth weight less than 750 g develop cerebral palsy and is 4.6% higher in twin pregnancies. Apart from risks of mortality and morbidity to the fetus, maternal risk of hypertension, other cardiovascular and pulmonary complications, gestational diabetes, and postpartum hemorrhage are also significantly increased in

Table 10.1: Risks of prematurity associated with multiple pregnancy[36]

Fetus	*Del. age*	*Perinat. mort.*	*RDS*	*ICH*	*Retinopathy*
Triplet	31 + 5	14%	23%	14%	10%
Quadru	29 + 5	36%	65%	15%	9%
Quintu	28 + 4	40%	75%	10%	25%

multiple pregnancies. While the best approach to reduce the prevalence of multiple pregnancies is to limit the number of embryos transferred to one or two, fetal reduction may be required in rare situations, where the conception is complicated with multiple pregnancies. Generally twin pregnancies are managed conservatively, but for triplets and higher-order pregnancies, fetal reduction is recommended and offered to the couple.

The procedure of fetal reduction may be done for two causes:

1. To reduce the number of fetuses (MFPR) to reduce prematurity and its complications: Karyotype by chorionic villus biopsy should be offered to all before performing MFPR. If not possible, at least nuchal translucency (NT) screening is performed. This is to assure that at the end of MFPR, the prognosis for the remaining fetus/es is/are good.
2. To eliminate the fetus with abnormality (selective reduction): As stated earlier, selective reduction is opted, when one of the fetuses of multifetal pregnancy is abnormal. When any such abnormality is detected by ultrasound, it must be confirmed by karyotyping before the procedure. Legally, confirmation after termination is also required for assurance that the abnormal fetus was terminated.

The procedure and technique of embryo reduction may change according to the age of the fetus and route of the procedure, but not because of its indication.

Preprocedure

Appropriate counseling must be done for every patient/couple before the procedure. That should include the risks of multiple pregnancies in terms of incidence of prematurity and associated complications of prematurity including miscarriage and neurological sequelae, on the other hand, procedure-related risks such as infection and miscarriage. It must be emphasized that miscarriage may occur even after 4–8 weeks of a successful procedure and pregnancy loss before 24 weeks is about 9–15%. The short-term and long-term sequelae of prematurity must also be discussed with the couple. They should be explained about immediate consequences of prematurity like respiratory distress syndrome, intracranial hemorrhage, necrotizing enterocolitis, and retinopathy and also about late consequences like neurological deficits, recurrent hospitalization in infancy, neonatal and infant mortality. Benefits of MFPR should be weighed against potential risks of procedure including fetal loss and maternal stress.

After the couple has consented for the procedure, a detailed ultrasound scanning of all the fetuses is done, to assess the fetal anatomy and growth in detail including NT if possible. Proper mapping of the sac positions by ultrasound is a must, if possible using 3D ultrasound. Laboratory investigations (blood and urine) for minor surgeries are done.

There are lots of views as to what is the best time and best method for the procedure. Some people may do embryo reduction as early as 8 weeks and claim that it causes less maternal psychological trauma and some may prefer waiting till 14 weeks arguing that MFPR can be done after ruling out anomalies in detail. We prefer to do it around 11–12 weeks as it is possible that before 9 weeks, a spontaneous miscarriage or missed miscarriage may occur even otherwise. There is also a scope to rule out major structural or chromosomal anomalies in the fetus before reduction.

Various methods and routes have been tried by different workers for the procedure. Choice depends on the gestational age, chorionicity, and the operator's expertise. The most widely used method for dichorionic twins is intracardiac/intrathoracic potassium chloride (KCl) injection. Methods like transcervical aspiration and mechanical trauma are used to reduce one of the fetuses as early as 7–8 weeks of pregnancy but are too crude and not widely accepted.

Embryo Reduction Using Potassium Chloride Injection

This can be done by transabdominal/transvaginal approach under ultrasound guidance. Preferred time to do this procedure is 9–11 weeks of gestation. Procedure done later than 12 weeks has no advantage; on the contrary, it leads to higher risk of coagulation disorders in mother according to some studies. When embryo reduction is done after 15 weeks,[37] preterm delivery at less than 33 weeks is three times higher. Asepsis is of prime importance. Embryo close to the probe is selected for reduction. Transcervical or transvaginal reduction may be safer very early in gestation and transabdominal safer in late first trimester.[38]

The procedure is preferably done under short GA, while some may prefer a local anesthesia with sedation. Patient is placed in lithotomy position. Parts are cleaned and painted with povidone-iodine solution or savlon and patient is draped with sterilized towels. Transvaginal ultrasound probe is cleaned and prepared for the procedure. It is covered by a sterile cover/jelly-free condom. The biopsy guide is attached to the probe and the probe is placed in vagina. Scanning is done to map the positions of the sacs and to find out the most easily approachable embryo. The biopsy guideline is switched on, on the scanner. The embryo desired to be reduced is brought in alignment with this line. A 20–21-gauge-long needle is introduced through the needle guide.

Attach needle to 2 cc syringe, filled with 1.3–2 mEq/L or 2–7 mmol of KCl to the needle and prefill the needle before it enters the gestational sac. Once the needle enters the sac, it is placed close to the embryo. Insert needle and with slight depression check that the needle is in the embryo. Gentle in and out movement of the probe will move the embryo also along with it, if the needle is in the embryo. The needle must enter the embryo in its thorax. Intracardiac location of the needle tip is the best but intrathoracic location would also do (Figs. 10.10A and B). In case of doubt, four-dimensional (4D) biopsy guide may be more useful. Once the position of the needle tip is confirmed to be in the heart or close to the heart of the embryo, slowly inject 1–2 mL of KCl. A forceful injection may push away the embryo. Injection jet can be seen on B-mode and confirmed by color Doppler. Sometimes injected KCl may also be seen as lucency in the fetal thorax as it creates hydrothorax. Wait patiently for a few minutes, without changing the position of the needle. Heart stops beating in few seconds. Monitor for asystole for 60 seconds. Remove needle. Fetus sinks in the amniotic cavity. Recheck after a few hours and on the next day. Close observation of the maternal heart must be done when KCl is injected.

Postoperative

Spotting is rare except for the transcervical approach. Observe for leakage of liquor amnii. Antibiotic cover is given for 7 days, tocolytics for 72 hours, and rest for 48 hours. Although some studies have shown that prophylactic antibiotics, tocolytics or cervical suturing has no role.

Risks of Procedure

- Premature rupture of membranes (PROM)
- Intra-amniotic infection—chorioamnionitis
- Clinical/lab evidence of disseminated intravascular coagulation, of which some cases may also require monitoring for decreasing fibrinogen levels and prolonged partial thromboplastin time (PTT) and heparin therapy.
- Rarely after initial asystole immediately after injection, the heart may again start beating and in such cases repeat KCl injection may be needed. Repeat procedure after 1 week may be required if the termination has not occurred. But this is a controversial issue.

When transabdominal approach is used, either free-hand technique or needle guide may be used, depending on operator's convenience. The procedure otherwise remains the same. Whatever route and whatever technique is used, extensive perinatal follow-up is essential to prevent premature delivery. Multifetal pregnancy reduction reduces but does not eliminate the risk of prematurity associated with higher-order pregnancies. Postprocedure prognosis is worse depending on the degree of higher-order pregnancies[39] and the number of pregnancies that are reduced (Figs. 10.11A to D).[37]

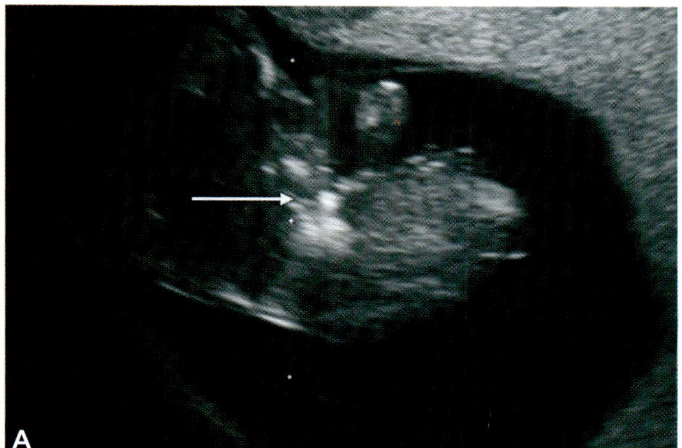

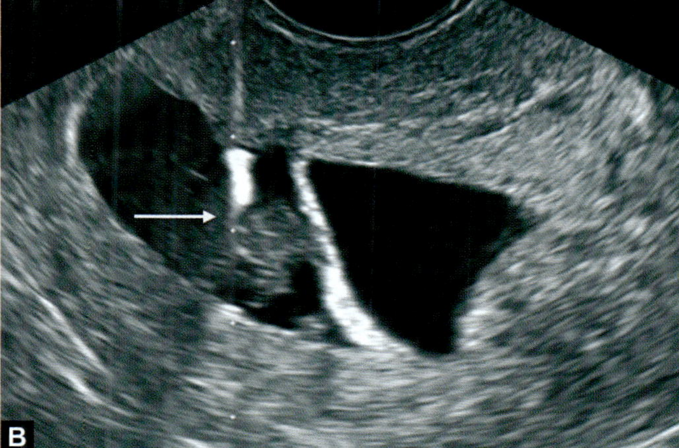

Figs. 10.10A and B: Fetal intrathoracic position of the needle tip is seen in both the images.

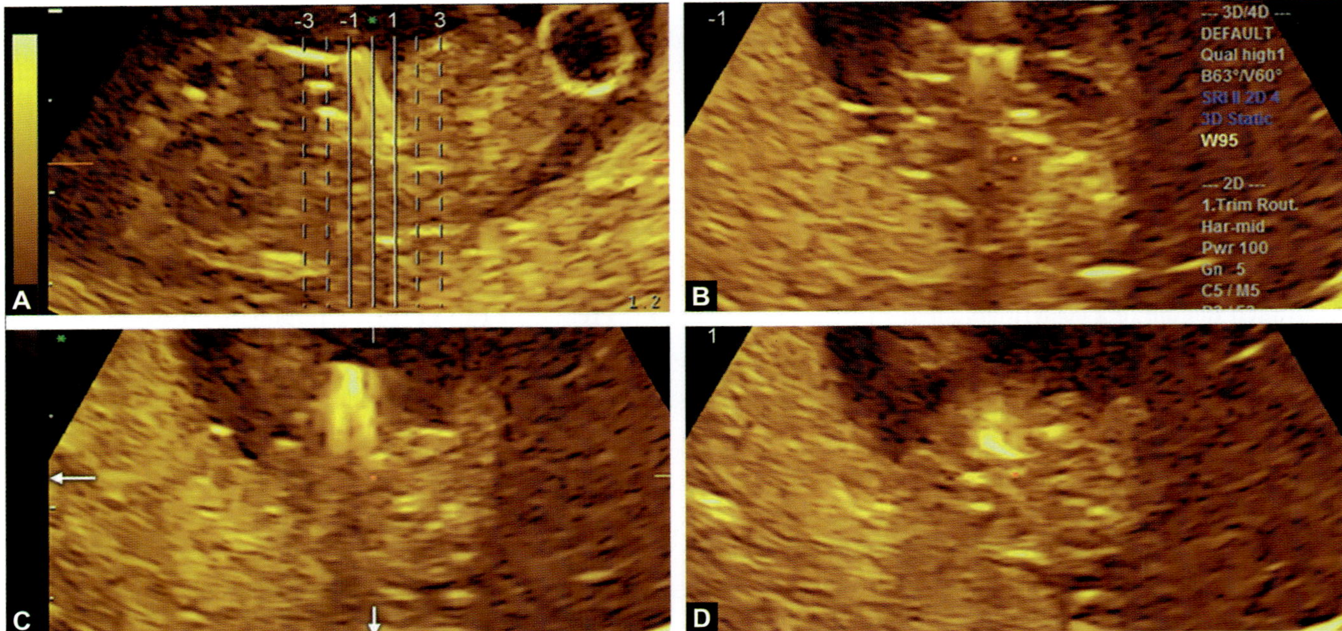

Figs. 10.11A to D: Embryo reduction: Needle position confirmed on three-dimensional (3D) ultrasound (US).

Reduction of triplets to twins significantly reduces the risk of prematurity in terms of gestational age at delivery, birth weight, overall pregnancy loss which makes it medically justifiable procedure.[40] In spite of all care taken, MFPR has been quoted as "a therapy to achieve most good for least harm." In spite of all available methods to reduce multifetal pregnancies, there is still a significant risk to the fetus and the mother. It is therefore insisted that single ET is the safest and the most desirable practice. The fact remains for all ultrasound-guided procedures. It has a steep learning curve, and success of the procedure increases with experience.

Though these procedures are not for monochorionic pregnancies. Specialized methods like laser coagulation of the cord is required for these fetuses to avoid damage to the remaining fetus.

KEY POINTS

- Ultrasound has proved to be reliable as a guiding tool for several procedures for managing the patients with subfertility
- Ultrasound-guided procedures are less invasive and have significantly reduced the postoperative hospital care
- Although minimally invasive, these procedures must be done in operation theatres and all emergency drugs and gadgets must be readily available
- Adequate asepsis, adequate anesthesia, and appropriate antibiotic cover are required
- It is essential to master the scanning technique before trying these procedures
- No ultrasound-guided procedure must be attempted if the ultrasound image quality is inadequate
- Transvaginal ultrasound-guided oocyte retrieval is a very simple and well-accepted method with very low complication rate
- Transabdominal route may be rarely needed for oocyte retrieval, if ovaries are placed high up in the pelvis, as in patients with absent uterus or if patient has had vaginoplasty
- Ultrasound-guided ET technique offers advantages over clinical touch or blind ET technique that it makes the procedure easier and improves the treatment outcome
- While the best approach to reduce multiple pregnancy rates is to limit the number of embryos transferred to one or two, fetal reduction may be required in rare situations, where the conception is complicated with multiple pregnancies

REFERENCES

1. Feichtinger W, Kemeter P. Laparoscopic or ultrasonically guided follicle aspiration for in vitro fertilization. J In Vitro Fertil Embryo Transf. 1984;1:244.
2. Lenz S, Lauritsen JG, Kjellow M. Collection of human oocytes for in vitro fertilization by ultrasonically guided follicular puncture. Lancet. 1981;1(8230):1163-4.
3. Kemeter P, Feichtinger W. Transvaginal oocyte retrieval using a transvaginal sector scan probe combined with an automated puncture device. Hum Reprod. 1986;1:21.
4. Hayes MF, Sacco AG, Savoy-Moore RT, Magyar DM, Endler GC, Moghissi KS. Effect of general anesthesia on fertilization and cleavage of human oocytes *in vitro*. Fertil Steril. 1987;48:975-81.
5. Wilhelm W, Biedler A, Hammadeh ME, Fleser R, Grüness V. Remifentanil for oocyte retrieval: a new single-agent monitored anaesthesia care technique. Anaesthesist. 1999;48:698-704.
6. Rosen MA, Roizen MF, Eger EI 2nd, et al. The effect of nitrous oxide on *in vitro* fertilization success rate. Anesthesiology. 1987;67:42-4.
7. Gonen O, Shulman A, Ghetler Y, et al. The impact of different types of anesthesia on *in vitro* fertilization-embryo transfer treatment outcome. J Assist Reprod Genet. 1995;12:678-82.
8. Raftery S, Sherry E. Total intravenous anaesthesia with propofol and alfentanil protects against postoperative nausea and vomiting. Can J Anaesth. 1992;39:37-40.
9. Cerne A, Bergh C, Borg K, et al. Pre-ovarian block versus paracervical block for oocyte retrieval. Hum Reprod. 2006;21:2916-21.
10. Bagtharia S, Haloob AR. Is there a benefit from routine follicular flushing for oocyte retrieval? J Obstet Gynaecol. 2005;25:374-6.
11. Kingsland CR, Taylor CT, Aziz N, et al. Is follicular flushing necessary for oocyte retrieval? A randomized trial. Hum Reprod. 1991;6:382-3.
12. Brown J, Buckingham K, Abou-Setta AM, et al. Ultrasound versus "clinical touch" for catheter guidance during embryo transfer in women. Cochrane Database Syst Rev. 2010;(1):CD006107.
13. Porter MB. Ultrasound in assisted reproductive technology. Semin Reprod Med. 2008;26(3):266-76.
14. Allahbadia GN, Kadam KS, Gandhi GN, et al. The stilette for a SureView. Fertil Steril. 2006;86(Suppl 3):S252.
15. Woolcott R, Stanger J. Potentially important variables identified by transvaginal ultrasound-guided embryo transfer. Hum Reprod. 1997;12(5):963-6.
16. Buckett WM. A meta-analysis of ultrasound-guided versus clinical touch embryo transfer. Fertil Steril. 2003; 80(4):1037-41.
17. Sallam HN, Sadek SS. Ultrasound-guided embryo transfer: a meta-analysis of randomized controlled trial. Fertil Steril. 2003;80(4):1042-6.
18. Gergely RZ, DeUgarte CM, Danzer H, et al. Three-dimensional/four-dimensional ultrasound-guided embryo transfer using the maximal implantation potential point. Fertil Steril. 2005;84(2):500-3.
19. Coroleu B, Carreras O, Veiga A, et al. Embryo transfer under ultrasound guidance improves pregnancy rates after in-vitro fertilization. Hum Reprod. 2000;15:616-20.
20. Wood EG, Batzer FR, Go KJ, et al. Ultrasound-guided soft catheter embryo transfers will improve pregnancy rates in in-vitro fertilization. Hum Reprod. 2000;15:107-12.
21. Karande V, Hazlett D, Vietzke M, et al. A prospective randomized comparison of the Wallace catheter and the Cook Echo-Tip catheter for ultrasound-guided embryo transfer. Fertil Steril. 2002;77(4):826-30.
22. Coroleu B, Barri PN, Carreras O, et al. Effect of using an echogenic catheter for ultrasound-guided embryo transfer in an IVF programme: a prospective, randomized, controlled study. Hum Reprod. 2006;21(7):1809-15.
23. Caanen MR, van der Houwen LE, Schats R, et al. Embryo transfer with controlled injection speed to increase pregnancy rates: a randomized controlled trial. Gynecol Obstet Invest. 2016;81:394-404.
24. Mansour R, Aboulghar M, Serour G. Dummy embryo transfer: a technique that minimizes the problems of embryo transfer and improves the pregnancy rate in human *in vitro* fertilization. Fertil Steril. 1990;54:678-81.
25. Henne MB, Milki AA. Uterine position at real embryo transfer compared with mock embryo transfer. Hum Reprod. 2004;19:570-2.
26. Blake DA, Farquhar CM, Johnson N, et al. Cleavage stage versus blastocyst stage embryo transfer in assisted conception. Cochrane Database Syst Rev. 2007;(4):CD002118.
27. Gupta P, Huria A. Management of ovarian cysts with percutaneous aspiration and methotrexate injection. Niger Med J. 2016;57(1):19-23.
28. Camus E, Poncelet C, Goffinet F, et al. Pregnancy rates after in-vitro fertilization in cases of tubal infertility with and without hydrosalpinx: a meta-analysis of published comparative studies. Hum Reprod. 1999;14(5):1243-9.
29. Hammadieh N, Coomarasamy A, Ola B, et al. Ultrasound-guided hydrosalpinx aspiration during oocyte collection improves pregnancy outcome in IVF: a randomized controlled trial. Hum Reprod. 2008;23:1113-7.
30. Thaler I, Yoffe N, Kaftory JK, et al. Treatment of ovarian hyperstimulation syndrome: the physiologic basis for a modified approach. Fertil Steril. 1981;36:110-3.
31. Al-Ramahi M, Leader A, Claman P, et al. A novel approach to the treatment of ascites associated with ovarian hyperstimulation syndrome. Hum Reprod. 1997;12:2614-6.
32. Abuzeid MI, Nassar Z, Massaad Z, et al. Pigtail catheter for the treatment of ascites associated with ovarian hyperstimulation syndrome. Hum Reprod. 2003;18:370-3.
33. Koike T, Araki S, Minakami H, et al. Clinical efficacy of peritoneovenous shunting for the treatment of severe ovarian hyperstimulation syndrome. Hum Reprod. 2000;15:113-7.

34. Aboulghar MA, Mansour RT, Serour GI, et al. Ultrasonically guided vaginal aspiration of ascites in the treatment of severe ovarian hyperstimulation syndrome. Fertil Steril. 1990;53(5):933-5.
35. Chauhan SP, Scardo JA, Hayes E, et al. Twins: prevalence, problems, and preterm births. Am J Obstet Gynecol. 2010;203(4):305-15.
36. Strauss A, Paek BW, Genzel-Boroviczeny O, et al. Multifetal gestation—maternal and perinatal outcome of 112 pregnancies. Fetal Diagn Ther. 2002;17(4):209-17.
37. Antsaklis A, Souka AP, Daskalakis G, et al. Pregnancy outcome after multifetal pregnancy reduction. J Matern Fetal Neonatal Med. 2004;16(1):27-31.
38. Evans MI, Dommergues M, Timor-Tritsch I, et al. Transabdominal versus transcervical and transvaginal multifetal pregnancy reduction: international collaborative experience of more than one thousand cases. Am J Obstet Gynecol. 1994;170(3):902-9.
39. Evans MI, Littman L, Richter R, et al. Selective reduction for multifetal pregnancy. Early opinions revisited. J Reprod Med. 1997;42(12):771-7.
40. Yaron Y, Bryant-Greenwood PK, Dave N, et al. Multifetal pregnancy reductions of triplets to twins: comparison with nonreduced triplets and twins. Am J Obstet Gynecol. 1999;180(5):1268-71.

Chapter

11

Assessing Complications of Assisted Reproduction Treatment

Miriam Baumgarten, Lukasz Polanski

Chapter Outline

FERTILITY TREATMENT BACKGROUND

Infertility has an increasing impact on health services worldwide due to the rising rate of fertility impairment among the general population, which often requires assisted reproduction treatment (ART). These techniques are expensive and frequently require multiple attempts to prove successful. With the birth of the first in vitro fertilization (IVF) baby in 1978, it became possible to give hope of a biologically own child to couples with various causes of infertility that otherwise would remain childless. Although throughout the years, these techniques have been used more commonly, there is still limited data on the, especially long-term, health effect for the women.

In the 1970s during the beginning of IVF treatment, oocyte retrievals were performed via the laparoscopic route in a natural cycle. Embryo and gametes were replaced into the Fallopian tubes. Over the last two decades, an enormous progress has been made aiming to improve the efficacy of all components of the IVF treatment process. Natural cycle IVF with laparoscopic oocyte retrievals and laparoscopic embryo transfers have been replaced by controlled ovarian stimulation with transvaginal oocyte retrieval (TVOR) and ultrasound-guided intrauterine embryo transfers. All these steps aim to make the treatment as patient-friendly and minimally invasive as possible. Although current IVF practice is generally safe, it is still not without associated complications.

In approximately 2% of ART cycles, various complications occur. Some of these can be prevented, some cannot. Complications of the ART process can be stimulation related, procedure related, or pregnancy related. Ovarian hyperstimulation syndrome (OHSS) is responsible for the majority of cycle-related complications, followed by bleeding and infection secondary to oocyte retrieval.

STIMULATION COMPLICATION

Ovarian Cysts

Although considered an adverse effect rather than a complication of stimulation, cysts can occur during pituitary downregulation with gonadotropin-releasing hormone (GnRH) agonists.[1] These cysts rarely cause symptoms, but can prevent optimal ovarian stimulation and influence treatment outcome. These cysts can be found during ultrasound assessment to confirm ovarian downregulation. Expectant or medical management can be attempted. However, an ultrasound-guided transvaginal cyst aspiration can be an option.

The incidence of functional cysts (Fig. 11.1) has been reported to be between 8% and 53%.[2] Qublan et al.[3] conducted a prospective study to assess the incidence and impact of ovarian cyst formation following administration of GnRH agonist on IVF cycle outcome. They concluded that the incidence of cyst formation during treatment is

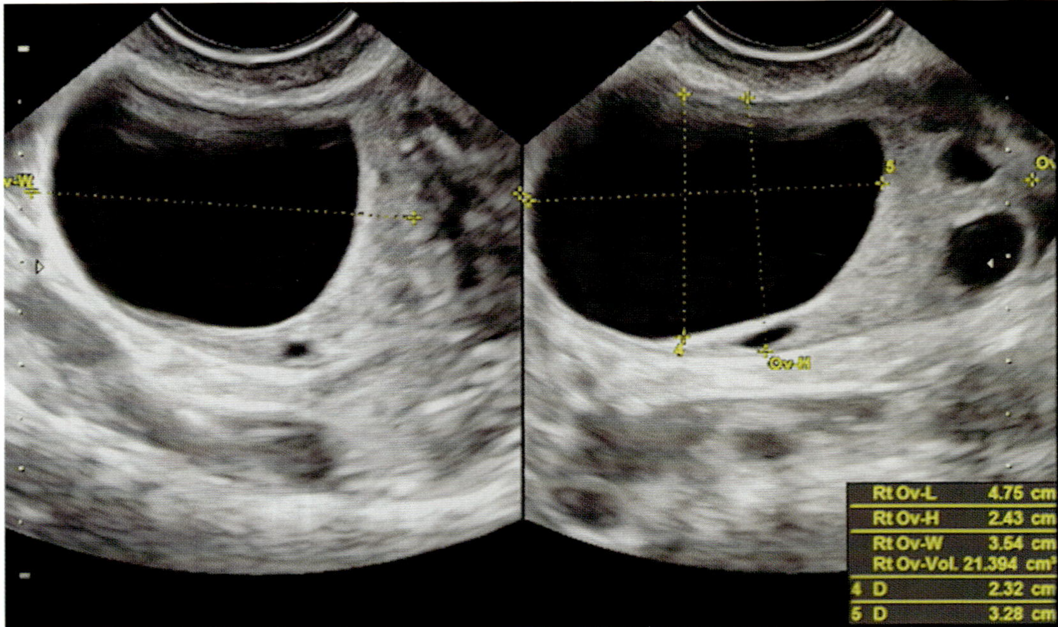

Fig. 11.1: Follicular cysts in ovary at downregulation scan.

lower than previously reported. In their study, the quality of oocytes and embryos was significantly compromised by the presence of a newly developed cyst, leading to a significant increase in cycle cancelation and a decrease in subsequent implantation and pregnancy rates. Neither conservative management nor cyst aspiration improved the IVF outcome.

Adnexal Torsion

Adnexal torsion is an infrequent but serious complication of ovarian stimulation. It should be suspected in every patient complaining of abdominal pain and nausea during, or after ovarian stimulation. Ovarian torsion is mainly caused by ovarian cysts, either pre-existing or being a direct result of the stimulation protocols.[4]

The incidence of simple cyst formation and associated torsion during stimulation is not well registered. The estimation of the prevalence is difficult, as most of the cysts remain asymptomatic. Kemmann et al.[5] described 4 cases of adnexal torsion among 648 menotropin-induced pregnancies. In a series of 154 women having 201 cycles complicated by OHSS, 75 got pregnant. Out of these 75 women with OHSS 12 (16%) presented with torsion of hyperstimulated ovary. Only 3 out of 126 nonpregnant cycles (2.3%) had a torsion.[6]

Diagnosis and Treatment

The diagnosis of adnexal torsion is usually difficult due to the nonspecific presenting symptoms, often leading to a delayed surgical intervention and loss of the affected ovary. Combination of ovarian enlargement, abdominal pain, nausea, progressive leukocytosis, and anemia might suggest adnexal torsion, especially given the history of previous ovarian cysts or ovarian hyperstimulation. On gray-scale imaging, the ovary is cystic and enlarged with heterogenous reduced echotexture (Fig. 11.2A). Follicles are often pushed toward the periphery. There may be small amount of free fluid in the pelvis. Doppler imaging may reveal reduced or absent Doppler signals with twisted ovarian pedicle (whirlpool sign) (Figs. 11.2B and C).

The only effective treatment of adnexal torsion can be achieved surgically. Although intraoperatively the adnexae appear dark, hemorrhagic, and/or ischemic, it is most likely that circulation will be restored by simply unwinding the torted pedicle in order to restore normal anatomy. This often is the only intervention required and allows for preservation of the ovary. In 11 cases of ovarian torsion following IVF, intraoperative unwinding of the adnexa was performed resulting in return of spontaneous circulation in eight patients. In the mentioned case series, no postoperative complications were reported and when the ovary

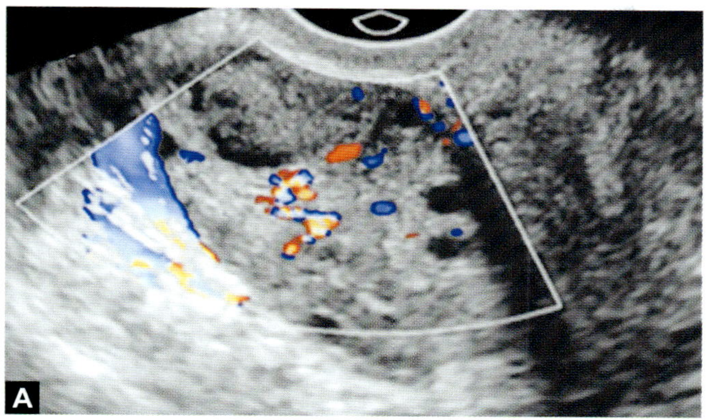

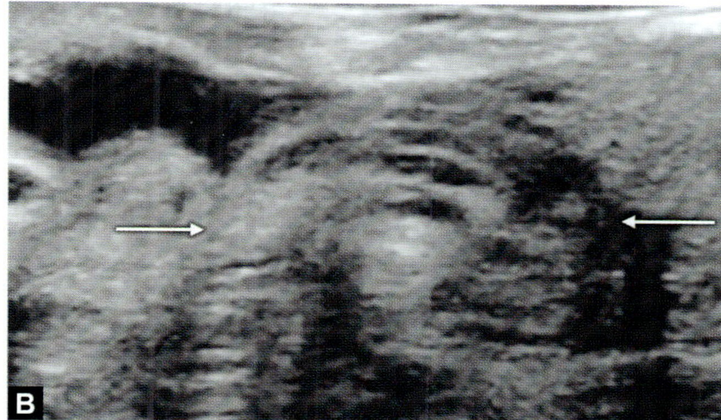

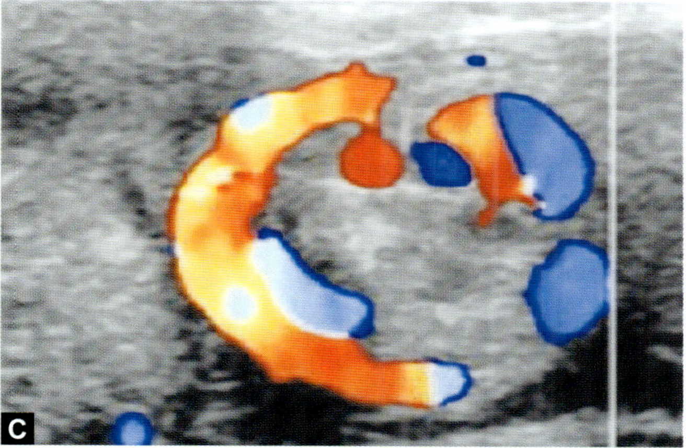

Figs. 11.2A to C: (A) Heterogenously hypoechoic ovary with reduced vascularity. (B) Free fluid in pelvis and whirlpool sign in adnexa seen on B-mode scan in a patient with ovarian torsion. (C) Whirlpool sign on color Doppler (*Courtesy:* Dr. Boopathy).

was spared, subsequent sonographic evaluation revealed its normal function. The authors concluded that torsion of hyperstimulated adnexa in patients that conceived after gonadotropin therapy is a special clinical entity requiring attention to achieve early diagnosis.[6]

Ovarian Hyperstimulation Syndrome

Ovarian hyperstimulation syndrome is by far the most important risk of ART stimulation. The complications resulting from OHSS, mainly thromboembolic events, are the cause of major morbidity and mortality.[7] Ovarian hyperstimulation syndrome is a condition inherently related with controlled ovarian stimulation. However, in extremely rare occasions, it can occur in a spontaneous ovulatory cycle.[8] The clinical symptoms of OHSS are most likely the result of increased vascular permeability of the gonadotropin-primed ovaries. The ovaries are bilaterally enlarged due to the presence of multiple follicular and theca lutein cysts. In addition to the physical enlargement of ovaries, an acute shift of intravascular fluid distribution occurs, causing clinical ascites leading to the development of abdominal distension, pain, and shortness of breath due to an upward diaphragm displacement.

Ovarian hyperstimulation syndrome occurs more typically as an iatrogenic complication in women undergoing IVF or intracytoplasmic sperm injection (ICSI), where supraphysiological doses of gonadotropin are used to induce multifollicular growth. Development of a large number of follicles, increasing ovarian size and serum estrogen levels, can cause serious complications and ultimately result in death.[9-12]

The first classification of OHSS used the measurement of hormones in 24 hours urine collections. When these tests became obsolete, Golan et al. adjusted the classification of OHSS in 1989.[13] A new component of ultrasound and its findings was introduced. Rizk and Aboulghar made the most recent classification of OHSS.[14]

Table 11.1: Classification of OHSS based on clinical and ultrasound features

OHSS	*Symptoms*	*Ultrasound features*
Mild	Abdominal bloating mild abdominal pain	Ovarian size usually less than 8 cm
Moderate	Moderate abdominal pain nausea ± vomiting	Evidence of ascites ovarian size usually 8–12 cm
Severe	Clinical ascites (occasionally hydrothorax) oliguria Hemoconcentration hematocrit more than 45% hypoproteinemia	Ovarian size usually more than 12 cm
Critical	Tense ascites or large hydrothorax Hematocrit more than 55% White cell count more than 25,000/mL Oligo/anuria Thromboembolism Acute respiratory distress syndrome	

Their classification included only two categories: (1) moderate OHSS and (2) severe OHSS. The aim of this classification was to make the diagnosis simple and clinically more relevant, as treatment and prognosis could be advised according to the category. The Royal College of Obstetricians and Gynaecologists (RCOG) provides us with a classification and advises on appropriate treatment including that for mild OHSS and moderate OHSS, modified as suggested by Mathur et al. in 2005.[15] Table 11.1 is the used classification of severity of OHSS in the United Kingdom (UK).

Incidence

The accurate incidence of OHSS is difficult to estimate due to different classifications of the condition used. The incidence also varies between different patient groups and treatments used. In IVF, up to 33% of cycles result in the development of mild OHSS. Although mild OHSS is considered clinically insignificant, it still has the potential to progress into the severe form, which is estimated to occur in 3.1–8.0% of cycles.[16]

Ultrasound Features

According to the most recent classification of OHSS by the RCOG, ovarian size estimation is used as one of the factors differentiating the clinical categories of this condition. The authors of the guidance notes advise caution, as ovarian size may not directly correlate with the clinical severity of OHSS in cases of assisted reproduction due to the effect of follicular aspiration. Using ultrasound, mild OHSS usually presents with a maximal ovarian dimension of less than 8 cm, moderate OHSS usually averages 8–12 cm with sonographic evidence of ascites (Figs. 11.3A to D), and in cases of severe OHSS the ovarian size usually exceeds 12 cm.[17]

Management

The clinical course of OHSS depends on its severity and the development of complications, and on the establishment of a pregnancy. It is considered a self-limiting disease, and treatment is mainly based on symptom management.[18] The critical cases remain a unique challenge for both fertility and intensive-care specialists.[14]

Moderate OHSS can be monitored on an outpatient basis. Monitoring would consist of follow-up by regular phone calls to the patient, and patient visits to the unit. During these visits assessment by ultrasound and full blood count, liver enzymes, and coagulation profile can be performed. Culdocentesis can be offered on an outpatient basis. In addition to alleviating discomfort, it should be considered for the prevention of disease progression in moderate or severe OHSS cases.[19]

Patients with tense ascites causing significant pain and/or respiratory compromise can benefit from paracentesis. Paracentesis will also improve oliguria which is secondary to reduced renal perfusion from ascites increasing intra-abdominal pressure and compromising the blood flow to the kidneys.[20,21]

If the situation of the patient requires hospitalization, her condition should be monitored by regular vital signs, daily weight, and girth measurement. Strict fluid balance is needed, particularly urine output. Minimal biochemical blood tests include electrolytes, kidney and liver functions test, coagulation, and a full blood count. An ultrasound

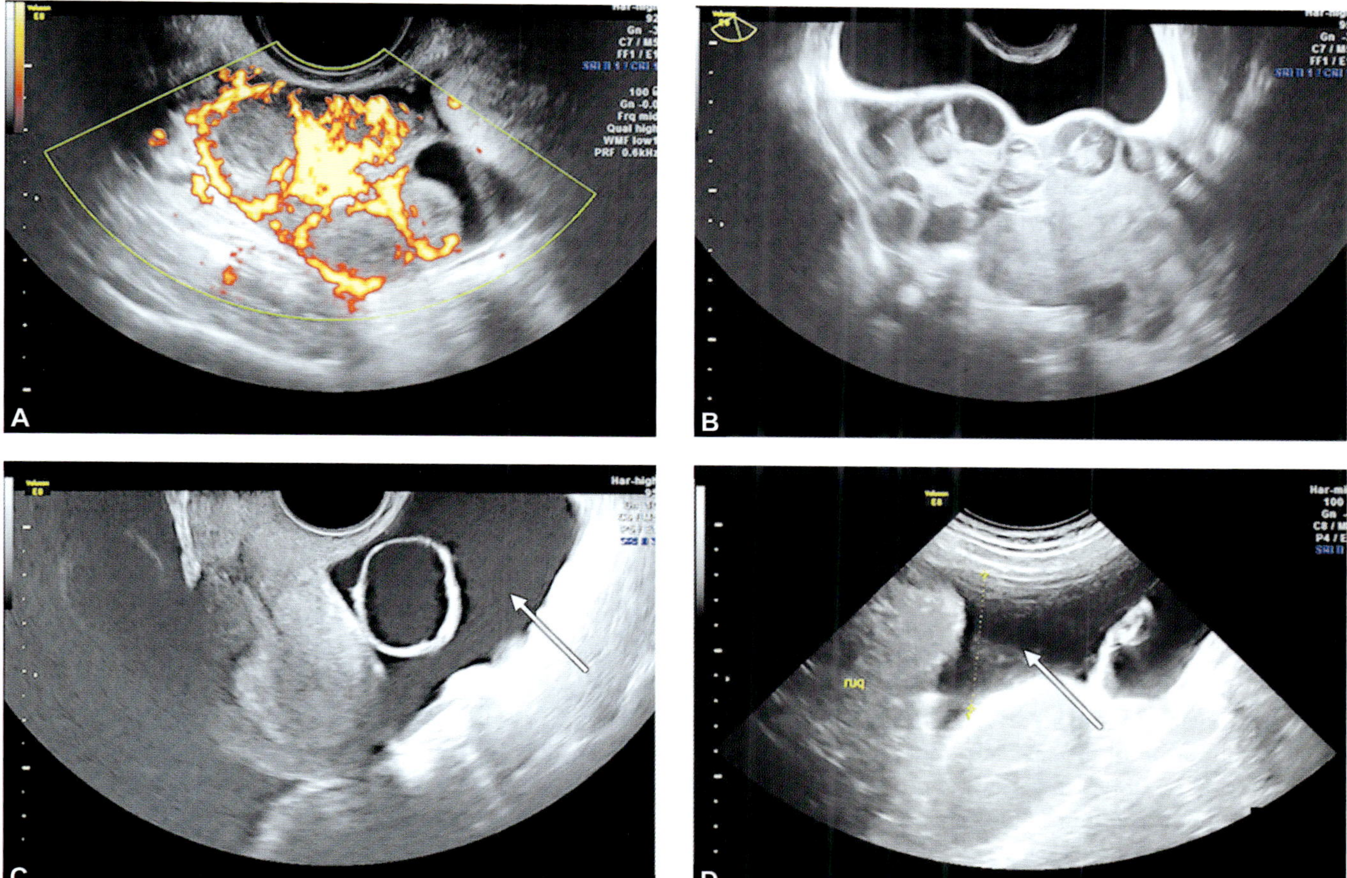

Figs. 11.3A to D: Ovarian hyperstimulation syndrome: (A) Power Doppler image demonstrates increased vascularity within the ovarian stroma of the postoocyte collection ovary. (B) Transvaginal ultrasound image demonstrating enlarged ovaries following transvaginal ultrasound-guided oocyte retrieval in a patient that developed OHSS ("kissing ovaries"). (C) Significant amount of free fluid in the pouch of Douglas (POD) (arrow). (D) Transabdominal ultrasound image of the right upper quadrant. Significant amount of free fluid in Morrison's pouch (arrow).

can be used to evaluate ovarian volumes and the presence of ascites. In addition, the diagnosis of a viable intrauterine pregnancy can be made. Chest X-ray should only be performed in the suspicion of a hydrothorax.

COMPLICATIONS OF OOCYTE RETRIEVAL

Transvaginal ultrasound-guided oocyte retrieval during IVF treatment was first described in 1985.[22] By virtue of its simplicity and effectiveness, it gained widespread popularity and has now become the gold standard for IVF therapy. Nevertheless, despite the obvious advantages, the aspiration needle may injure the adjacent pelvic organs and structures leading to serious complications. The most common complications are hemorrhage, trauma and injury to pelvic structures, and subsequent pelvic infection. Other complications described in association with ultrasound-guided oocyte retrieval include adnexal torsion, rupture of endometriotic cysts, and even vertebral osteomyelitis. Puncturing the ovary under the guidance of ultrasound by introducing the needle into the field of vision manually is a difficult technique requiring a lot of experience. It becomes considerably simpler and safer with the use of fixed needle guides.

The transvaginal egg collection was studied in 1988 by Evers et al.[23] describing complications and problems in the first 181 transvaginal scan-guided follicle aspirations. No major complications occurred. In 3% of patients, it appeared impossible to aspirate the follicles because of a method-related problem such as localization of ovaries being too high above the vaginal fornix or the ovaries being too mobile. The method was found to be easily mastered with short learning curve and the oocyte yield of this method was already high, even in the early learning phase of the procedure. The mean duration of the procedure decreased from more than 30 minutes to less than 20 minutes in the first 7 months after the introduction of this technique in the IVF program.

On rare occasions when the ovary is located high as in certain cases of Rokitansky syndrome or due to other pelvic pathologies, or in case of cervical cancer, one may need to use laparoscopic-guided oocyte retrieval. Laparoscopic egg collection has similar complications to those described earlier, but the risk of injury to internal organs is higher when compared to ultrasound guidance. In addition, there is the risk of complications associated with the use of a general anesthetic, although this is a rare event in healthy young women.

Bergh et al. in 1991 conducted a survey of 12 large IVF clinics in Denmark, Finland, Norway, and Sweden. The questionnaire sent to the Nordic centers asked mainly about the numbers of clinical complications. The number of cycles in the 12 clinics in total was 10,125 with 7,331 embryo transfers performed and 1,116 clinical pregnancies.[24] At the time of the article publication, most oocyte collections were done by transvaginal ultrasound-guided aspirations, but less than 700 oocyte retrievals were still performed via the laparoscopic route. Of the commenced cycles 0.7% were complicated by OHSS requiring hospitalization. In this group, one patient had an ovarian torsion requiring surgery. Complications during the laparoscopic oocyte collection occurred in two patients, both of whom had subsequent laparotomy. In one case, injured intestine necessitated repair. In the other case, no intraperitoneal damage could be found. Complications were reported in the transvaginal ultrasound-guided follicle aspirations in 35 cases. They all involved bleeding. Most of the bleeding was vaginal which was successfully managed conservatively. In two cases, laparotomy was required to stop intraperitoneal hemorrhage (Fig. 11.4) from the ovarian veins. A retroperitoneal hematoma was suspected in two patients, but they were managed conservatively with full regression of symptoms. The overall complication rate of ultrasound-guided puncture was 0.7% (35 complications out of 5,122 embryo transfers). The authors chose to calculate the complication rate per embryo transfer because the collected data did not permit analysis per oocyte retrieval.

Deaths related to IVF were described by Braat et al.[25] Maternal mortality directly linked to IVF treatment in the Netherlands between 1984 and 2008 was investigated. Six deaths occurred in the period of 1990–1997. Three women suffered from severe OHSS, two died as a result of respiratory distress syndrome and multiorgan failure. One woman died of cerebrovascular thrombosis 3 days after oocyte retrieval. Two other women died of sepsis 31 and 62 days after oocyte retrieval. The last fatal case was related to a dose error of local anesthetic medication administered just before oocyte retrieval.[25]

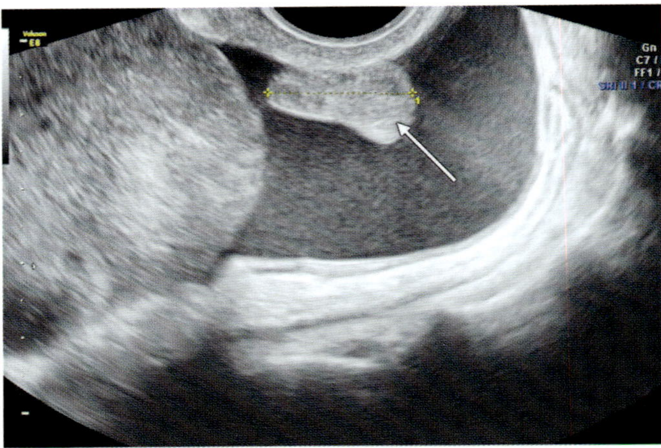

Fig. 11.4: Blood in the pouch of Douglas noted soon after egg collection with an organized blood clot (arrow), managed conservatively.

Limited evidence suggests that TVOR risks might be related to the number of previous oocyte collections via the transvaginal route. A vaginal perforation occurred when pressure was applied to the ultrasound probe in a 41-year-old woman undergoing her sixth ovarian stimulation cycle. The authors of this case report suggested that difficult access on the side of the injury, multiple previous oocyte collections, advanced age, and associated poor wound healing contributed to the complication.[26]

In the retrospective analysis of Roest et al.,[27] 2,495 consecutive cycles resulting in oocytes retrieval were assessed for major clinical complications. Around 0.7% of cycles were complicated by severe OHSS (grades 4 and 5) requiring hospitalization. Adnexal torsion occurred in two cases. In one case, torsion and ovarian rupture were diagnosed requiring an adnexectomy due to the inability to stop the bleeding following detorsion. One serious visceral injury was diagnosed when appendicitis developed a week after the IVF procedure. On day 8 after TVOR, a laparoscopic appendectomy was performed and on histological examination multiple puncture wounds were demonstrated.[28] In the series of Roest et al.,[23] pelvic inflammatory disease was diagnosed in 0.24% of cases, with an increase in body temperature to more than 38°C and signs of pelvic peritonitis on physical examination, accompanied by elevated leukocyte count and erythrocyte sedimentation rate.

Overall, injuries to internal organs such as bowels, bladder, or blood vessels during the transvaginal ultrasound-guided oocyte retrieval are an extremely rare complication with a historically quoted estimated incidence of approximately 1 in 1,000 cases.

Bleeding

Background

Bleeding during or after oocyte collection from the ovary or from the vagina is usually minimal and is very rarely a significant problem. The need for blood transfusion is rare and estimated to be around 1 in 500.

Incidence

In a report concerning 600 ultrasound-guided follicle aspirations, intraperitoneal bleeding was reported in 0.5% of cases, vaginal bleeding in 0.8%, and postoperative infection in 0.5% of the patients.[29]

Infection

Every invasive procedure carries the risk of introducing pathogens and subsequent development of localized or generalized infection. Infection following TVOR usually occurs within days of the intervention. Although a case report by Sharpe et al. illustrated the possibility of infection as a complication of TVOR presenting months after the procedure. In the case report, the authors describe a patient who did not become acutely ill despite the formation of a pelvic abscess because of a spontaneous development of a vaginal fistula, which allowed drainage of the abscess.[30]

Incidence

In the Nordic study, postoperative infections of clinical significance (pelvic abscesses) were reported in 20 patients, 0.3% per embryo transfer. Six of these patients had to be treated surgically. Two patients required drainage, two a bilateral salpingectomy, and two a unilateral salpingo-oophorectomy. In the other 14 cases, antibiotic treatment gave adequate result. In the clinics that performed ultrasound-guided aspiration, this resulted in postoperative infection of 0.2% per embryo transfer.[24]

In a cohort of 3,656 patients, Dicker et al.[31] reported 14 cases of acute abdomen (0.4%) following TVORs due to pelvic infections or bleeding.

Kelada et al.[32] performed a literature review stating incidences of pelvic infection between 0.4[32] and 1.3%.[33] They state that routine prophylactic administration of antibiotics remained controversial and of unproven benefit. It can be considered in patients with known adhesions, endometriosis, and pseudocysts.

MULTIPLE PREGNANCIES

While the ultimate aim of ART is to achieve a singleton pregnancy (Figs. 11.5A and B), ARTs have contributed to the increasing rate of multiple gestations over the past

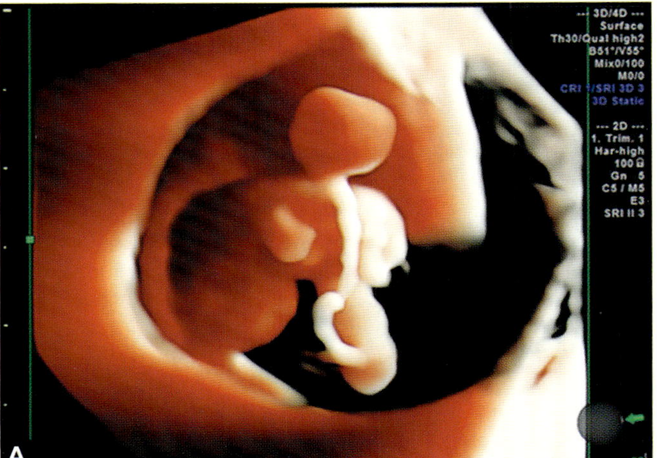

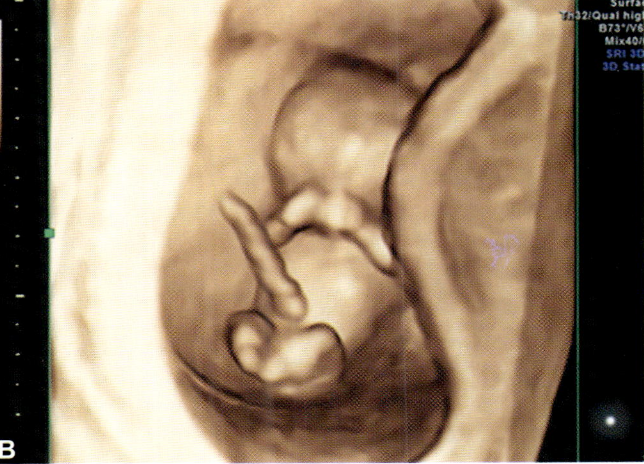

Figs. 11.5A and B: Three-dimensional (3D) reconstruction of a singleton intrauterine pregnancy: (A) 6–7 weeks and (B) 10 weeks.

two decades. Recent figures indicate approximately one in five IVF pregnancies are multiple gestations. This is in stark contrast to the spontaneous conception background rate of 1 in 80.[34] Higher-order pregnancies (triplet or more) in approximately two-thirds of cases are the result of ovulation induction without the use of IVF or any similar procedure.[35] Prevention of multiple gestations in the ovulation induction population should commence at the treatment stage. Development of three or more follicles of 10 mm or more on the day of human chorionic gonadotropin (hCG) injection is the leading cause of increased risk of multiple pregnancies, and multifollicular development should be avoided when stimulated ovulation induction is used.[36] During IVF treatment, irrespective of age, transfer of a single blastocyst stage embryo carries a less than 2% multiple gestation risk. For a double blastocyst embryo transfer, the risk approximates 39%, whereas a double cleavage stage embryo transfer carries a 27% risk of multiple gestation.[34]

Ultrasound is a very useful tool in the diagnosis of multiple gestations. Two terms require clarification before a description of sonographic diagnosis of multiple gestations can be attempted. These terms are zygocity and chorionicity. Depending on the type of conception, two types of twin pregnancies can be distinguished. Dizygotic (DZ) twins are a result of implantation of two fertilized ova; monozygotic (MZ) twins arise when a single embryo splits during the initial weeks following fertilization.[37,38] Chorionicity refers to the type of placentation. In a monochorionic (MC) placenta, the separating membrane between the twins consists of two adjacent amnions. Dichorionic (DC) twin pregnancies are separated by two layers of chorion and amnion, each originating from one of the twins.[39] Dizygotic twins are always DC, monochorionic twins are always MZ.[39] Depending on the time of the embryo division different types of MZ twins can occur. Embryo division up until 4 days following fertilization leads to formation of a DC diamniotic (DCDA) MZ pregnancy. Division 4–8 days following fertilization leads to formation of a MC diamniotic (MCDA) MZ pregnancy which is the most common type of MZ twins. Monochorionic monoamniotic (MCMA) MZ twin gestations account for up to 4% of MZ twins and occur when a zygote splits 8–12 days following fertilization. Later division of the embryo leads to development of conjoined twins.[39] Prior to the eighth week of pregnancy, identification of two distinct gestation sacs within the endometrial cavity diagnoses a DC gestation. Chorionicity can be detected by identification of the "lambda sign" or "twin peak sign" (Figs. 11.6A and B) which is present in up to 99–100% of DC pregnancies between 10th and 14th completed week of gestation.[40,41] As the pregnancy progresses, the "lambda sign" might disappear, so that determination of chorionicity in the second and third trimesters is not reliable. The "lambda sign" signifies the presence of chorion frondosum between the two layers of amniotic membranes.[39] The amniotic membranes can be identified at around the eighth week of pregnancy; hence, accurate determination of amnionicity in MC twins can be performed at this time. Earlier in pregnancy, presence of two distinct yolk sacs in the extraembryonic coelom predicts the twin pregnancy to be diamniotic (Figs. 11.7A to F). Presence of a single yolk sac indicates the pregnancy that can form an MC monoamniotic gestation,

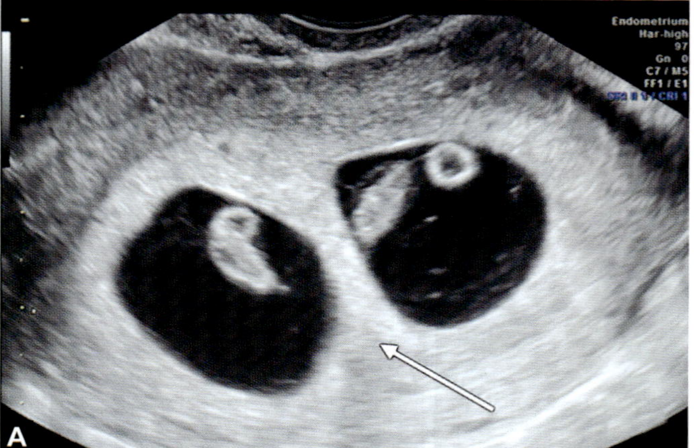

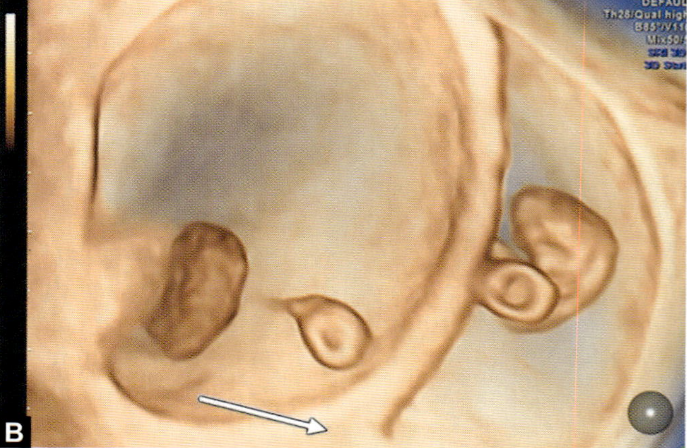

Figs. 11.6A and B: Dichorionic, diamniotic twin gestation (7–8 weeks of gestation). A "lambda sign" is clearly distinguishable on the two-dimensional (2D) and 3D ultrasound images (arrows).

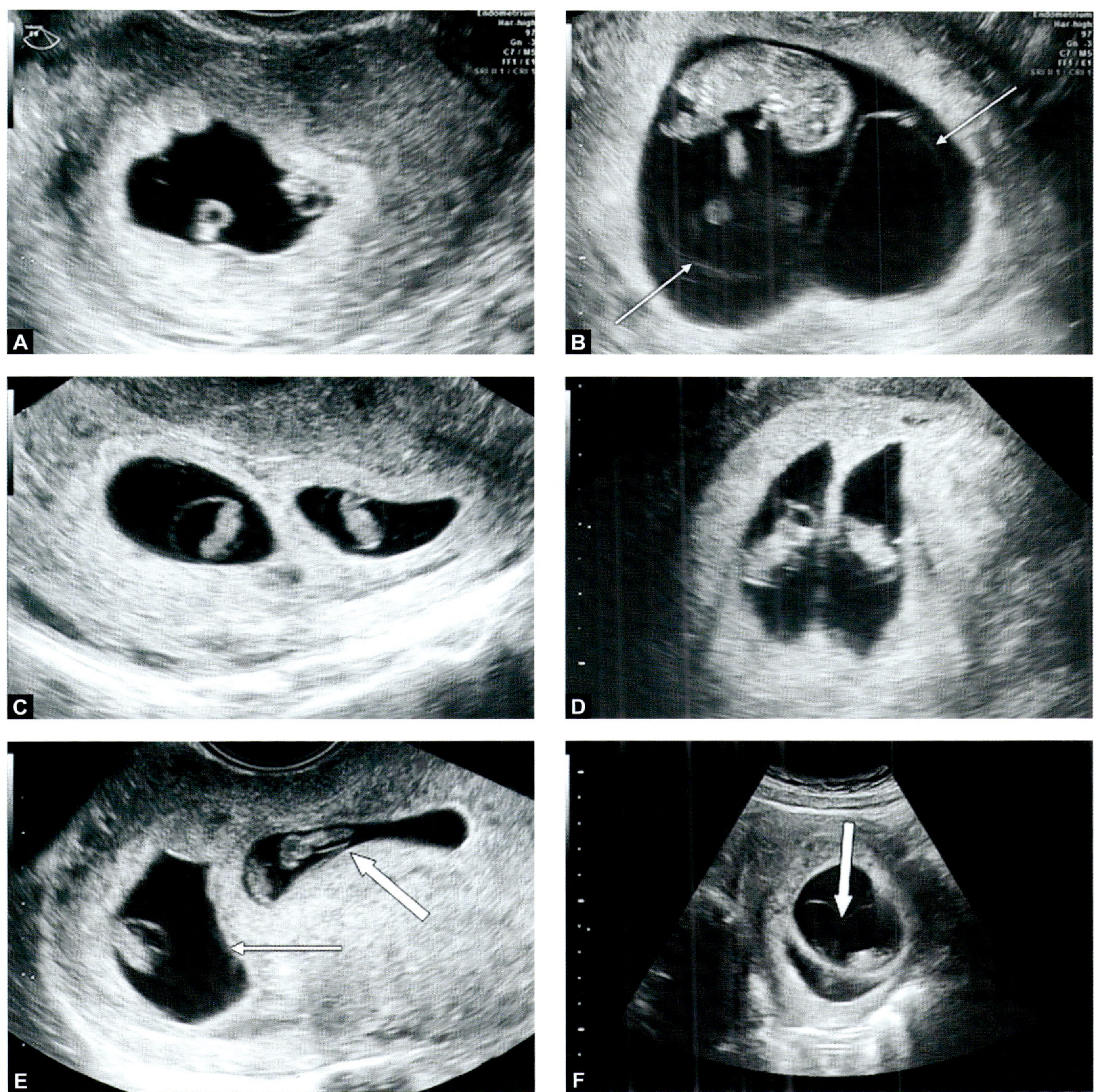

Figs. 11.7A to F: Multiple gestations: (A) Monochorionic, diamniotic twins at 5–6 weeks of gestation. The separating membrane is not yet distinguishable. (B) Same pregnancy at 9–10 weeks of gestation. Both amnions are clearly visible (arrows). (C and D) Various appearances of septae separating DCDA twins (6–7 weeks of gestation). (E) Triplet pregnancy: Two gestation sacs are visible, on containing a single fetus (thin arrow); second one containing two fetuses (thick arrow). (F) A thin separating membrane is visible, characterizing the twins as MCDA (arrow) in a triplet pregnancy. (*Abbrivation:* DCDA, dichorionic diamniotic; MCDA, monochorionic diamniotic)

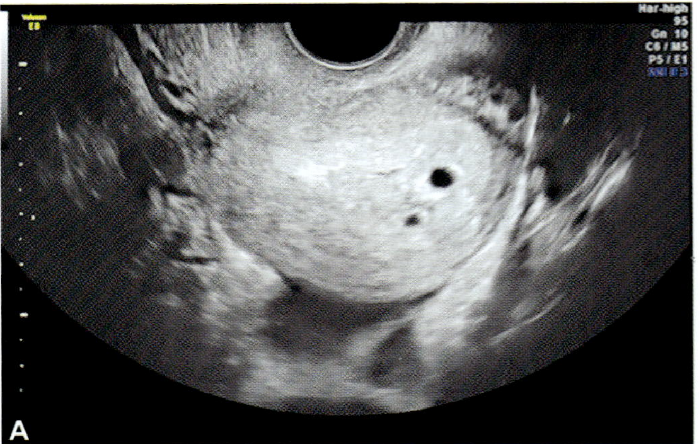

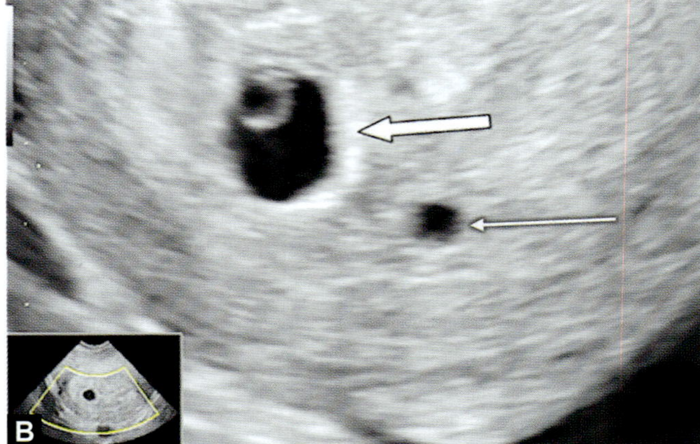

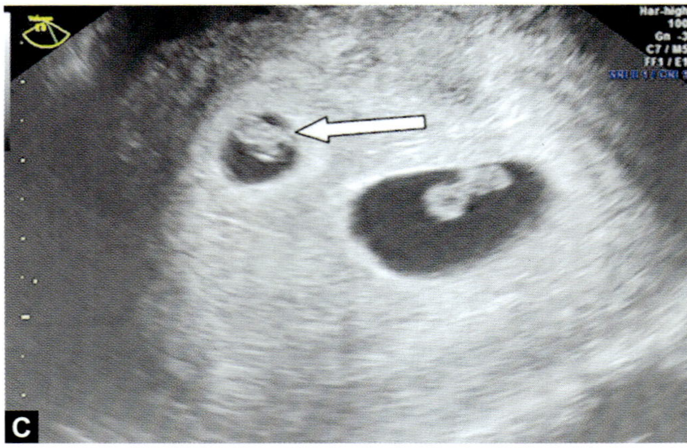

Figs. 11.8A to C: (A) Early onset twin growth discrepancy, "vanishing twin syndrome." (B) Gestation sac of the affected twin is smaller eliciting a less pronounced decidual reaction (thin arrow) compared to the normally developing twin (large arrow). There is no content within the affected gestation sac (5–6 weeks of gestation). (C) Gestation sac is smaller, no fetal cardiac activity is noted within the twin affected by growth restriction (arrow) (missed miscarriage) (6–7 weeks of gestation).

and this warrants a rescan in the latter half of the first trimester to accurately diagnose the type of a twin gestation.[39,42]

First trimester growth discrepancy has been associated with an increased risk of miscarriage of one or both the twins (Figs. 11.8A to C). Irrespective of chorionicity, an early first trimester (7 + 0 to 9 + 6 weeks) crown-rump length (CRL) discrepancy of less than 20% predicts both viable fetuses with a likelihood of 97% on a subsequent scan at 11th–14th week of gestation. A discrepancy of more than 60% has been related to a loss of both twins.[43] The so-called "vanishing twin syndrome," where a pregnancy commences as a twin pregnancy and ends in the delivery of a single fetus is relatively common in the ART setting. Around 10.4% singleton pregnancies resulting from IVF treatment were conceived as a twin pregnancy. Observational studies suggest that if spontaneous twin reduction to a singleton pregnancy occurred later than the eighth week of pregnancy, significant obstetric and neurological sequelae are more prevalent in the live born sibling.[44] This data can be used to counsel couples considering double embryo transfers in an ART cycle.

Higher-order gestations are diagnosed and described in a similar fashion as twin pregnancies. In triplet pregnancies, the chorionicity and amnionicity of each triplet is described in relation to the other: fetus 1 with fetus 2, 1 with 3, and 2 with 3. Monochorionic triplets are always MZ. Dichorionic triplets can be MZ or DZ, whereas trichorionic triplets can be MZ, DZ, or trizygotic.[45] If doubt regarding chorionicity and amnionicity exists, a repeat ultrasound scan should be arranged. Sonographic assessment of higher-order pregnancies should follow the same principals as is used in triplet pregnancies.

The clinical management and risks related to high-order pregnancies are beyond the scope of this chapter and will not be considered further.

ECTOPIC PREGNANCY

Development of a pregnancy outside of the endometrial cavity can be broadly termed as an ectopic pregnancy (EP). Multiple sites of implantation of an early pregnancy are possible, including the Fallopian tubes, ovaries, the cervix, cesarean section scar, interstitial portions of the tube, and the abdominal cavity, with Fallopian tubes being the most frequent site of implantation. Contemporaneous existence of an ectopic and an intrauterine gestation is termed a heterotopic pregnancy. Approximately 1% of all spontaneously conceived pregnancies develop as an EP. The incidence of heterotopic pregnancies in the general population is estimated to be 1 in 20,000 to 1 in 50,000 pregnancies. In the ART setting, this can be as frequent as 1 in 100.[46]

The overall trend of ectopic gestations is on the increase. This is thought to be related to an increasing prevalence of pelvic infections caused by such pathogens as *Chlamydia trachomatis* and *Neisseria gonorrhea,* as well as the wide spread use of ART. Incidence of EPs associated with ART, where an embryo transfer was performed, is approximately 1–3%.[47] In view of the high frequency of occurrence of this potentially fatal condition, an early transvaginal scan is recommended in all women undergoing IVF or ICSI. This should be routinely performed between 6 and 8 weeks of gestation.[47] The clinical manifestations of an EP can vary greatly, with the initial symptoms developing as early as the fifth week of gestation, or as late as the 12th week of gestation.[48] Asymptomatic patients are diagnosed during an ultrasound scan; however, symptomatic cases can present with a significant intra-abdominal hemorrhage and signs of hypovolemic shock requiring immediate surgery.

With current ultrasound equipment, transvaginal ultrasound is the basic diagnostic tool for identification of ectopic gestations. Upon presentation, two-thirds of ectopic gestations should be diagnosed at the initial transvaginal ultrasound scan, and up to 91% of EPs should be reliably diagnosed using ultrasound alone prior to instigating any treatment.[48,49] When no pregnancy tissue is identified on an ultrasound scan, either inside or outside of the uterus, this clinical state is termed a "pregnancy of unknown location (PUL)." It is estimated that approximately 10% of PUL patients will have an EP visualized on a subsequent ultrasound.[48] Prior to the advent of high-definition transvaginal ultrasound, a "pseudosac" has been related with EPs. Current sonographic equipment should be able to distinguish an early gestation sac, located eccentrically in the endometrial cavity and surrounded by a decidual response, from blood or fluid within the cavity, this however can be operator dependent (Fig. 11.9).[48] Use of the term "pseudosac" is no longer recommended, and if doubt as to the nature of the transonic area within the cavity exists, a second opinion and appropriate follow-up should be arranged.

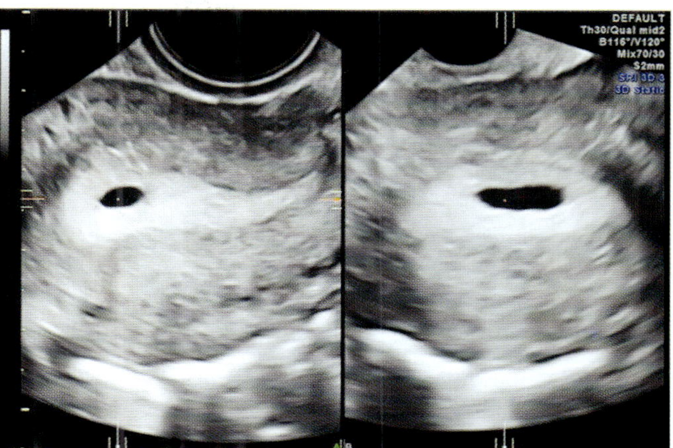

Fig. 11.9: Pseudosac: A cystic structure with regular outline, filled with anechoic fluid displacing the midline of the endometrial cavity. Note absence of decidual reaction around the pseudosac.

Classical approach to sonographic diagnosis of EPs consisted of a transabdominal ultrasound scan followed by a transvaginal approach. The abdominal route does not provide much useful information for the diagnosis of EPs, hence its routine use is currently not recommended.[48] The transvaginal approach is generally well tolerated and allows for tactile assessment of pelvic organs under sonographic "vision."

Systematic and thorough assessment of the pelvic organs is necessary to exclude an EP, especially when no gestation is visualized within the endometrial cavity. A measurement of the endometrium and comment on its appearance needs to be made in the ultrasound report. A detailed assessment of the adnexa should follow. Normal Fallopian tubes should not be visible on an ultrasound scan; however, any intra-Fallopian pathological process can lead to collection of fluid within the lumen of the oviduct, its distention, and wall thickening, allowing for visualization of the diseased tube.[50]

In spontaneous conceptions, majority of EPs (70–85%) are located on the ipsilateral side to the corpus

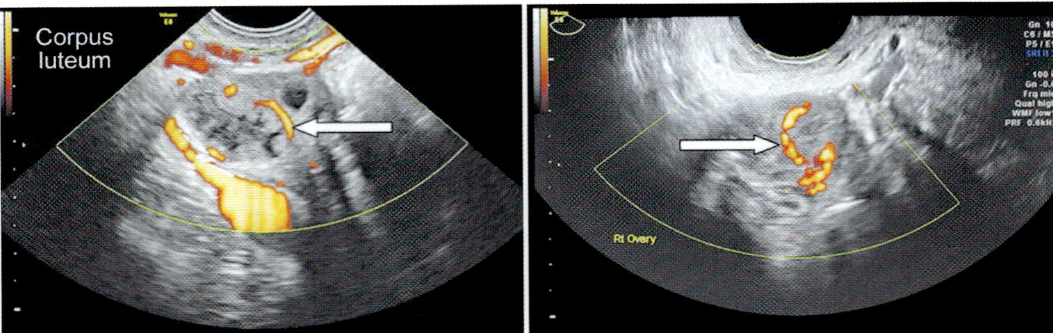

Fig. 11.10: Corpus luteum: A heterogenous mass within the boundaries of the ovary surrounded by increased Doppler signal (arrows), suggesting significant vascularity.

luteum (CL) which can be identified as a heterogenous mass within the boundaries of the ovary, and surrounded by a ring of increased vascularity as demonstrated by power Doppler sonography ("ring of fire") (Fig. 11.10).[48] In an embryo transfer ART cycle; no single CL can be identified, so the mentioned association does not apply. Approximately 60% of tubal EPs have an appearance of a heterogenous mass located between the uterine corpus and the ovary. With gentle pressure applied by the operator via the sonographic probe, this mass moves separately to the mentioned organs. Presence of pain in the region containing the suspicious lesion provides additional clinical information, increasing the suspicion of an EP. Twenty percent of EPs have an appearance of a hyperechogenic ring, or a "bagel sign," and 13% resemble a normally developing pregnancy with a gestation sac containing a yolk sac, fetal pole with or without fetal cardiac activity (Figs. 11.11A to C).[48] A concomitant finding might be presence of particulate fluid (ground-glass appearance) within the pouch of Douglas (POD). This signifies an intra-abdominal blood collection which can be either a sign of tubal rupture or leakage of blood from the fimbrial end of the affected tube. When free fluid is identified in the POD, a transabdominal scan can be performed to assess the presence of fluid in the upper abdomen, namely in the space between Glisson's capsule of the liver and Gerota's fascia of the right kidney (the Morison's pouch). Positive finding signifies at least 670 mL intra-abdominal hemorrhage.[51,52]

Interstitial EP is characterized by absence of trophoblastic tissue within the endometrial cavity, which however can be identified within the myometrial (interstitial) part of the tube. A thin, continuous rim of myometrium is present.[48] At an early stage of development, three-dimensional (3D) assessment of the uterus in the coronal plane can aid in diagnosis of an interstitial pregnancy located within the myometrial part of the Fallopian tube. High vascularity of the site of implantation makes them a significant health risk, if rupture occurs.

Cervical EPs are rare, but if undiagnosed and instrumented, can be a cause of a significant hemorrhage often requiring an emergency hysterectomy. Sonographic findings in case of this EP consist of an empty endometrial cavity and presence of trophoblast below the internal cervical os (Fig. 11.12). Lack of a "sliding sign" when gentle pressure is applied to the cervix differentiates an implanted cervical ectopic from a miscarrying intrauterine pregnancy.[48] Cesarean scar pregnancy is diagnosed in a similar way, with an empty endometrial cavity and gestation tissue located within the anterior myometrium in the region of the previous surgical scar (Fig. 11.13).

Rare ovarian EPs can pose a diagnostic dilemma, especially in the IVF setting. Follicles of stimulated ovaries post-TVOR, often refill with fluid and demonstrate an increased peripheral vascularity. This on occasions can mimic an ectopic gestation. Ovarian EPs have a thick outer hyperechogenic ring differentiating it from a benign ovarian cyst, or a postoocyte collection follicle.[48] Thorough assessment in combination with Doppler ultrasonography and experience allows for differentiation of these two different conditions.

Improvement in the quality and resolution of sonographic equipment allows transvaginal ultrasound to be the gold standard of diagnosis of all EPs, but only when used by appropriately trained medical personnel. If diagnostic doubt exists, appropriate follow-up consisting of a second opinion, serial serum beta-hCG, and repeat ultrasound scan can be suggested depending on the patient's clinical condition and access to out of hours of emergency services. Septate uterus is a concomitant finding.

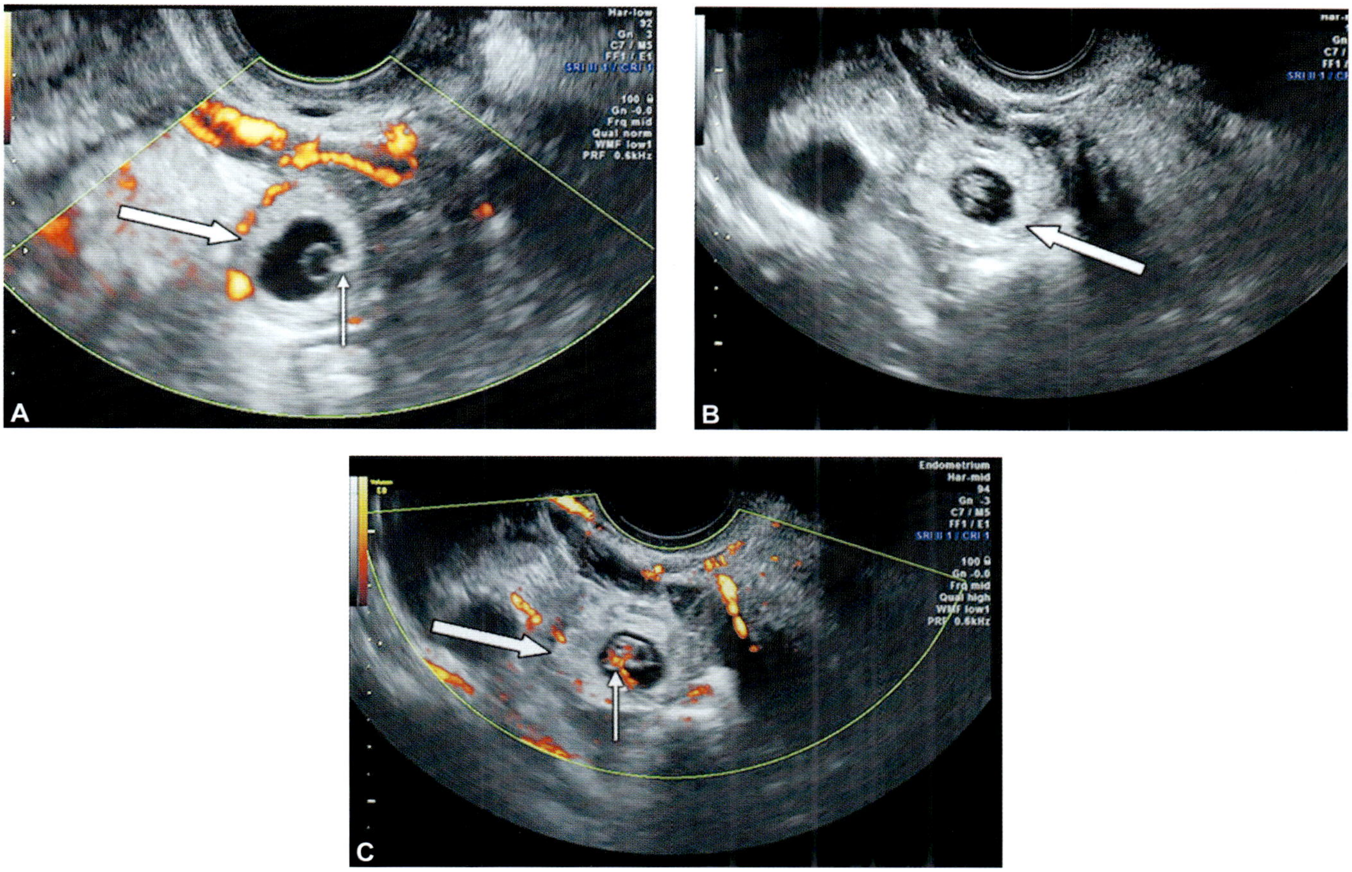

Figs. 11.11A to C: Tubal ectopic pregnancy (EP): A hyperechoic ring is distinguishable (gestation sac) (thick arrows) between the uterus and the ovary. The ectopic gestation sac contains a yolk sac and a fetal pole. Doppler image demonstrates fetal cardiac pulsatility (thin arrows). No free fluid is visible in the pelvis.

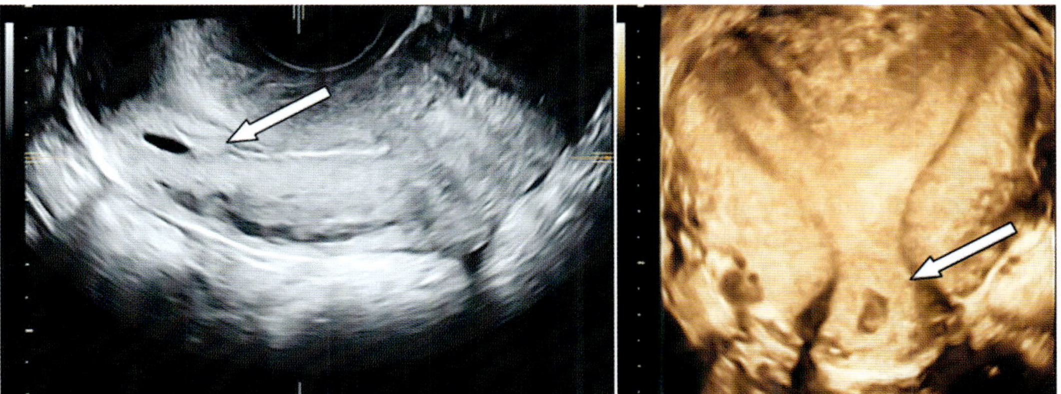

Fig. 11.12: Cervical ectopic pregnancy (EP) in retroverted uterus. Ectopic trophoblast (arrows) is located below the internal cervical os.

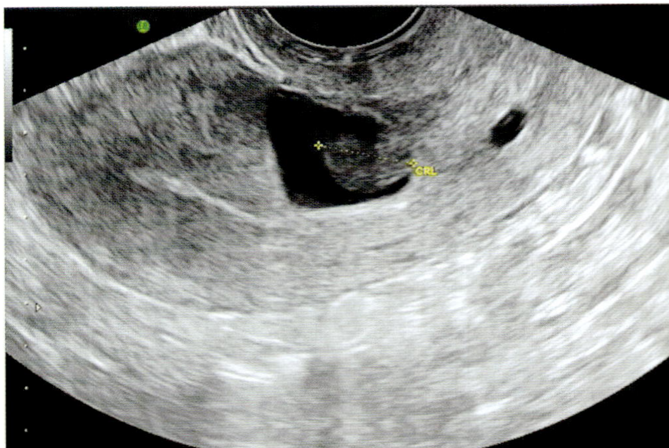

Fig. 11.13: Cesarean scar pregnancy: Gestational sac with fetus above the cervix, located in the previous cesarean scar, thin endometrium in the fundus of the uterus.

KEY POINTS

- Introduction of ultrasound has made ART more patient-friendly, minimally invasive, and less risky
- Complications of the ART process can be stimulation related, procedure related, or pregnancy related
- Adnexal torsion is an infrequent but serious complication of ovarian stimulation. The diagnosis is made clinically, but ultrasound features complement its diagnosis
- On ultrasound in a typical torsed ovary, follicles are often pushed toward the periphery. There may be small amount of free fluid in the pelvis. Doppler imaging may reveal reduced or absent Doppler signals with twisted ovarian pedicle (whirlpool sign)
- Ovarian hyperstimulation syndrome is by far the most important risk of ART stimulation
- Ultrasound pictures of OHSS (ovarian size and presence of free fluid in the pelvis and upper abdomen) help to classify and categorize its severity
- Ultrasound helps to diagnose the complications of oocyte retrieval such as internal bleeding and ovarian abscess
- Sonographic diagnosis of multiple gestations is easy but should define its zygocity and chorionicity for appropriate management of multiple pregnancies
- Systematic and thorough assessment of the pelvic organs is necessary to exclude an EP, especially when no gestation is visualized within the endometrial cavity
- While Fallopian tube is the most common site of EP, rarely cervical and cesarean EPs can also occur after ART
- Heterotopic pregnancies are more common after ART

REFERENCES

1. Jenkins JM, Anthony FW, Wood P, et al. The development of functional ovarian cysts during pituitary down-regulation. Hum Reprod. 1993;8(10):1623-7.
2. Biljan MM, Lapensée L, Mahutte NG, et al. Effects of functional ovarian cysts detected on the 7th day of gonadotropin-releasing hormone analog administration on the outcome of IVF treatment. Fertil Steril. 2000;74(5):941-5.
3. Qublan HS, Amarin Z, Tahat YA, et al. Ovarian cyst formation following GnRH agonist administration in IVF cycles: incidence and impact. Hum Reprod. 2006;21(3):640-4.
4. Hibbard LT. Adnexal torsion. Am J Obstet Gynecol. 1985;152(4):456-61.
5. Kemmann E, Ghazi DM, Corsan GH. Adnexal torsion in menotropin-induced pregnancies. Obstet Gynecol. 1990;76(3 Pt 1):403-6.
6. Mashiach S, Bider D, Moran O, et al. Adnexal torsion of hyperstimulated ovaries in pregnancies after gonadotropin therapy. Fertil Steril. 1990;53(1):76-80.
7. Chan WS, Dixon ME. The "ART" of thromboembolism: a review of assisted reproductive technology and thromboembolic complications. Thromb Res. 2008;121 (6):713-26.
8. Dieterich M, Bolz M, Reimer T, et al. Two different entities of spontaneous ovarian hyperstimulation in a woman with FSH receptor mutation. Reprod Biomed Online. 2010;20(6):751-8.
9. Beerendonk CC, van Dop PA, Braat DD, et al. Ovarian hyperstimulation syndrome: facts and fallacies. Obstet Gynecol Surv. 1998;53(7):439-49.
10. Mozes M, Bogokowsky H, Antebi E, et al. Thromboembolic phenomena after ovarian stimulation with human gonadotrophins. Lancet. 1965;2(7424):1213-5.
11. Semba S, Moriya T, Youssef EM, et al. An autopsy case of ovarian hyperstimulation syndrome with massive pulmonary edema and pleural effusion. Pathol Int. 2000;50(7):549-52.
12. Cluroe AD, Synek BJ. A fatal case of ovarian hyperstimulation syndrome with cerebral infarction. Pathology. 1995;27(4):344-6.
13. Golan A, Ron-el R, Herman A, et al. Ovarian hyperstimulation syndrome: an update review. Obstet Gynecol Surv. 1989;44(6):430-40.
14. Rizk B, Aboulghar M. Modern management of ovarian hyperstimulation syndrome. Hum Reprod. 1991;6(8):1082-7.
15. Mathur R, Evbuomwan I, Jenkins J. Prevention and management of ovarian hyperstimulation syndrome. Current Obstet Gynaecol. 2005;15:132-8.
16. Delvigne A, Rozenberg S. Epidemiology and prevention of ovarian hyperstimulation syndrome (OHSS): a review. Hum Reprod Update. 2002;8(6):559-77.
17. Navot D, Bergh PA, Laufer N. Ovarian hyperstimulation syndrome in novel reproductive technologies: prevention and treatment. Fertil Steril. 1992;58(2):249-61.
18. Delvigne A, Rozenberg S. Review of clinical course and treatment of ovarian hyperstimulation syndrome (OHSS). Hum Reprod Update. 2003;9(1):77-96.

19. Fluker MR, Copeland JE, Yuzpe AA. An ounce of prevention: outpatient management of the ovarian hyperstimulation syndrome. Fertil Steril. 2000;73(4):821-4.
20. Abramov Y, Elchalal U, Schenker JG. Pulmonary manifestations of severe ovarian hyperstimulation syndrome: a multicenter study. Fertil Steril. 1999;71(4):645-51.
21. Borenstein R, Elhalah U, Lunenfeld B, et al. Severe ovarian hyperstimulation syndrome: a reevaluated therapeutic approach. Fertil Steril. 1989;51(5):791-5.
22. El-Shawarby S, Margara R, Trew G, et al. A review of complications following transvaginal oocyte retrieval for in-vitro fertilization. Hum Fertil. 2004;7(2):127-33.
23. Evers JL, Larsen JF, Gnany GG, et al. Complications and problems in transvaginal sector scan-guided follicle aspiration. Fertil Steril. 1988;49(2):278-82.
24. Bergh T, Lundkvist O. Clinical complications during in-vitro fertilization treatment. Hum Reprod. 1992;7(5):625-6.
25. Braat DD, Schutte JM, Bernardus RE, et al. Maternal death related to IVF in the Netherlands 1984-2008. Hum Reprod. 2010;25(7):1782-6.
26. Cho MM, McGovern PG, Colon JM. Vaginal perforation during transvaginal ultrasound-guided follicle aspiration in a woman undergoing multiple cycles of assisted reproduction. Fertil Steril. 2004;81(6):1695-6.
27. Roest J, Mous HV, Zeilmaker GH, et al. The incidence of major clinical complications in a Dutch transport IVF programme. Hum Reprod Update. 1996;2(4):345-53.
28. Van Hoorde GJ, Verhoeff A, Zeilmaker GH. Perforated appendicitis following transvaginal oocyte retrieval for in-vitro fertilization and embryo transfer. Hum Reprod. 1992;7(6):850-1.
29. Baber R, Porter R, Picker R, et al. Transvaginal ultrasound directed oocyte collection for in vitro fertilization: successes and complications. J Ultrasound Med. 1988;7(7):377-9.
30. Sharpe K, Karovitch AJ, Claman P, et al. Transvaginal oocyte retrieval for in vitro fertilization complicated by ovarian abscess during pregnancy. Fertil Steril. 2006;86(1):219.e11-3.
31. Dicker D, Ashkenazi J, Feldberg D, et al. Severe abdominal complications after transvaginal ultrasonographically guided retrieval of oocytes for in vitro fertilization and embryo transfer. Fertil Steril. 1993;59(6):1313-5.
32. Kelada E, Ghani R. Bilateral ovarian abscesses following transvaginal oocyte retrieval for IVF: a case report and review of literature. J Assist Reprod Genet. 2007;24(4):143-5.
33. Tureck RW, Garcia CR, Blasco L, et al. Perioperative complications arising after transvaginal oocyte retrieval. Obstet Gynecol. 1993;81(4):590-3.
34. A Statistical Report: Human Fertilization & Embryology Authority. (2011). Improving outcomes for fertility patients: multiple births. [online]. Available from http://www.hfea.gov. uk/docs/2011-12-01_-_Multiple_Births_Publication_2011_-_Rationalising_Register_Data_-_FINAL_L2.DOC.pdf. [Accessed March, 2013].
35. Wilcox L, Kiely J, Melvin C, et al. Assisted reproductive technologies: estimates of their contribution to multiple births and newborn hospital days in the United States. Fertil Steril. 1996;65(2):361-6.
36. Tur R, Barri P, Coroleu B, et al. Risk factors for high-order multiple implantation after ovarian stimulation with gonadotrophins: evidence from a large series of 1878 consecutive pregnancies in a single centre. Hum Reprod. 2001;16(10):2124-9.
37. Bajoria R, Kingdom J. The case for routine determination of chorionicity and zygosity in multiple pregnancy. Prenat Diagn. 1997;17(13):1207-25.
38. Benirschke K. The biology of the twinning process: how placentation influences outcome. Semin Perinatol. 1995;19(5):342-50.
39. Sperling L, Tabor A. Twin pregnancy: the role of ultrasound in management. Acta Obstet Gynecol Scand. 2001;80(4):287-99.
40. Sepulveda W, Sebire NJ, Hughes K, et al. The lambda sign at 10-14 weeks of gestation as a predictor of chorionicity in twin pregnancies. Ultrasound Obstet Gynecol. 1996;7(6):421-3.
41. Sepulveda W, Sebire NJ, Nicolaides KH. The lambda sign in twin pregnancies. Ultrasound Obstet Gynecol. 1996;8(6):429.
42. Bromley B, Benacerraf B. Using the number of yolk sacs to determine amnionicity in early first trimester monochorionic twins. J Ultrasound Med. 1995;14(6):415-9.
43. Bora S, Bourne T, Bottomley C, et al. Twin growth discrepancy in early pregnancy. Ultrasound Obstet Gynecol. 2009;34(1):38-42.
44. Pinborg A, Lidegaard O, la Cour Freiesleben N, et al. Consequences of vanishing twins in IVF/ICSI pregnancies. Hum Reprod. 2005;20(10):2821-9.
45. Guilherme R, Drunat S, Delezoide AL, et al. Zygosity and chorionicity in triplet pregnancies: new data. Hum Reprod. 2009;24(1):100-5.
46. Ludwig M, Kaisi M, Bauer O, et al. Heterotopic pregnancy in a spontaneous cycle: do not forget about it! Eur J Obstet Gynecol Reprod Biol. 1999;87(1):91-3.
47. Kennedy R. (2005). Risks and complications of assisted conception. British Fertility Society Factsheet. [online]. Available from http://www.britishfertilitysociety.org.uk/public/factsheets/docs/BFS-risks%20and%20complications%20of%20assisted%20conception%20.pdf. [Accessed March, 2013].
48. Winder S, Reid S, Condous G. Ultrasound diagnosis of ectopic pregnancy. Australas J Ultrasound Med. 2011;14(2):29-33.
49. Condous G, Okaro E, Khalid A, et al. The accuracy of transvaginal ultrasonography for the diagnosis of ectopic pregnancy prior to surgery. Hum Reprod. 2005;20(5):1404-9.
50. Merz E. Gynecology. Ultrasound in Obstetrics and Gynecology, 2nd edition. Stuttgart, New York: Thieme; 2007.
51. Condous G, Okaro E, Bourne T. The conservative management of early pregnancy complications: a review of the literature. Ultrasound Obstet Gynecol. 2003;22(4):420-30.
52. Abrams BJ, Sukumvanich P, Seibel R, et al. Ultrasound for the detection of intraperitoneal fluid: the role of trendelenburg positioning. Am J Emerg Med. 1999;17(2):117-20.

Chapter

12

Application of Ultrasound in Evaluation of Male Infertility

S Boopathy Vijayaraghavan, G Swapna

Chapter Outline

INTRODUCTION

Male factors form one-third of the causes for infertility in a couple. Evaluation and effective management of male infertility has always been difficult due to lack of standard tests for functional assessment of sperm and inadequate knowledge of etiological factors and pathophysiology. While advances in the field of assisted reproduction in the form of intracytoplasmic sperm injection (ICSI) have revolutionized management of male infertility, there is limited progress in developing an effective treatment strategy to correct its etiopathogenesis. Causes of male infertility can be due to defects in sperm production, storage and maturation, transport, secretions of accessory organs, and delivery. Defects in production (testicular dysfunction) can result in either decreased quantity or abnormal function of the spermatozoa. Transport is affected by obstruction at various levels, i.e. epididymis, vas deferens, or ejaculatory duct. Disease of prostate and seminal vesicles can result in faulty secretion affecting the fertility. Delivery of the semen may be affected by stricture of urethra or retrograde ejaculation. A physical cause can be identified in one-third of these patients[1] and it is idiopathic in the rest. Causes include congenital or acquired urogenital abnormalities, genetic and immunological factors, endocrine factors, genital tract infection, and retrograde ejaculation. Imaging plays a role in identifying potentially correctable causes. An imaging investigation is useful when one of the following is suspected as the cause:

- Varicocele when there is abnormal sperms
- Nonpalpable (undescended) testes
- Obstructive causes

Abdominoscrotal scan is preferred when there are abnormal sperm parameters, undescended testes, or varicocele. Transrectal ultrasonography (TRUS) is performed when obstructive cause is considered. Sonography is almost always the initial imaging method, as it is noninvasive, safe, widely available, and is able to define many of the causes. It is useful in the evaluation of testicular morphology and vascular perfusion, patency of the efferent ducts and prostatic pathology.

SONOGRAPHY OF SCROTUM

Scrotal ultrasound (US) is excellent for the evaluation of the scrotum and demonstrates abnormalities of the testis, peritesticular abnormalities such as varicocele, epididymal pathology and also to visualize secondary changes caused by distal vasal obstruction.

Technique

The US examination should begin with the patient in supine position. The scrotum is supported by a towel between

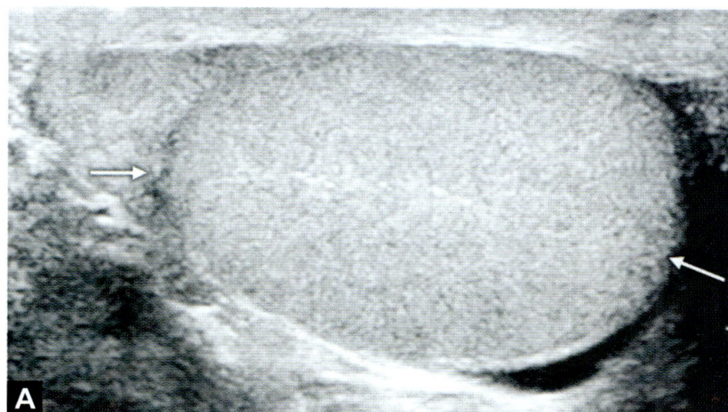

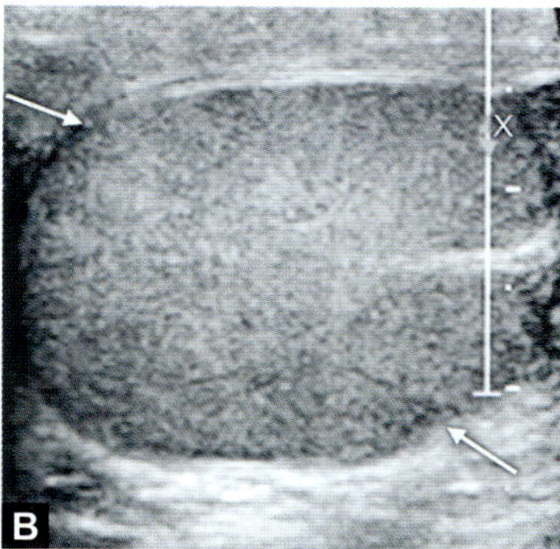

Figs. 12.1A and B: (A) Longitudinal and (B) transverse scans of the normal testis (arrows) showing the uniform granular appearance.

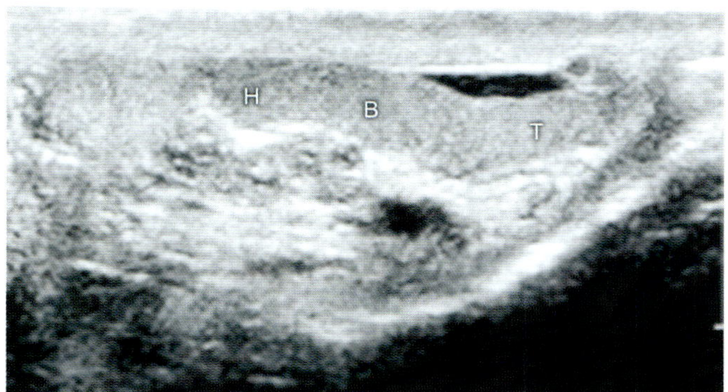

Fig. 12.2: Longitudinal scan of posterolateral aspect of testis showing the head (H), body (B), and tail (T) of normal epididymis.

the thighs. A towel covers the penis, which is placed over the abdomen to keep it out of the scanning field. Generous amount of gel is applied to the scrotum to avoid artifacts due to scrotal hair. The examination starts on the asymptomatic side, if there is any scrotal pain or discomfort. A high-frequency probe of 7–12 MHz with short focal zone and large footprint is used to cover the length of the testis in a single image. Each testis and epididymis should be examined separately in longitudinal and transverse planes. Study is done using gray scale, color and spectral Doppler techniques.

Normal Sonographic Anatomy

The normal testis is an ovoid or slightly rounded structure. It is homogeneously granular with uniformly distributed medium level echoes (similar to thyroid echotexture) (Figs. 12.1A and B). Both the testes are symmetrical in size, shape, and echotexture. So it is always important to compare both the testes side by side. Volume of the testis is calculated as length × width × height × 0.523. A total volume (both testes) of greater than 30 mL and a single testicular volume of 12–15 mL are generally considered as normal.[2] Mediastinum testis is a linear echogenic strand that runs craniocaudally within the testis. The rete testis at the mediastinum testis is sometimes seen as a hypoechoic area in the posterosuperior aspect of the testis in transverse section. Scanning from the lateral aspect of the scrotum may allow visualization of the entire epididymis (Fig. 12.2). The body and tail are better appreciated in the presence of hydrocele. Head of epididymis is isoechoic or slightly more echogenic than testis. It is about 10–12 mm in diameter. The body and tail are isoechoic or slightly less echogenic than the head. On color Doppler study, fine vessels coursing through the normal testis is seen and normal intratesticular flow is symmetrical on both sides (Figs. 12.3A and B). Normally, there is very minimal flow or no flow in the epididymis (Fig. 12.4).

TRANSRECTAL ULTRASONOGRAPHY

In recent years, high-resolution TRUS has been a very important safe, accurate noninvasive imaging technique for evaluating the distal male reproductive tract that helps to identify the patients with potentially correctable causes of infertility. Transrectal ultrasonography enables high-resolution imaging of the prostate, seminal vesicle, and vas deferens. It is the method of choice for investigating the cause of obstructive azoospermia (OA) which is indicated by:

- Low volume or normal volume semen with azoospermia and normal testicular size
- Low ejaculatory volume with severe oligozoospermia
- Enlarged epididymis with numerous cystic spaces on scrotal scan

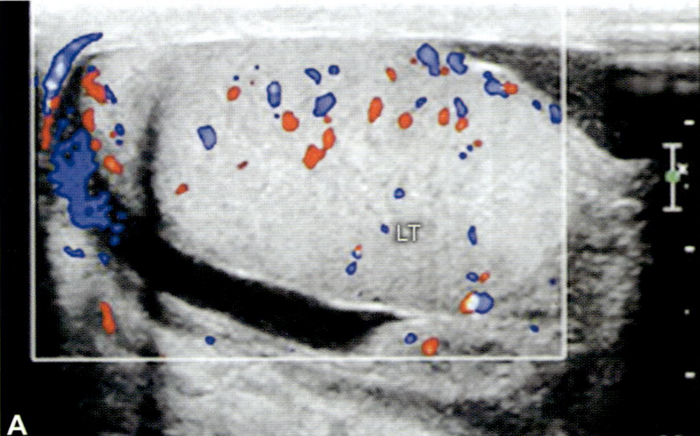

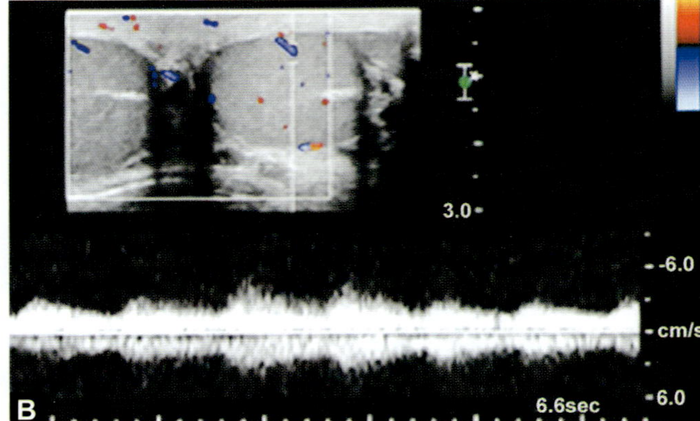

Figs. 12.3A and B: (A) Color and (B) spectral Doppler study of the normal testis (LT, left testis).

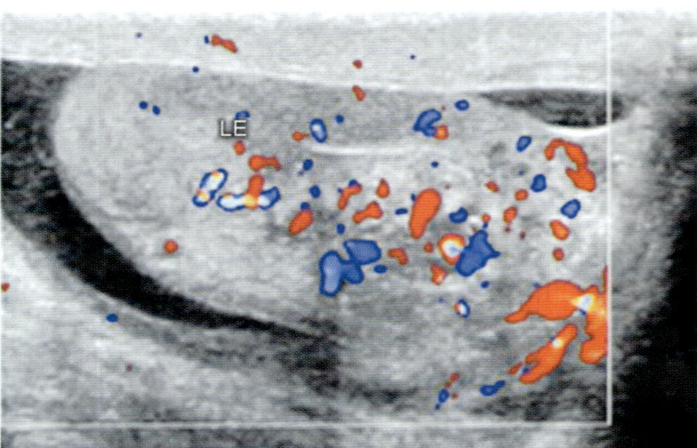

Fig. 12.4: Color Doppler study of normal epididymis showing sparse flow in it (LE, left epididymis).

- Abnormal digital rectal examination
- Normal gonadotropin [follicle-stimulating hormone (FSH) and luteinizing hormone (LH)] levels. Transrectal ultrasonography is also used to guide prostatic biopsy and cyst aspiration.

Technique

Transabdominal scan should be done before TRUS. A high-frequency transrectal probe of 6–10 MHz is used. Patient should empty the bladder first. Patient should lie in left lateral decubitus position with flexion of his right hip and knee. A sterile cover with gel inside it is placed over the probe. Gel is applied over the sterile cover. The probe is inserted gently into the rectum through the anus to relax the sphincter. Systematic survey of prostate, seminal vesicle, and vas deferens has to be done in axial, sagittal, and oblique planes. On sagittal plane, base and apex of prostate, urethra, seminal vesicles, and ejaculatory ducts are assessed (Video 12.1). On transverse plane, prostate gland, lateral gland margin, neurovascular bundle, and seminal vesicles are assessed (Video 12.1). Oblique scan is done mainly to visualize the long axis of the vas deferens and seminal vesicles.

Normal Sonographic Anatomy

Normal prostate is a symmetric triangular and ellipsoid structure with homogeneous echogenicity (Figs. 12.5 and 12.6). Normal seminal vesicles are paired, well-defined, saccular, elongated hypoechoic organs situated cranial to the prostate and posterior to urinary bladder with bow-tie appearance on axial images (Fig. 12.7). Vas deferens appears as round or oval tubular structures cranial to prostate and medial to seminal vesicles (Fig. 12.7). Ejaculatory ducts are difficult to visualize in normal men.

NONOBSTRUCTIVE CAUSES OF MALE INFERTILITY

These may be varicocele or various testicular pathologies.

Varicocele

Varicocele is a pathological dilatation of veins of the pampiniform plexus in the spermatic cord.[3] Varicoceles develop from a reversal of blood flow within the internal spermatic and cremasteric veins.[4] There are three main anatomic explanations for the origin of varicoceles.[5] The first theory emphasized the fact that the drainage of the

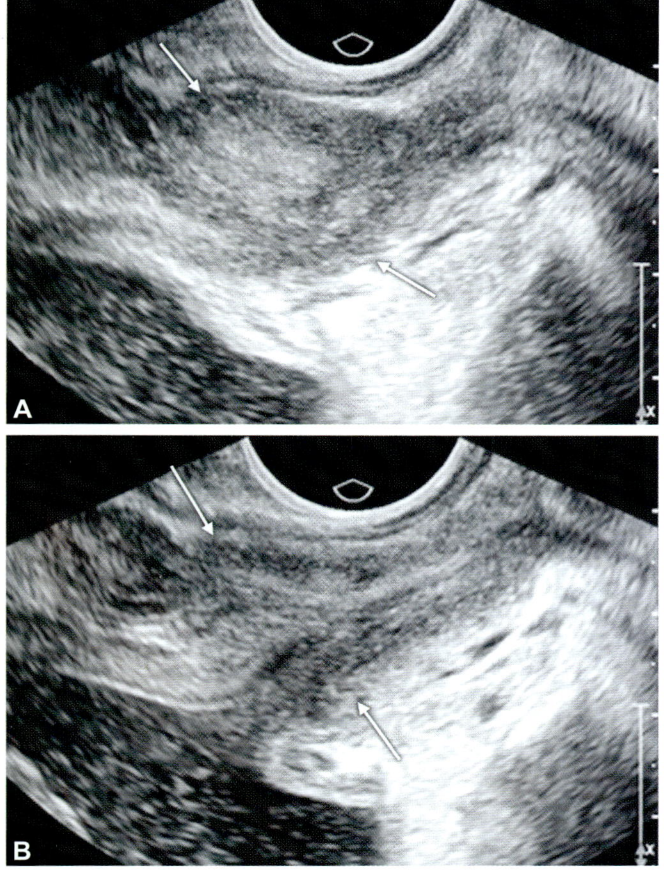

Figs. 12.5A and B: (A) Midline sagittal and (B) parasagittal transrectal ultrasonography (TRUS) scan of the normal prostate (arrows).

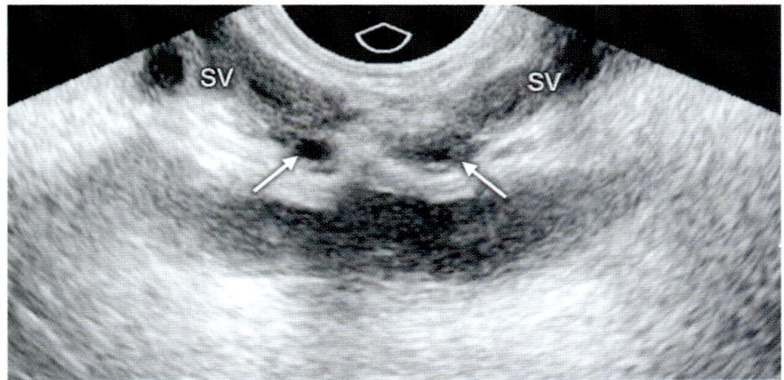

Fig. 12.7: Axial transrectal ultrasonography (TRUS) scan of the normal seminal vesicles (SV) with bow-tie appearance and ampulla of the vasa deferentia (arrows) of both sides.

testicular veins differs between the right and left. While the right testicular vein enters directly into the inferior vena cava at an oblique angle, the left testicular vein join the left renal vein at right angle. This difference is thought to result in increased hydrostatic pressure in the left testicular vein

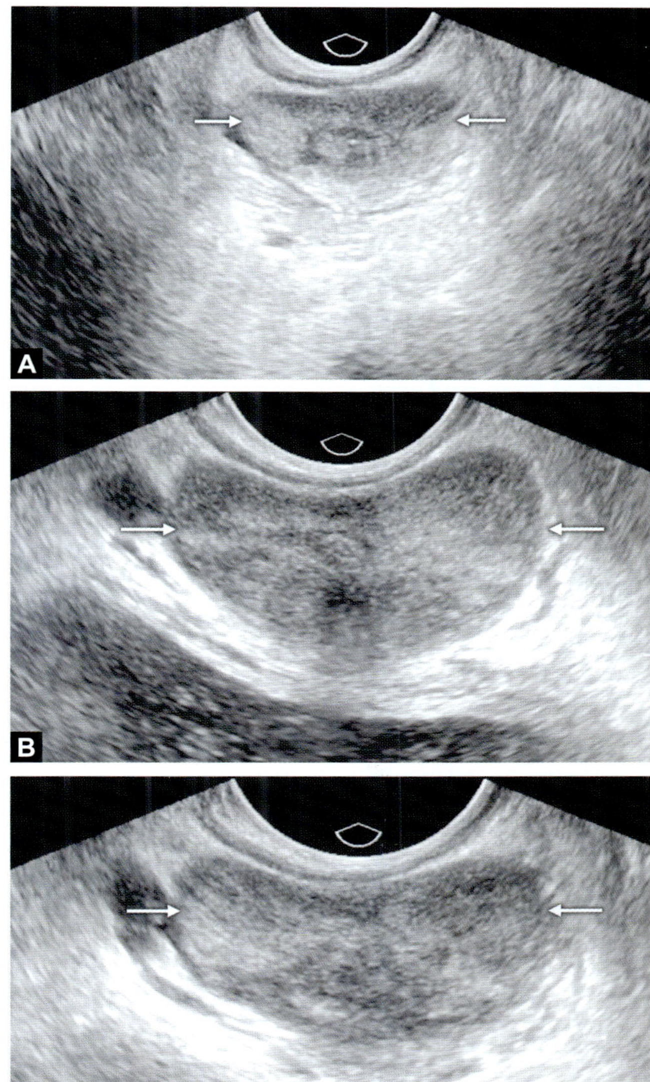

Figs. 12.6A to C: Axial transrectal ultrasonography (TRUS) scan of the normal prostate (arrows) through the (A) apex, (B) middle, and (C) base.

resulting in dilatation of the pampiniform plexus. The second theory postulates that an absence of competent valves leads to varicoceles. The final theory suggests that compression of the renal vein between the aorta and superior mesenteric artery increases the hydrostatic pressure in the testicular vein via a "nutcracker" effect.[5] Epidemiologic studies suggest that approximately 15% of all men in the general population have a clinical varicocele. In contrast, between 19% and 41% of men evaluated for infertility are found to have varicoceles.[5] Interestingly, the rate of varicocele is increased in men with secondary infertility to approximately 70%, suggesting that varicoceles may cause a progressive decline in fertility potential.[6] The pathophysiology of varicocele as a cause of infertility is controversial. The primary proposed hypotheses involve hyperthermia, venous pressure, testicular blood flow, hormonal imbalance, toxic substance, and reactive oxygen species.[4,5,7-9] It is difficult to identify a single or dominant factor, and it is likely that many of these etiological causes contribute to infertility seen in clinical practice.

Clinical Presentation

The clinical presentation of varicocele is highly variable. Most patients are asymptomatic. Besides infertility, the other symptoms include swelling, discomfort, and scrotal pain particularly after standing for a few hours. Clinical examination for varicocele is done in erect position, in resting state and with Valsalva maneuver. It is felt as a bag of worms and increase in caliber with Valsalva maneuver. It reduces in recumbent position. If it does not reduce, it may indicate a secondary obstructive cause. Clinical evaluation of varicocele has limitation since it is subjective. It is also complicated by coexistent pathology like hydrocele, obesity, cremasteric contraction, and hernia, which result in low sensitivity and specificity.

Sonographic Technique

The patient is examined in supine and erect positions, in resting state and with Valsalva maneuver. Study is performed with gray scale and repeated with color and spectral Doppler. The pulse repetition frequency (PRF) is kept low since venous flow is studied but it should be high enough to avoid movement artifact due to Valsalva maneuver.

Sonographic Features

On gray scale, varicocele appears as multiple serpiginous, tubular vascular structures measuring over 2.5 mm in diameter (Fig. 12.8). It is seen usually adjacent to or proximal to the upper pole of the testis and head of epididymis. When large, it extends lateral, posterior, and inferior to testis. It can be seen to extend within the testis (Figs. 12.9A and B). The caliber of the vein increases with Valsalva maneuver. On color Doppler study, there is usually no flow seen in resting state. On Valsalva maneuver, there is reflux of flow in the veins (Video 12.2). The color will be a mixture of red and blue, since the veins are tortuous and direction of flow is different (Fig. 12.10A). In spectral Doppler, the

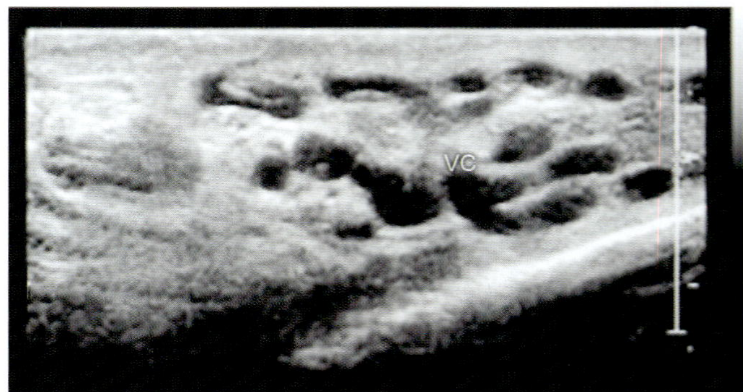

Fig. 12.8: Oblique scan of the scrotum showing varicocele (VC) containing dilated, tortuous veins of pampiniform plexus.

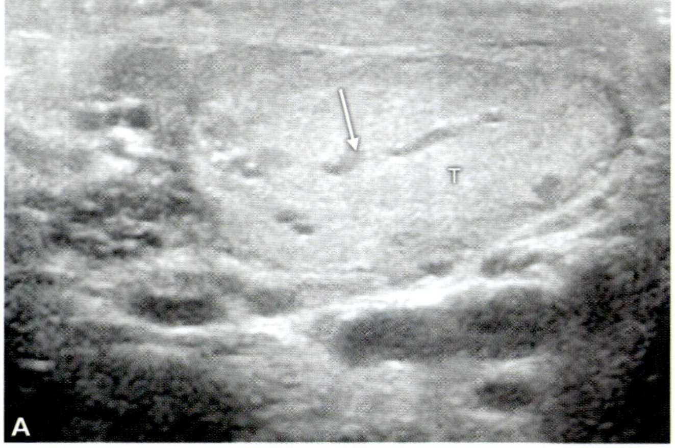

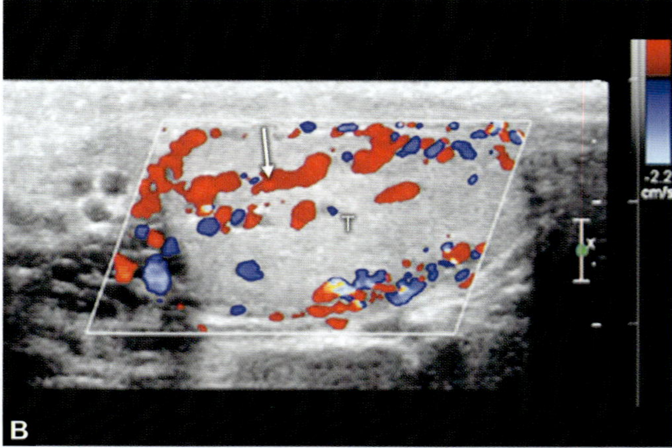

Figs. 12.9A and B: (A) Oblique scan of testis and (B) color Doppler study of the testis (T) showing intratesticular varicocele (arrow).

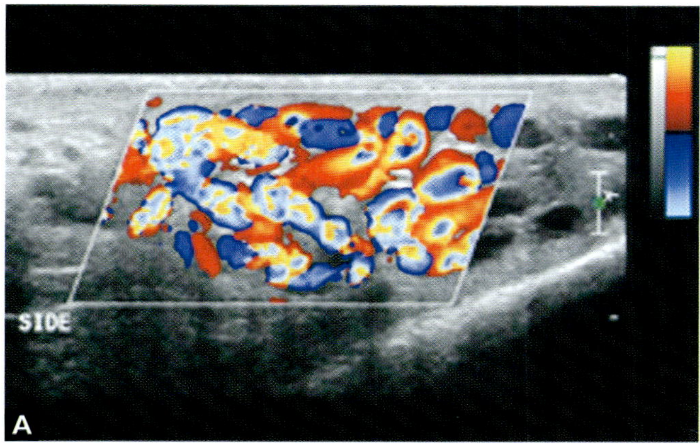

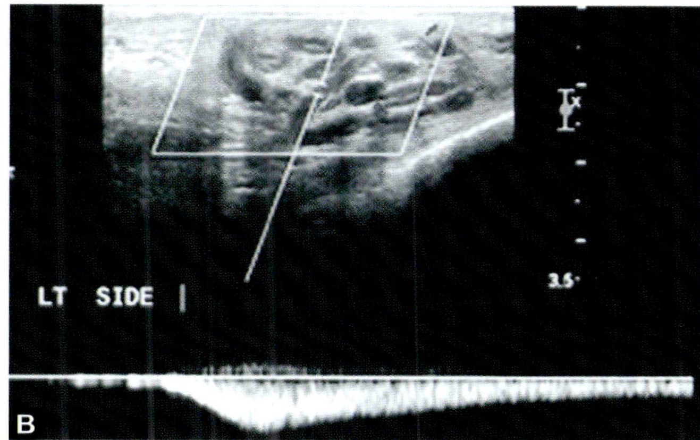

Figs. 12.10A and B: (A) Color and (B) spectral Doppler study showing reflux of venous flow in the veins of varicocele.

sample volume has to be kept small since there are multiple tortuous veins. This has to be checked on gray scale to see if the sample volume remains in the lumen with Valsalva maneuver. In spectral Doppler, the reflux is elicited with Valsalva maneuver both in supine and erect positions (Fig. 12.10B) (Video 12.3).

Differential Diagnosis

Lymph varix mimics varicocele since it also shows dilated tortuous vascular structures. It usually does not show immediate change when position of patient is changed from supine to erect and with Valsalva maneuver on gray scale. It fails to show reflux of venous flow with Valsalva maneuver. Occasionally, the "microfilaria dance sign" can be seen as wriggling movement in the lumen of the dilated lymphatics on gray scale and color Doppler study (Video 12.4). Ectasia of rete testis can mimic intratesticular varicocele. It will not show reflux of flow on Valsalva maneuver and there will be lack of dilated veins outside the testis.

Classification of Varicocele

The clinical and ultrasound (USG) classification of varicocele are reviewed here. Dubin and Amelar[10] devised a clinical grading system for varicocele that has the advantage of being universally accepted and easy to use. Grade 1 varicoceles are palpable only during the Valsalva maneuver, Grade 2 are readily palpable without the need for the Valsalva maneuver, and Grade 3 are visible on inspection.[11,12] A significant step forward in varicocele characterization comes from Solbiati[13] and more recently Sarteschi and colleagues.[14] These authors suggest that varicocele should be defined on the basis of the following USG features: extension, size and number of dilated veins, affected side, duration of retrograde flow during Valsalva maneuver, presence of spontaneous retrograde flow in the upright position, volume and echotexture of the affected testicle (in comparison to the contralateral), and demonstration of retrograde flow in the inguinal canal of the affected side. Recently, Isidori and Lenzi[14] have proposed a revised integrated classification of varicocele that offers a comparison between the clinical (Dubin) and US classifications (Solbiati) (Table 12.1).

Management

The impact of varicocele and its treatment in male infertility has been a matter of debate for the past 20 years and is not yet resolved. The discrepancies among the several small, inadequately controlled studies in the literature depend on five major issues:[11] (1) there is no unequivocal correlation between the size of the varicocele and the degree of sperm-quality impairment; (2) in some patients, sperm quality improves after varicocele ablation, but in others it remains the same, due to other concomitant disorders; (3) most studies do not assess whether the varicocele repair was actually successful; (4) the final outcome of delivered pregnancies is strongly affected by female factor infertility; and (5) most studies used a clinical rather than US classification of varicoceles; therefore, accuracy in staging of the disease cannot be compared objectively.

National Institute of Clinical Excellence (NICE) guidelines (2013) in the UK states that men should not be offered surgery for varicoceles as a form of fertility treatment because it does not improve pregnancy rates as has

Table 12.1: Ultrasound classification of varicocele

Grade	*B-mode*	*Reflux-Doppler*
Grade 1	Dilated vessels (>2.5 mm) in inguinal region only	Inguinal reflux only during Valsalva maneuver (lasting 2–3 seconds)
Grade 2	Supratesticular vessel dilation (>3 mm)	Supratesticular reflux only during Valsalva maneuver, lasting more than 3 seconds
Grade 3	Supra- and peritesticular vessel dilation (>3 mm)	Supra- and peritesticular reflux at rest which increases during Valsalva maneuver, lasting more than 3 seconds
Grade 4	Peritesticular vessel dilation with further dilatation during functional maneuver, testicular hypotrophy	Peritesticular reflux at rest which may or may not increase during Valsalva maneuver
Grade 5	Peritesticular vessel dilation that does not increase with functional maneuver, or intratesticular vessels, and testicular hypotrophy	Peritesticular reflux at rest which increases minimally during Valsalva maneuver or dilated intratesticular vessels which refill with Valsalva maneuver

been shown in a systematic review of seven randomized controlled trials (RCTs) compared pregnancy rates of varicocele repair in men with normal semen (two RCTs), subclinical varicoceles (three RCTs), and clinical varicoceles with abnormal semen (two RCTs). The review found that varicocele repair did not improve pregnancy rates in couples with male fertility problems or unexplained fertility problems pregnancies among 281 treated couples versus 50 pregnancies among 259 controls [relative risk (RR) 1.01, 95% confidence interval (CI) 0.73–1.40 using a fixed effects model; RR 1.04, 95% CI 0.62–1.75 using a random effects model]. The guidelines of European Association of Urology on male infertility(2016) has described the following recommendations for management of varicocele:

1. Treat varicoceles in adolescents with progressive failure of testicular development documented by serial clinical examination.
2. Do not treat varicoceles in infertile men who have normal semen analysis and in men with a subclinical varicocele.
3. Treat varicoceles in men with a clinical varicocele, oligospermia and otherwise unexplained infertility in the couple.

Undescended Testis or Cryptorchidism

Undescended testis, also known as cryptorchidism, refers to the condition in which the testis fails to reach the scrotum. The testis develops intra-abdominally and moves toward the scrotum during fetal development. Normally, the descent of testis into the scrotum occurs by the ninth month of gestational age or a few weeks of postnatal life. The descent may be arrested at any level along the path from the retroperitoneum to the scrotum. Although most of the patients with nonpalpable testis (NPT) present during childhood, there are a few patients who present in adulthood with infertility. The descent of testis is very important for normal spermatogenesis. Progressive germ cell damage occurs in undescended testis secondary to increased temperature at its extra scrotal location and untreated postpubertal undescended testis may be completely devoid of germ cells. In bilateral cryptorchidism, the rate of paternity is approximately 50% but unilateral condition results in little, if any, impairment of fertility.[1] Other complications are testicular malignancy, torsion, and inguinal hernia. The rationale of management of this condition is to place the testis in the scrotum to maximize its potential for spermatogenesis, screen for occurrence of malignancy, or remove a nonviable testis. Preoperative localization of the testis by an imaging study will be beneficial, since it will modify the surgical procedure. So the aims of an imaging method are: (1) to localize the testis, including ectopic locations; (2) to know if the testis is viable or atrophic; and (3) to know if the testis is absent. On clinical examination, 80% of undescended testis are palpable and do not need any imaging investigation. The rest 20% of undescended testes are nonpalpable.[15,16] Nonpalpable testis is due to undescended canalicular and abdominal testis, or rarely due to absent, ectopic, or atrophic testis.

All these years the imaging was targeted toward visualizing the testis and hence there was difficulty in visualizing the atrophic, absent, and ectopic testis. This resulted in low sensitivity and specificity of the imaging method.[17,18] Tracking the spermatic cord is a new technique to locate the testis.[19] The spermatic cord, being an accompanying structure of the testis, helps to locate the testis.

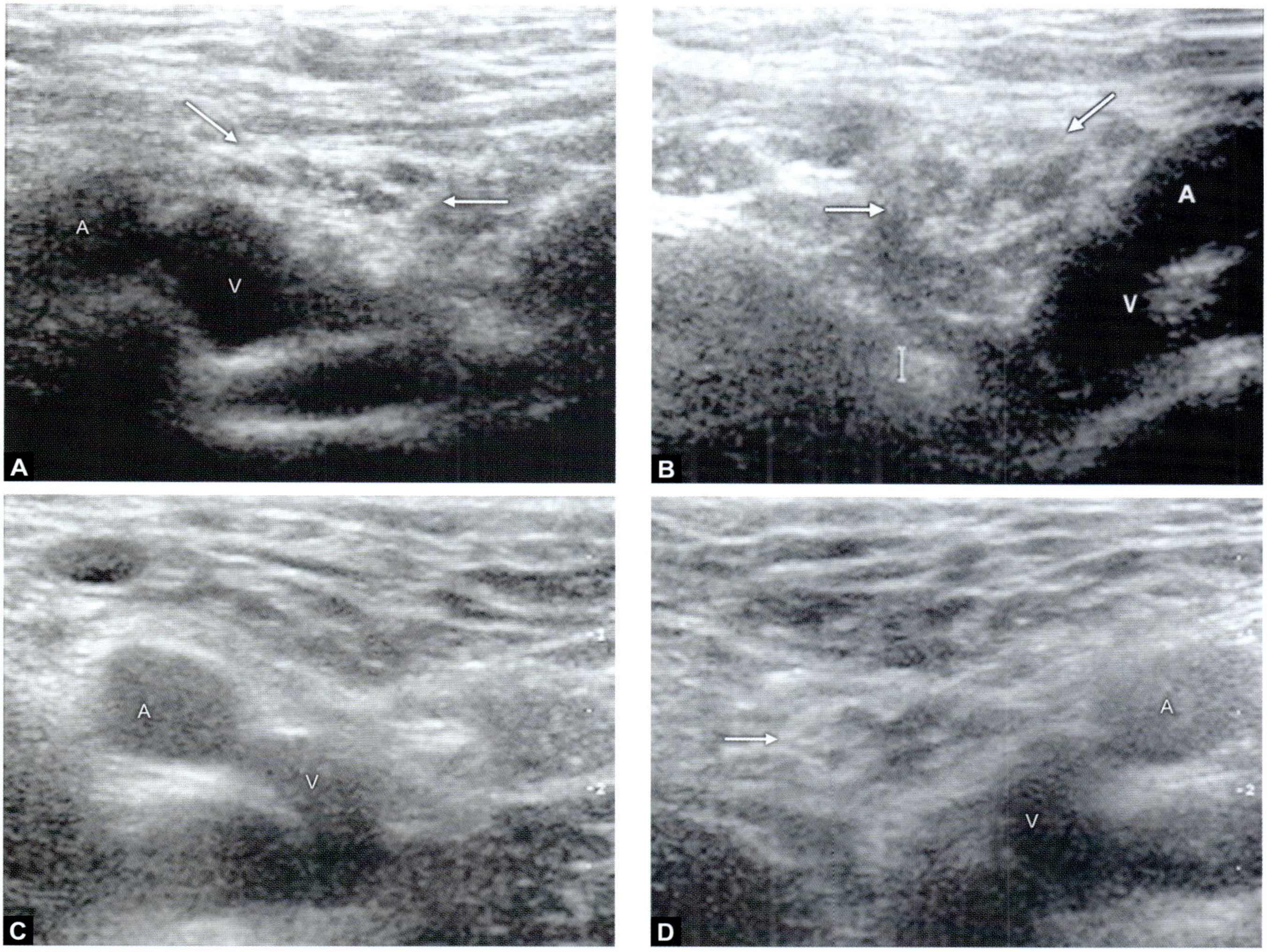

Figs. 12.11A to D: Transverse scan of the (A) right and (B) left inguinal regions of a normal patient showing the oblique section of spermatic cord (arrows) anteromedial to the common femoral artery (A) and vein (V). (C and D) Similar sections in a patient with a right nonpalpable testis (NPT) revealing a nonvisualization of the spermatic cord on right side and normal cord (arrow) on left side.

The high-resolution of the recent US scanners helps to visualize the spermatic cord in the inguinal canal. On a transverse scan of inguinal region, it is seen as an oval echogenic structure with a few round echopoor areas, representing the vas deferens and vessels (Figs. 12.11A to D). It is seen anteromedial to the common femoral vessels. When it is seen, it can be traced down as shown in Video 12.5. The visualization and tracing the cord helps to locate the NPT in the following ways:

1. When the cord is visualized, it can be traced down and that can lead to a testis of normal size located either in the inguinal canal (Fig. 12.12) or in the scrotum.

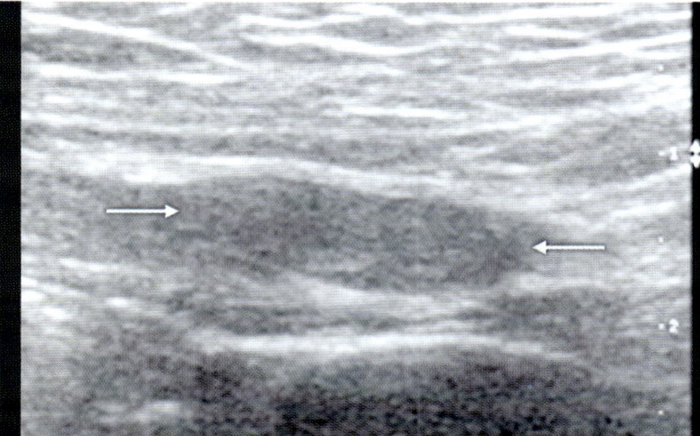

Fig. 12.12: Oblique section showing the testis (arrows) in the inguinal canal.

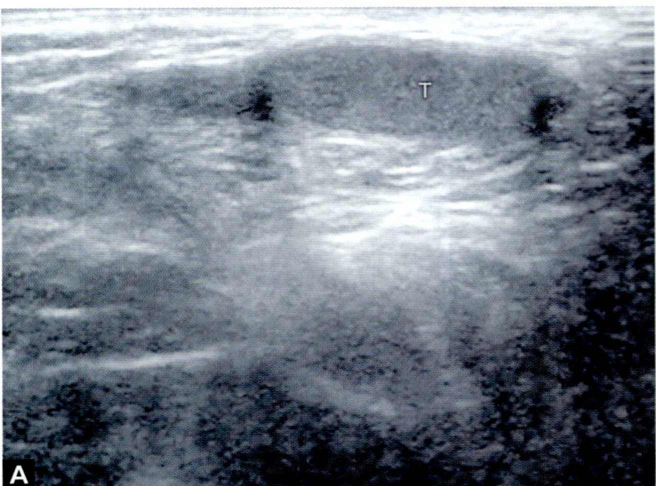

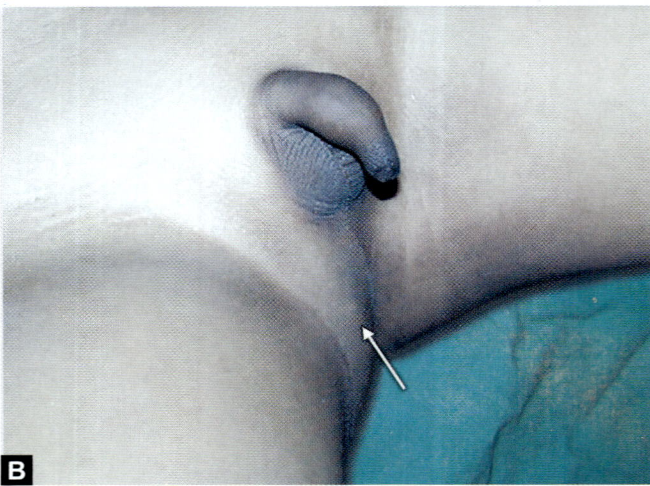

Figs. 12.13A and B: (A) Perineal testis image showing the testis (T) in subcutaneous plane in the perineum posterolateral to the scrotum; (B) photograph showing the site of the located testis (arrow).

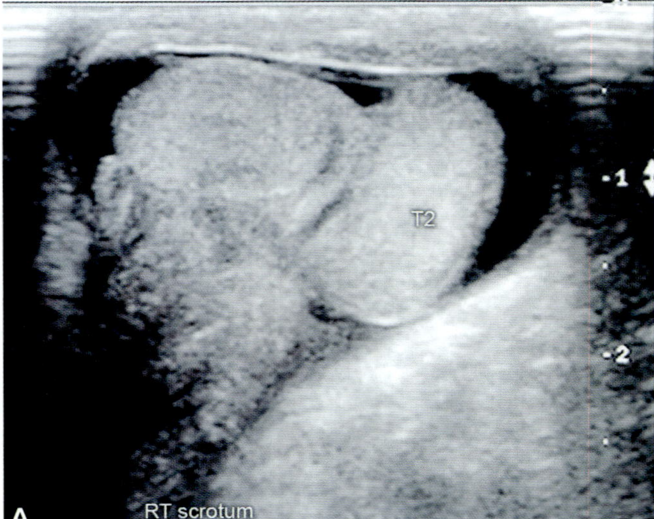

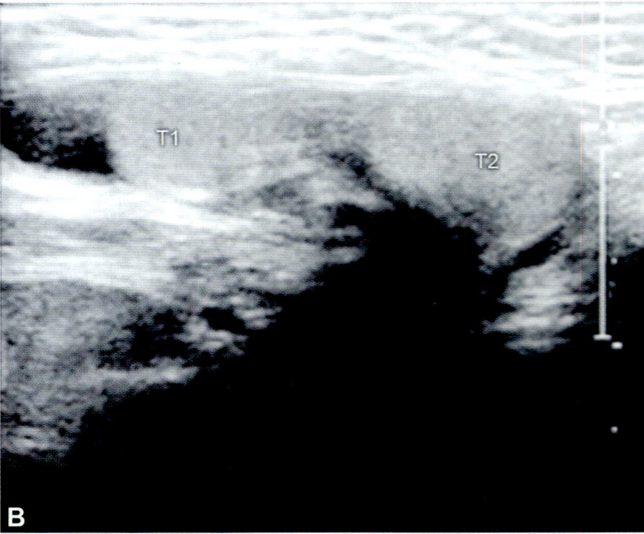

Figs. 12.14A and B: Transverse testicular ectopia: (A) Image showing both testes (T1 and T2) in the right side of scrotum; (B) image showing both testes (T1 and T2) in the same inguinal canal.

2. The visualized cord can be traced to an ectopic testis, which otherwise would have evaded detection. Ectopic testis is the condition where the testis is located outside the path of its descent. It can be located in the following locations: (a) superficial inguinal pouch, (b) anterior abdominal wall, (c) prepenile region, (d) perineal region (Figs. 12.13A and B), and (e) femoral region.[20,21]

   In all these situations, the spermatic cord is seen in the inguinal canal and it acts as a guide to the ectopic testis. Transverse testicular ectopia is the condition where both the gonads migrate toward the same hemiscrotum. The testis may lie in the opposite hemiscrotum (Fig. 12.14A), in the opposite inguinal canal (Fig. 12.14B), or at the opposite deep inguinal ring.
3. Tracing the visualized cord leads to an atrophic testis in the canal or scrotum that can be easily missed otherwise due to its very small size. The smallest atrophic testis can be 3–4 mm. Such a small testis can be missed on routine USG, but with the technique of tracking the spermatic cord, it can be easily identified and confirmed. The atrophic testes may have varied appearance, being echopoor, echogenic, or showing central/eggshell calcification (Figs. 12.15A to E).

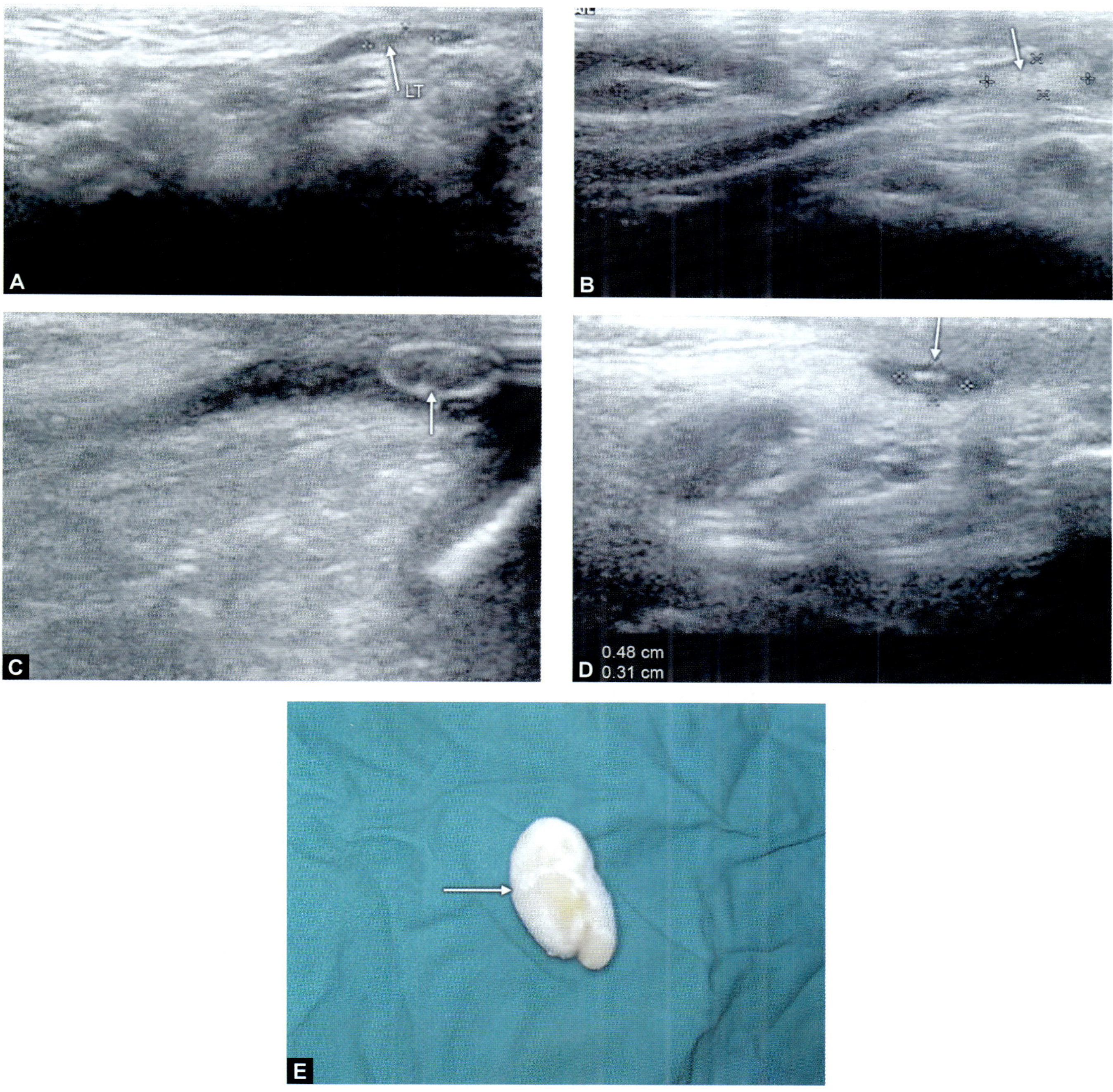

Figs. 12.15A to E: Images showing varying appearance of atrophic testis (arrow): (A) echopoor, (B) echogenic, (C) eggshell calcification, and (D) central calcification; (E) photograph of an atrophic testis (arrow) removed at exploration.

4. The cord can be looped in the inguinal canal in ascended testis where the returning loop can be traced to the intra-abdominal testis. Ascended testis is defined as a condition where the testis is initially thought to be normally descended but is later found to be outside of the scrotum[22] (Figs. 12.16A to G) (Video 12.6).
5. If the testis is not visualized in spite of the spermatic cord being visualized in inguinal canal, it would indicate a vanished testis. Vanished testis occurs

when the testis has descended into the scrotum but has atrophied totally due to torsion or an ischemic event during prenatal or early postnatal life. In this situation, the spermatic cord will be seen in the inguinal canal, but when tracked down it does not lead to a testis. USG predicts vanished testis accurately.

6. If the spermatic cord is not visualized in the inguinal canal it rules out an extra-abdominal location of the testis and the search can be extended up to look for an abdominal, retroperitoneal, or pelvic location of the testis (Figs. 12.17A to E).

If necessary, a lower-frequency probe can be used. The intraabdominal testis is differentiated from a bowel loop by the presence of peristalsis in the bowel (Video 12.7) and the mobility of the testis. In conclusion, high-resolution sonography, with tracking the spermatic cord technique, is a cost-effective and sensitive preoperative imaging method in NPT. It is useful in selecting the ideal therapeutic surgical approach and avoids diagnostic laparoscopy in most of the patients (Flow Chart 12.1).

Testicular Atrophy

Testicular atrophy is associated with reduced spermatogenesis and a reduction in fertility. Atrophy may occur following previous inflammation, ischemia, trauma, torsion, liver cirrhosis, estrogen treatment, hypopituitary disorders, and aging. On US, there is a global reduction in the volume of the testis (Figs. 12.18A and B). A decrease in both testicular reflectivity and vascularity is common findings. The epididymis usually appears normal.[2]

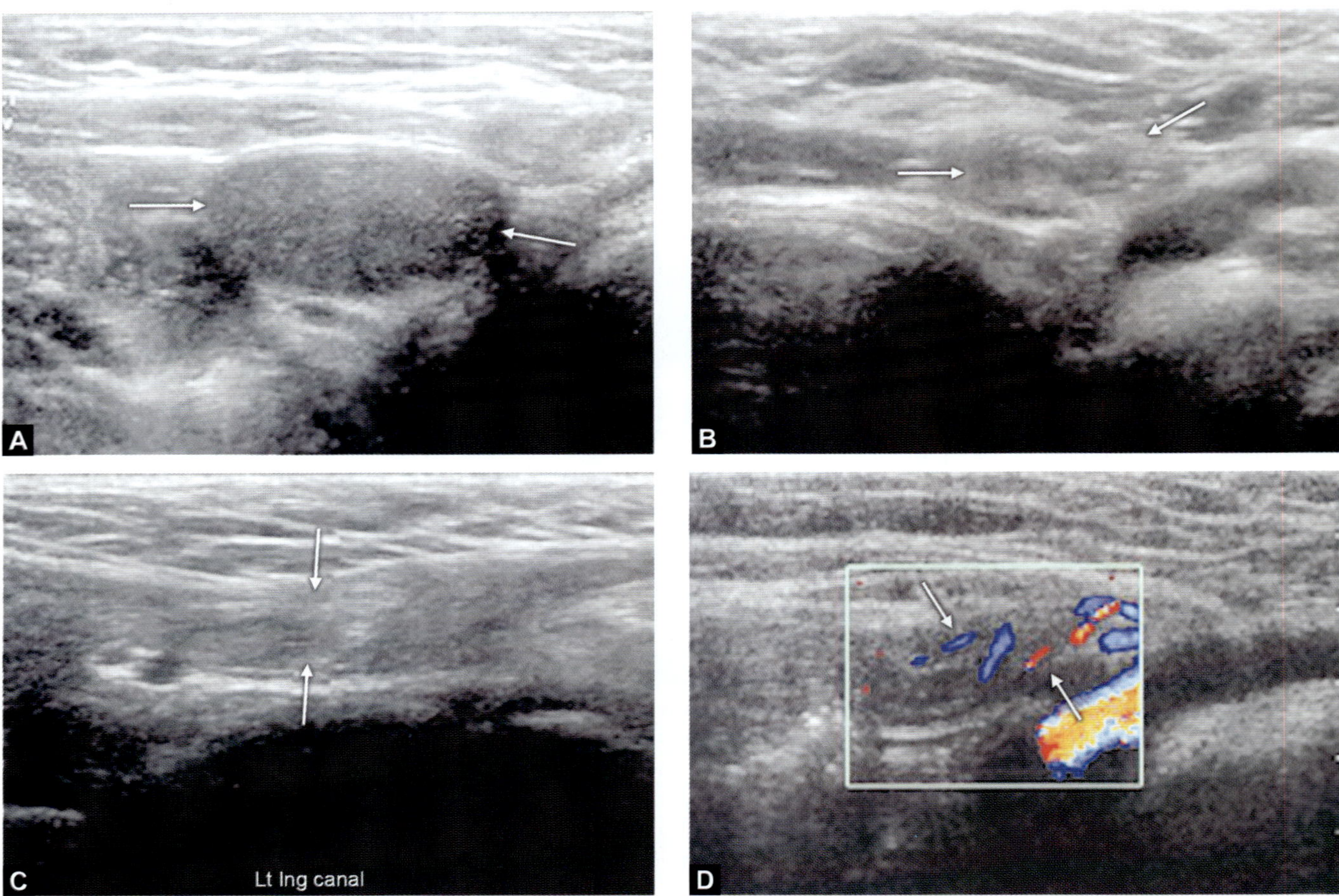

Figs. 12.16A to D: Ascended testis. (A) Image of the lower abdomen showing the intra-abdominal testis (arrows); (B) transverse and (C) longitudinal sections of inguinal region showing the two loops (arrows) of the spermatic cord in the inguinal canal; (D) color Doppler image showing the testicular artery (arrows) in the two loops of the cord confirming the looping of the cord.

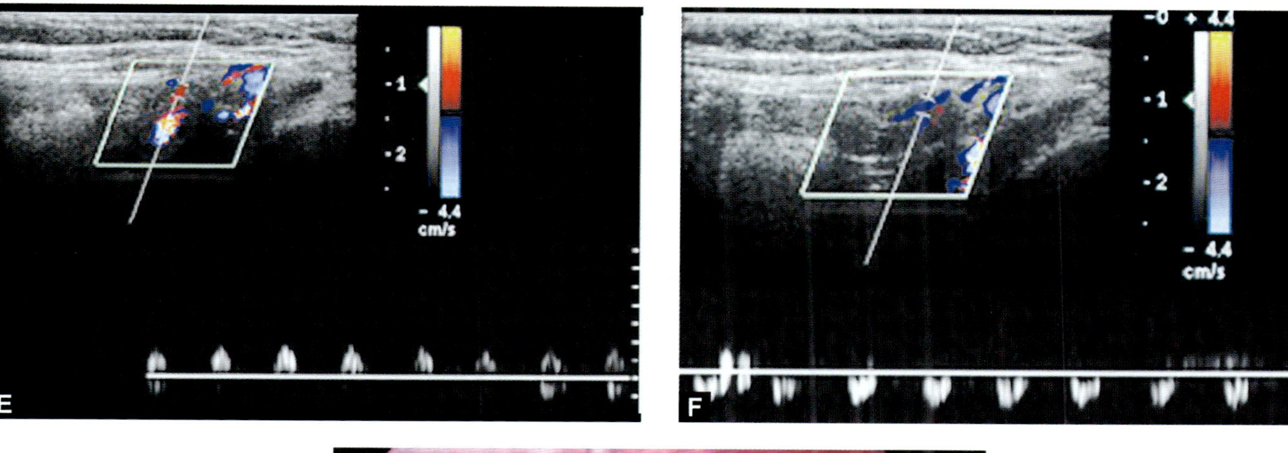

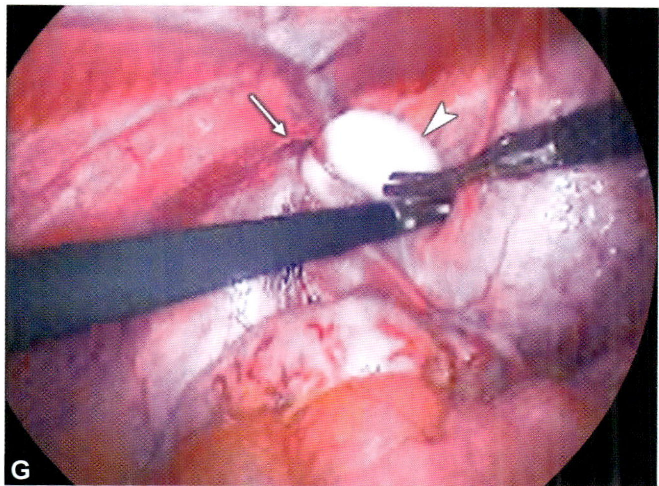

Figs. 12.16E to G: (E and F) spectral Doppler images of testicular artery in the two loops showing flow in opposite directions; (G) laparoscopic picture shows the intra-abdominal testis (arrowhead) with spermatic cord (arrow) emerging out of the internal ring. (Continued)

Orchitis and Epididymo-orchitis

Even though there is not enough conclusive epidemiological data, infections and inflammations of the genital tract are considered frequent cause of reduced male fertility.[23] Both clinical and pathological evidences exist to support the theory that chronic inflammatory conditions of the testes disrupt spermatogenesis and irreversibly alter both the quantity and quality of sperm.[23] Chronic epididymitis and epididymo-orchitis can also result in testicular atrophy. Pure orchitis is uncommon and is most often associated with mumps virus.[24] Epididymitis may also result in postinflammatory obstruction of the epididymis causing OA. When the inflammation is unilateral, the impact on fertility is minimal. However, if it is bilateral, it becomes significant. Bilateral inflammation is common in tuberculosis, which is discussed later. If bilateral nonspecific infection is seen, congenital anomaly like ectopic ureteric opening or fistula between urinary tract and colorectum should be considered.

Adrenal Rests in Testis

It is a rare cause of infertility and is due to increased adrenocorticotropic hormone (ACTH) due to congenital adrenal hyperplasia, adrenogenital syndrome, or Addison's disease. In these conditions, glucocorticoid synthesis is defective. As a result, there is increased ACTH, which prevents involution of aberrant adrenal rests in the testes. These intratesticular nodules of adrenal rests can enlarge

Flow Chart 12.1: Algorithm for management of nonpalpable testis (NPT) after sonography using the tracking the cord technique.

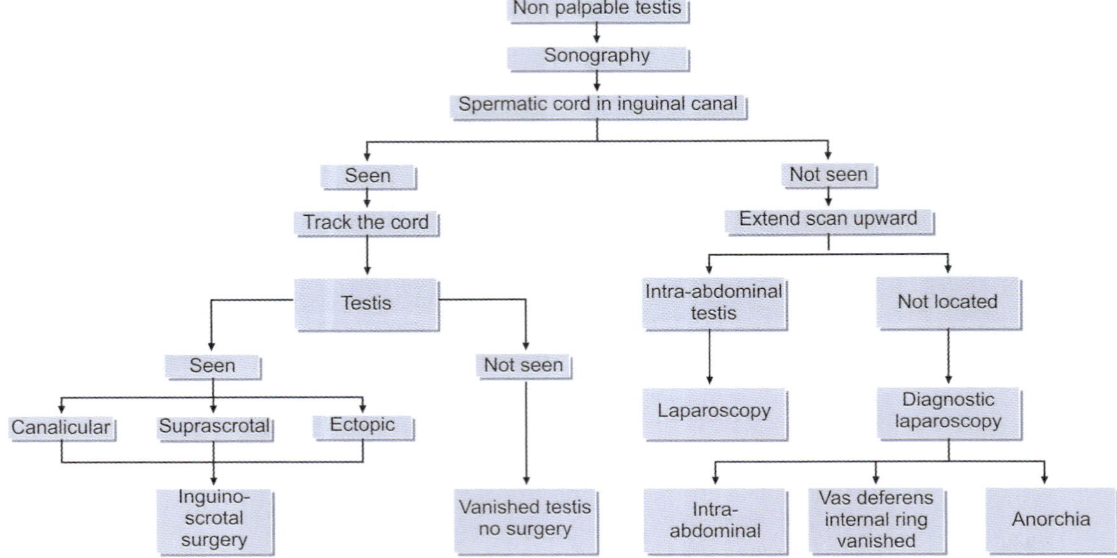

gradually, thereby destroying the testicular parenchyma which results in low testosterone production and infertility. These lesions are not premalignant and tend to regress with hormone replacement.[25] On USG, it appears as rounded heterogeneous solid masses and is multifocal in origin. They may be bilateral. They usually originate near the hilum and extend peripherally (Figs. 12.19A to G). On color Doppler study, the masses show normal, hypovascularity, or hypervascularity. The vessels course through the masses which differentiate the condition from tumors.[26]

Testicular Tumors

Testicular cancer is one of the leading cancers in young men aged between 15 and 34 years. It is also widely accepted that men with infertility have an increased risk of testicular cancer, even after excluding the common risk factors for testicular cancer and infertility, such as a history of undescended testes and chromosomal aberrations.[27-29] Similarly, patients presenting with a primary testicular tumor often have decreased semen quality and reduced fertility that appears to be specific for germ cell tumors.[1] Peterson et al.,[30] using patients with testicular lymphoma as a control group, demonstrated a reduction in fertility in patients with a germ cell tumor compared with preserved fertility in the control group.[30] Scrotal US is the modality of choice for assessment of testicular tumors. The features of testicular malignancy are varied but most tumors are seen as irregular echopoor masses in the testis. They may show increased vascularity on color Doppler study[2] (Figs. 12.20A and B). As testicular cancer usually affects young men, preservation of semen prior to therapy (either surgery or radiotherapy) is an important consideration, and semen cryopreservation may be indicated.

OBSTRUCTIVE CAUSES OF MALE INFERTILITY

Ultrasonography is used to detect the level and cause of obstruction. Evaluation of the entire genital tract from the testis to the urethra is essential. In patients with OA, testicular US is often abnormal. In a study performed by Moon et al.,[31] 86% of cases of OA had an abnormal US. The abnormalities associated with obstruction included tubular ectasia of the epididymis (Fig. 12.21), tapering of the epididymal tail[17] (Fig. 12.21), absence of the epididymis, epididymal calcifications (Figs. 12.22A and B) and the presence of heterogeneous mass along the epididymal course.[17,31] This study also demonstrated a larger testicular volume in OA than nonobstructive azoospermia (NOA). Thus, scrotal US is a useful preliminary test in diagnosing OA and differentiating it from NOA. However, TRUS is the modality of choice for assessing the actual cause of OA. Using TRUS, a systematic evaluation of the

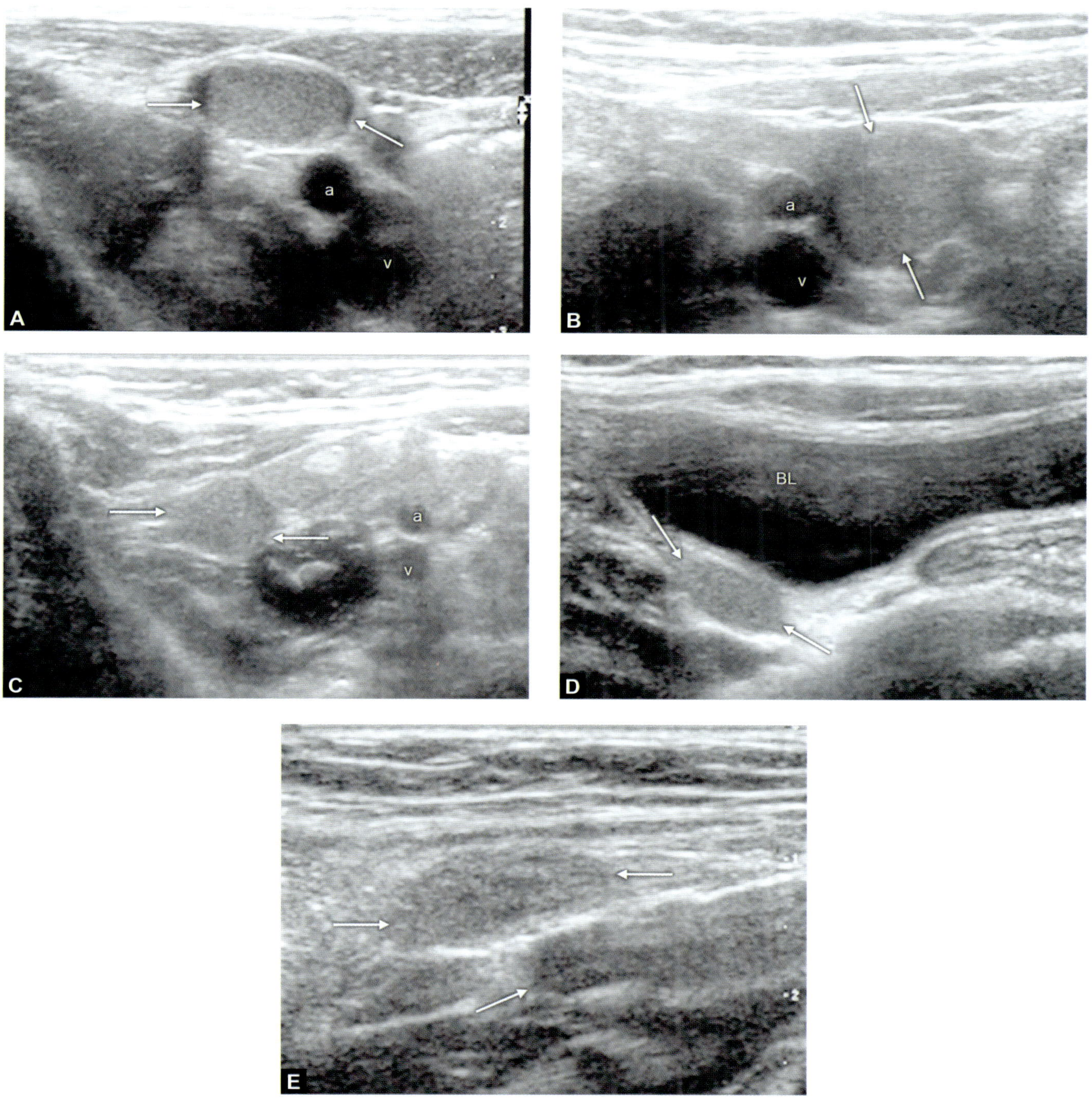

Figs. 12.17A to E: Sections of the lower abdomen showing the location of intra-abdominal testis (arrows): (A) anterior, (B) medial, and (C) lateral to external iliac vessels (a and v). (D) Testis is located along the right side wall of pelvis (arrows) and (E) anterior to the bifurcation of the common iliac artery (arrowhead) (*Abbreviation:* BL, urinary bladder).

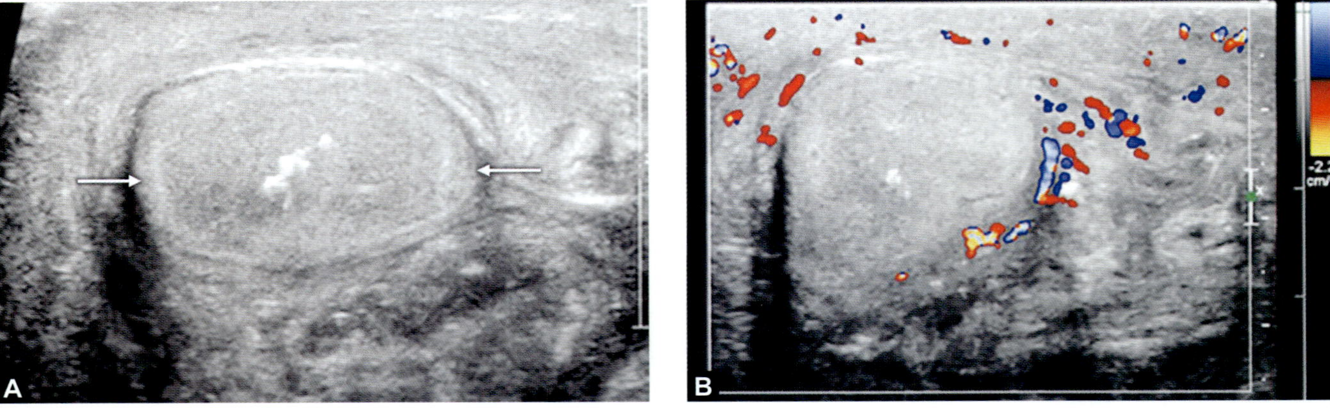

Figs. 12.18A and B: (A) Longitudinal scan of testis (arrows) showing global decrease in volume of the testis in testicular atrophy; (B) color Doppler study showing sparse flow in the atrophic testis.

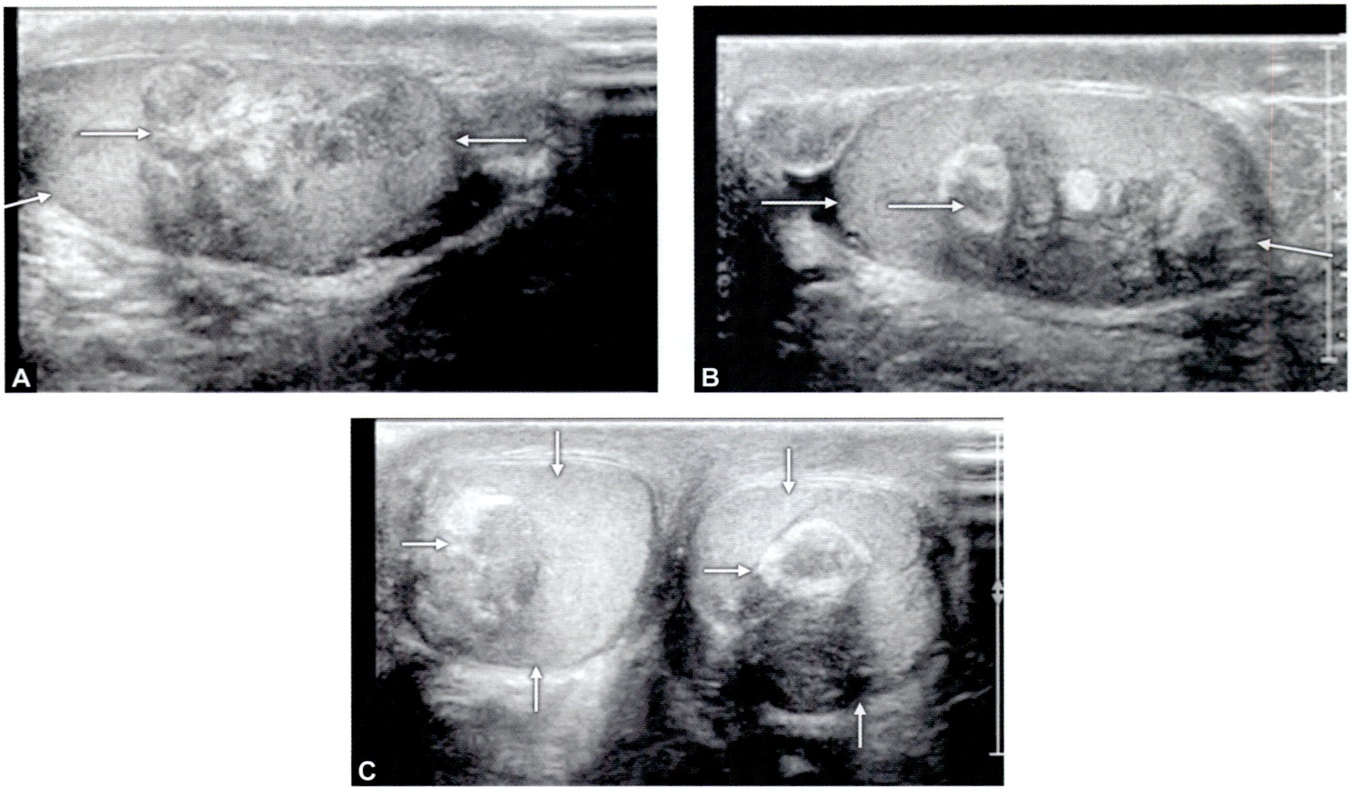

Figs. 12.19A to C: (Contd.)

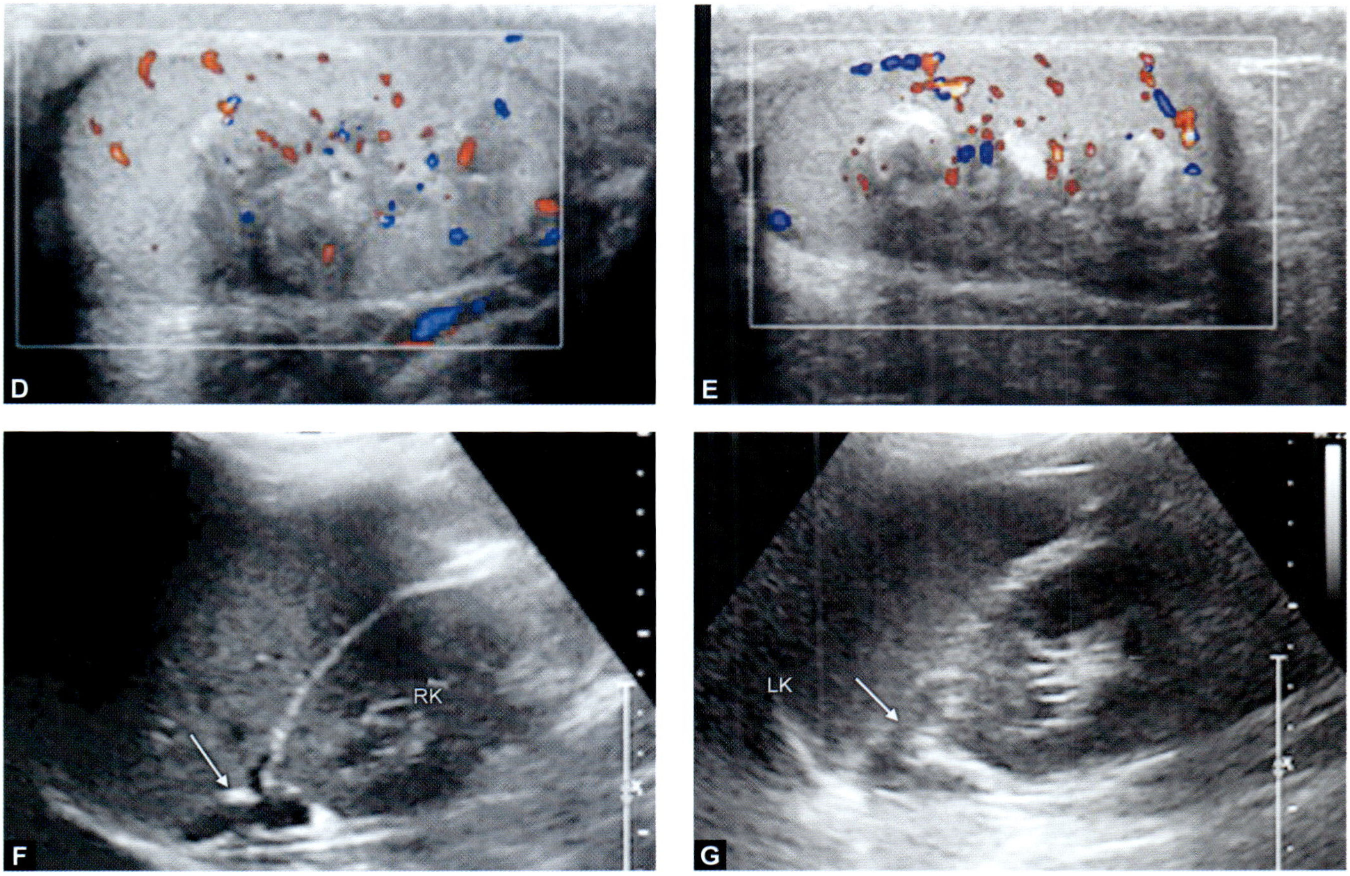

Figs. 12.19A to G: (Contd.) Adrenal rest in the testis. (A and B) Longitudinal and (C) transverse images of both testis (arrows) showing multiple rounded heterogeneous solid masses (arrowheads) in both testes; (D and E) color Doppler image shows vessels coursing through the masses; (F and G) coronal scan of both adrenals (arrows) showing bilateral adrenal hyperplasia (*Abbreviations:* RK, right kidney; LK, left kidney).

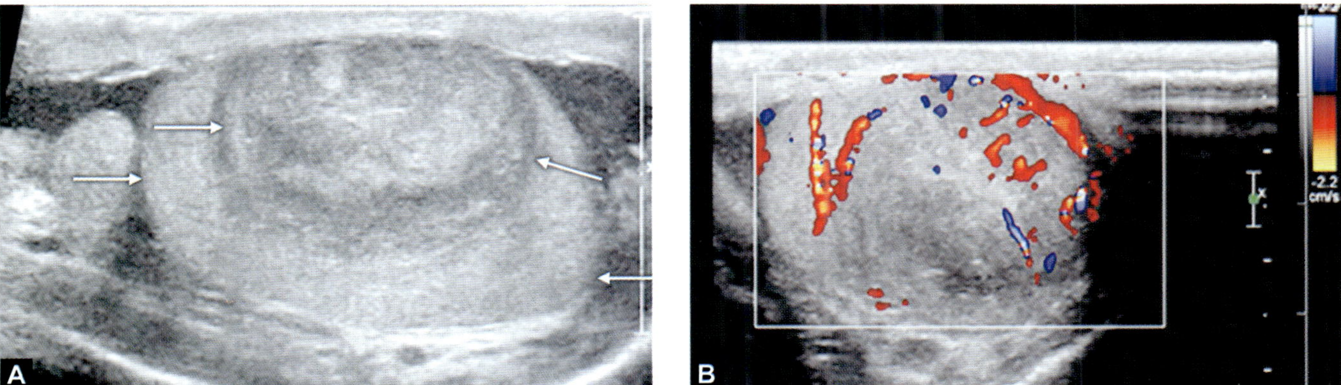

Figs. 12.20A and B: Testicular tumor. (A) Gray-scale and (B) color Doppler images showing an echopoor mass (arrowheads) with flow in the testis (arrows).

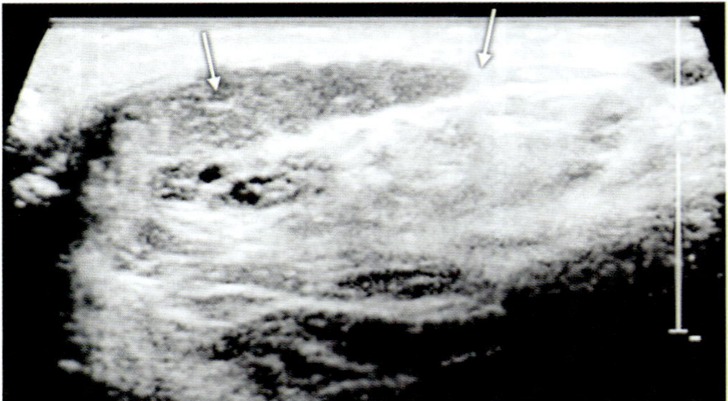

Fig. 12.21: Image showing tubular ectasia of epididymis (arrowhead) and tapering of the epididymis (arrow).

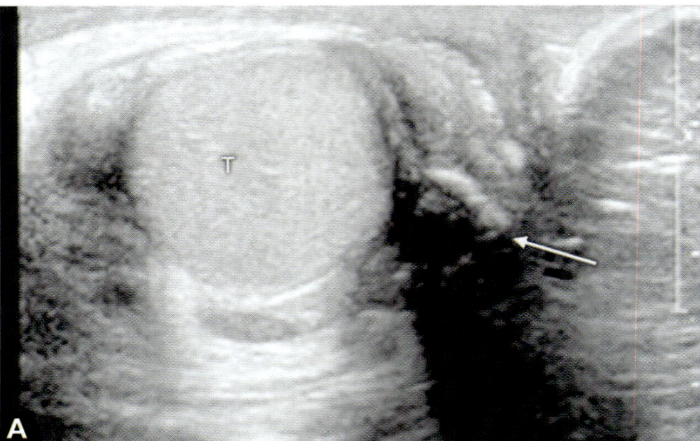

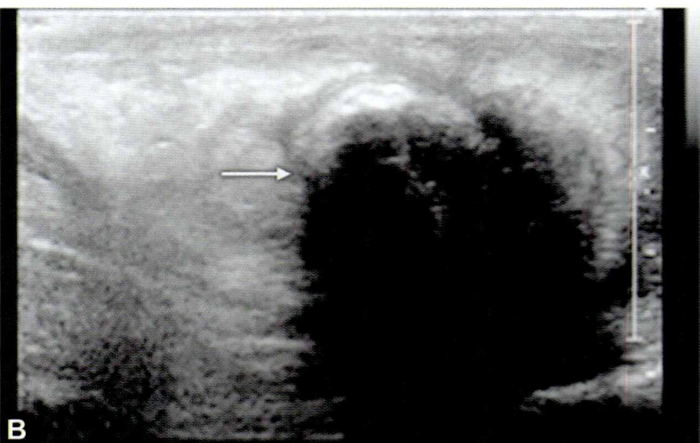

Figs. 12.22A and B: Axial and oblique scans showing epididymal calcification (arrows) (*Abbreviation:* T, testis).

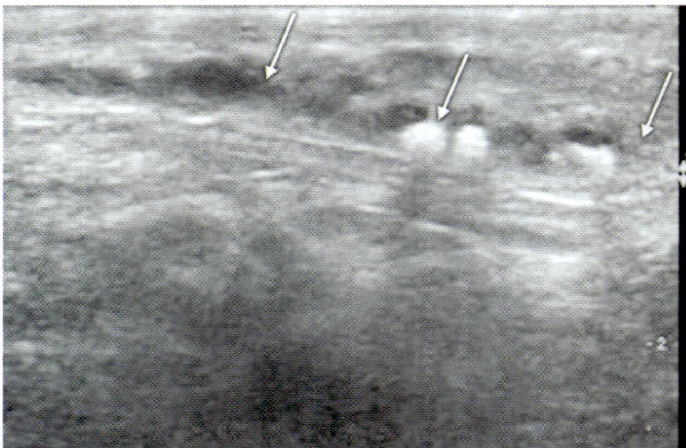

Fig. 12.23: Long-axis scan of the vas deferens (arrowheads) showing obstructing calculus (arrow).

terminal vas deferens, seminal vesicles, ejaculatory ducts, and prostate can be carried out in both axial and sagittal planes. Kuligowska et al.[32] assessed 276 patients with OA using TRUS: 25% were found to have a normal TRUS, 34% congenital bilateral absence of the vas deferens (CBAVD), 15% absent seminal vesicles and ejaculatory ducts, 9% obstructing cysts, and 4.4% obstructing calculi (Fig. 12.23). The level of obstruction may be anywhere along the tract from epididymis to the urethra. The level of obstruction determines the possible treatment of correctable causes—vasoepididymal anastomosis for proximal level and transurethral resection of the ejaculatory ducts or cyst for distal cause. The cause at each level can be congenital or acquired. Infection is a common cause anywhere along the tract, especially epididymitis. In India, tuberculosis is still a common cause of infection and is discussed later.

Vas Deferens Obstruction

Vas deferens obstruction can be congenital or acquired. The most common cause of congenital vas deferens obstruction is CBAVD, which is seen in 2% of patients under investigation for infertility. Up to 82% of patients with CBAVD have at least one mutation within the cystic fibrosis gene.[33] Therefore, patients with CBAVD must be considered for cystic fibrosis screening and genetic counseling prior to sperm retrieval/ICSI treatment.[34] In patients with CBAVD, scrotal US demonstrates dilatation of the tubules in epididymis (Fig. 12.24) with the epididymis stopping abruptly at the junction of the body and tail beyond which the vas deferens is not seen. Transrectal ultrasonography shows absence of the ampulla of the vas deferens[35] (Figs. 12.25A to C). Congenital bilateral absence of the

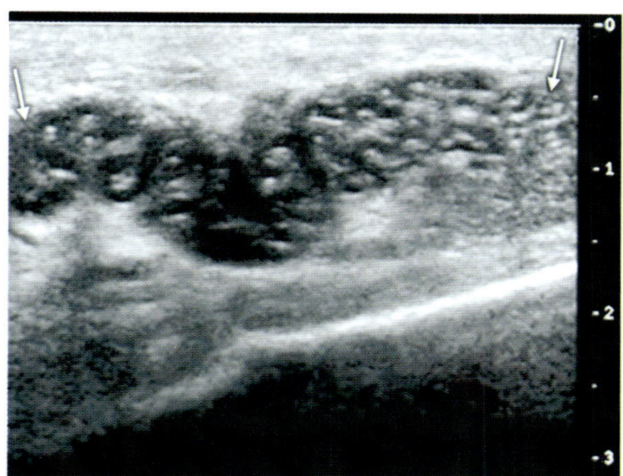

Fig. 12.24: Longitudinal scan of epididymis (arrows) shows dilated tubules in it in a case of distal vasal obstruction.

vas deferens is nearly always associated with abnormalities of the seminal vesicle, mostly agenesis (Figs. 12.26A and B) (Video 12.8) and ejaculatory duct.[32,36] Agenesis of vas deferens is known to be associated with renal anomalies, including agenesis, cross-fused ectopia, and ectopic pelvic location. In view of this, renal US is advised when agenesis of the vas deferens is diagnosed. Obstruction of vas deferens may also be amenable to microsurgical reconstruction.[37] The common acquired causes of vasal obstruction are tuberculosis, which is discussed later, and vasectomy. Sonography reveals a characteristic dilated inhomogeneous appearance on US described as ectasia of the epididymis (Fig. 12.24) with distended lumen of vas deferens (Figs. 12.27A and B).

Ejaculatory Duct Obstruction

Ejaculatory duct obstruction (EDO) is relatively uncommon, with the incidence of complete bilateral EDO reported as less than 1% in infertile men.[38] Congenital causes of EDO include duct atresia or stenosis as well as compression by midline prostatic cystic lesions, e.g. cysts of the prostatic utricle (previously named Mullerian duct cysts), and ejaculatory duct cysts.[39] Cystic obstruction of the ejaculatory ducts is usually congenital and acquired lesions are rare.[2] It is difficult to differentiate the cyst of prostatic utricle and ejaculatory duct cyst, since both are seen as pyriform cysts in midline—even though the latter can be paramedial and become very large extending beyond the prostate (Figs. 12.28A to F). Ejaculatory duct cysts are prostatic cysts derived from the Wolffian duct and urogenital sinus, into which the ejaculatory ducts empty, and therefore these

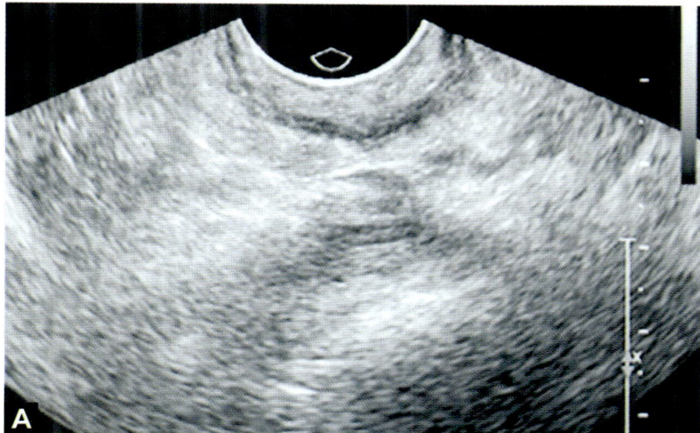

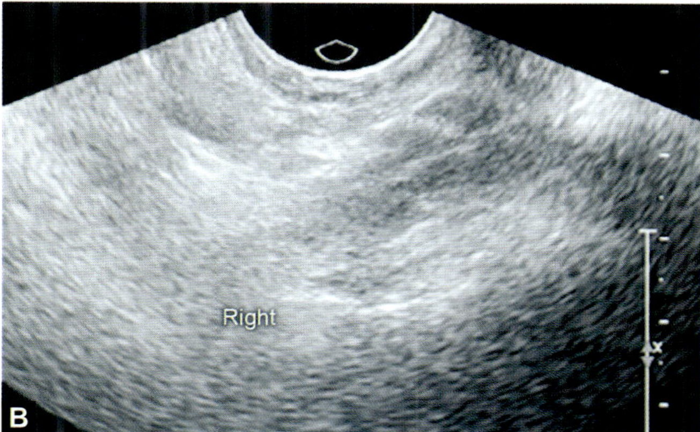

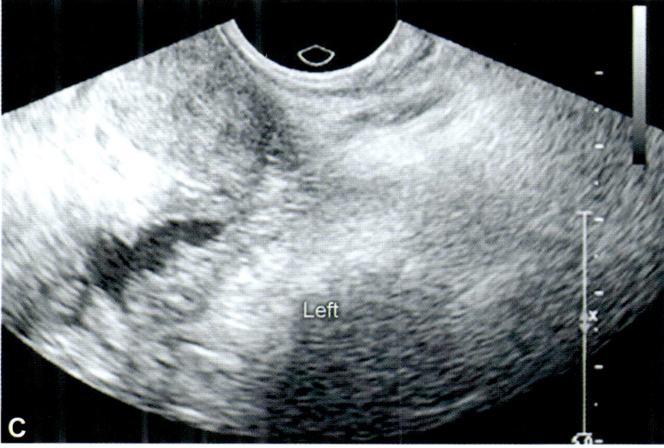

Figs. 12.25A to C: (A) Axial and (B and C) right and left oblique transrectal ultrasonography (TRUS) sections showing absence of ampulla of vas deferens and seminal vesicles.

cysts will contain sperm. Confirmation of the diagnosis of an ejaculatory duct cyst can be obtained by demonstrating spermatozoa from cyst fluid on US-guided cyst aspiration. Despite the low overall incidence of EDO, correct diagnosis is important as it can be treated by transurethral resection

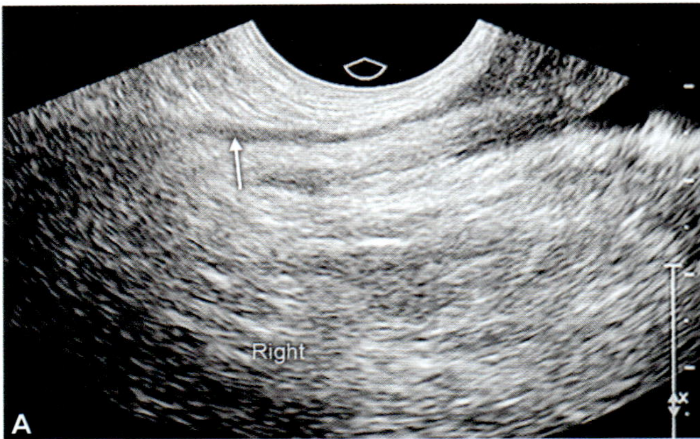

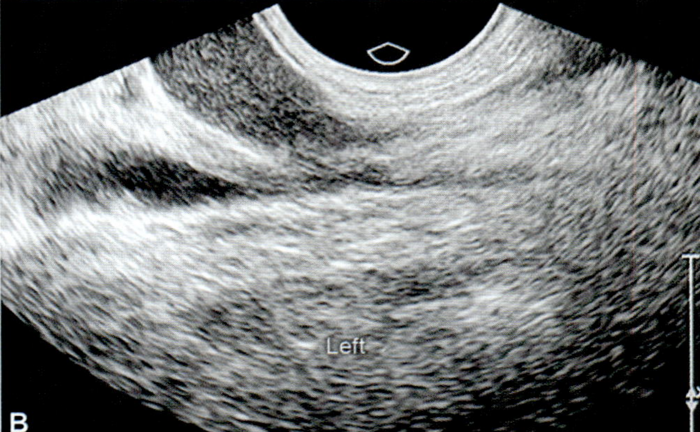

Figs. 12.26A and B: Oblique transrectal ultrasonography (TRUS) sections showing absence of seminal vesicles on both sides (right and left).

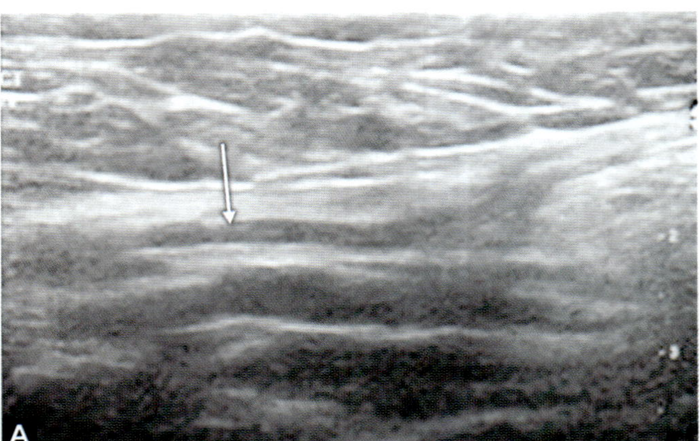

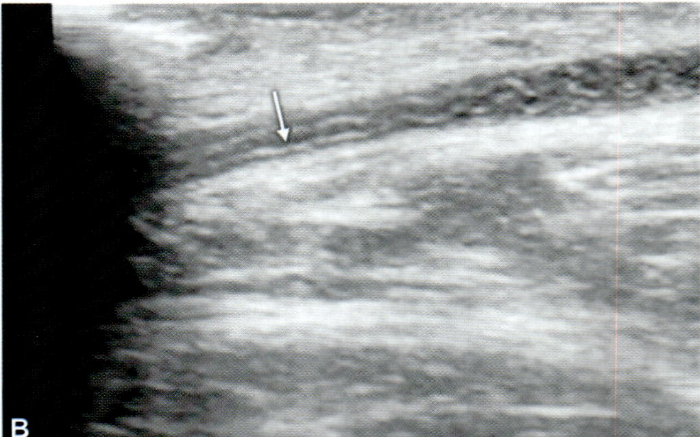

Figs. 12.27A and B: (A) Longitudinal scan of normal vas deferens (arrowhead) and (B) showing distended lumen (arrow) of vas deferens in distal obstruction.

of the ejaculatory duct. This is followed by the appearance of sperm in the ejaculate in approximately 50–73% of cases with a 25% pregnancy rate.[37] When the cyst causes obstruction to the ejaculatory ducts, US will show dilated seminal vesicles (Figs. 12.29A and B) associated with dilated tubules in the epididymis (Fig. 12.24). There may be ectasia of the rete testis (Figs. 12.30A and B) and epididymal cyst (Figs. 12.31A and B). Acquired causes include calculi in the distal ejaculatory ducts at the level of the ampulla, which may be associated with dilatation of the proximal duct and evidence of obstruction.[32] Iatrogenic causes include surgery to the base of the bladder and infections acquired following catheterization.[1]

Genital Tract Tuberculosis

The incidence of tuberculosis as the cause of male infertility cannot be assessed since the disease causes infertility by a chronic process of destruction and fibrosis and the lesions are rarely seen when the patient presents for infertility.[40] However, different stages of tuberculosis are characteristically seen in the same patient and occasionally the active lesions may be seen along the tract indicating the cause. Hence, all the features of tuberculosis are described here.

The primary site for infection of the male genital tract is often the epididymis. Spread is via the hematogenous route with the infection spreading to adjacent organs by direct extension. The sexual transmission of genital tuberculosis is very rare despite the fact that a man with genital tuberculosis can have the organisms in his semen. Direct extension of the disease from urinary tuberculosis has not been established as yet. The disease is characterized pathologically by areas of focal necrosis with caseation and cavitation, with the lesions healing by fibrosis and calcification. The fibrosis around the ejaculatory ducts can result in their obstruction, leading to dilatation of seminal

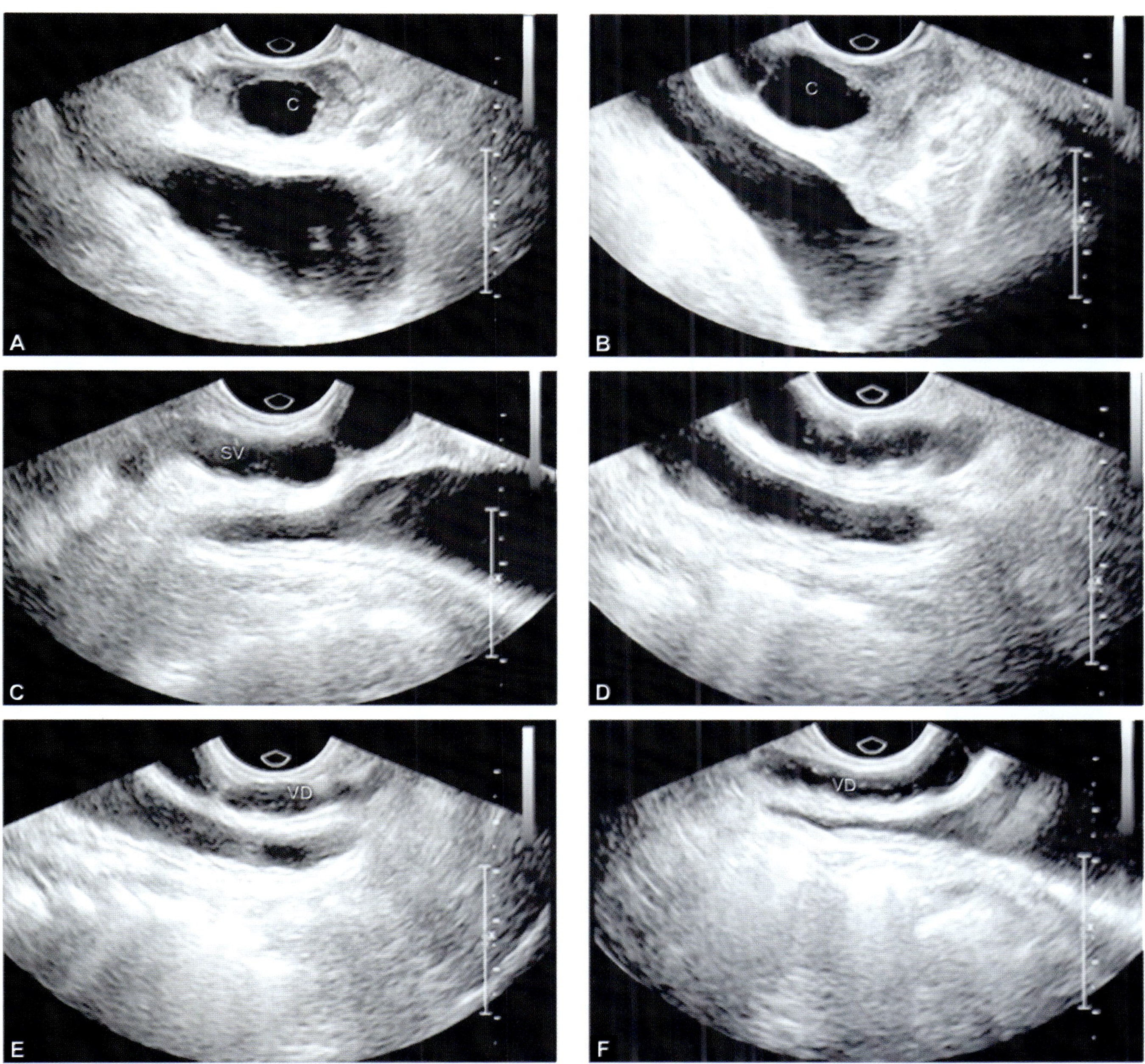

Figs. 12.28A to F: (A and B) Axial and sagittal transrectal ultrasonography (TRUS) sections of prostate showing a midline pyriform cyst (C) with obstruction of ejaculatory ducts resulting in dilated (C and D) seminal vesicles (SV) and (E and F) vasa deferentia (VD).

vesicles associated with dilated tubules in the epididymis. There may be ectasia of the rete testis and epididymal cysts. Rarely, particularly in immunocompromised patients [such as those suffering from acquired immunodeficiency syndrome (AIDS)], there may be tuberculous abscesses of prostate which can extend to the periprostatic region or develop into fistulae.[41] Most patients with tuberculosis of the prostate are asymptomatic while some may develop hemospermia, many present with infertility, mostly with azoospermia. A rare manifestation is that of fever secondary to an abscess.

Ultrasound of the prostate performed via the transrectal route often fails to reveal any abnormality in the prostate. Occasionally, focal areas of decreased

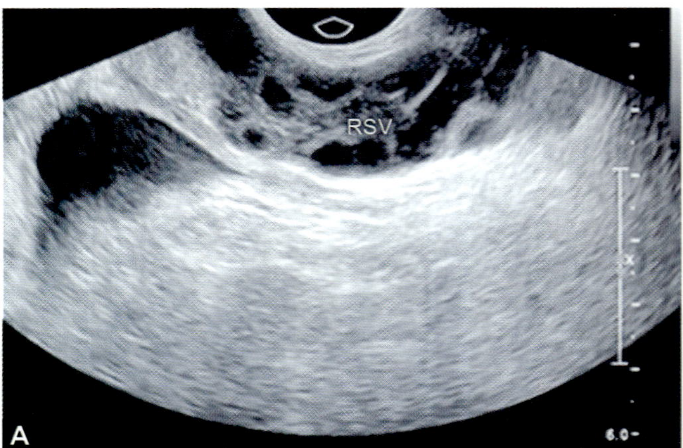

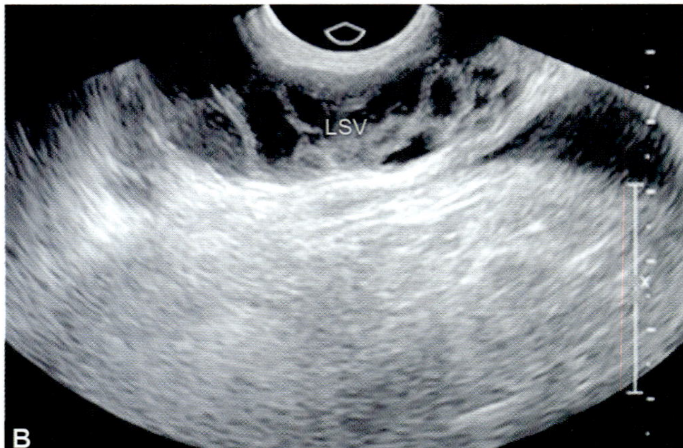

Figs. 12.29A and B: Right and left oblique transrectal ultrasonography (TRUS) scans showing dilated seminal vesicles (RSV and LSV) in a case of obstruction to epididymis (*Abbreviations:* RSV, right seminal vesicle; LSV, left seminal vesicle).

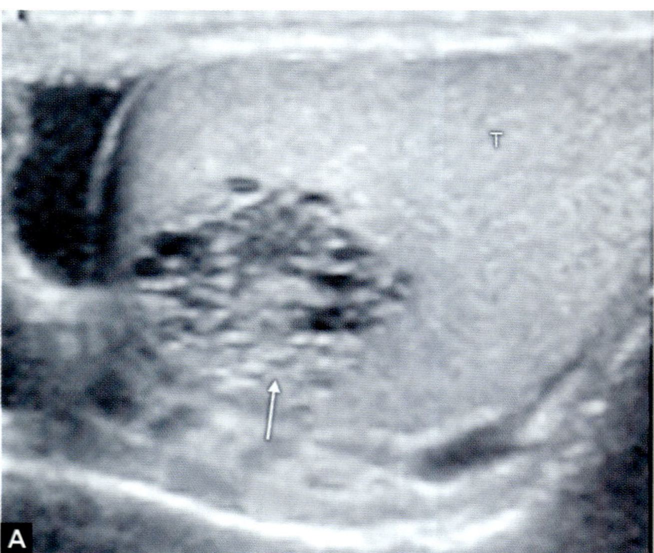

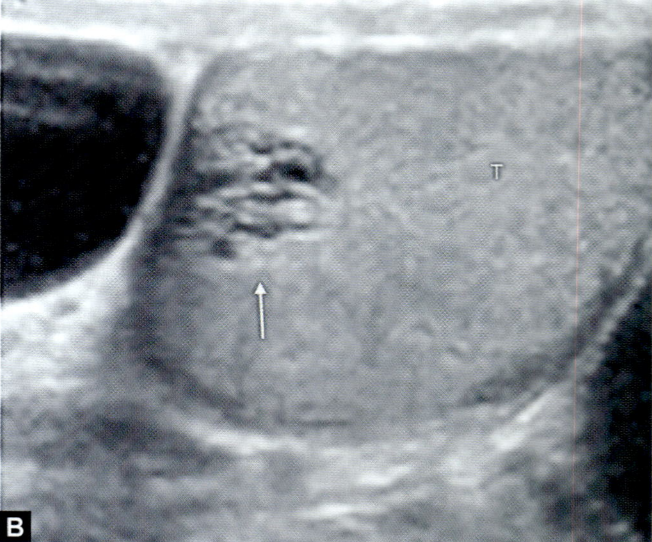

Figs. 12.30A and B: Transverse scan of both testes (T) showing ectasia of rete testis (arrow).

echogenicity (Fig. 12.32)[42,43] can be seen, as areas of dystrophic calcification (Fig. 12.33). Rarely, there may be an abscess in the prostate with or without a periprostatic collection (Fig. 12.34), which can mimic a pyogenic abscess particularly in an immunocompromised patient.[44] Very rarely, there may be a fistulous tract to the perineum or an air-filled tract extending from the prostate to the anal canal indicating an anourethral fistula.

When patients present with infertility due to obstruction of the ejaculatory ducts, US will show dilated seminal vesicles (Figs. 12.29A and B) associated with dilated tubules in the epididymis (Fig. 12.24). There may be ectasia of the rete testis (Figs. 12.30A and B) and epididymal cysts (Figs. 12.31A and B). The development of prostatic lesions can be nonspecific and may mimic the appearances of malignancy or other infections. When the symptoms are chronic or there are additional features of urinary tuberculosis, a biopsy may not be necessary. Otherwise a guided biopsy or aspiration is necessary to prove tuberculosis. In chronic lesions that develop fibrosis and calcification, it may be impossible to prove the existence of the infection and indeed may not even be necessary, as the treatment is directed more toward alleviating the patient's symptoms by relieving any obstruction which may also be useful in

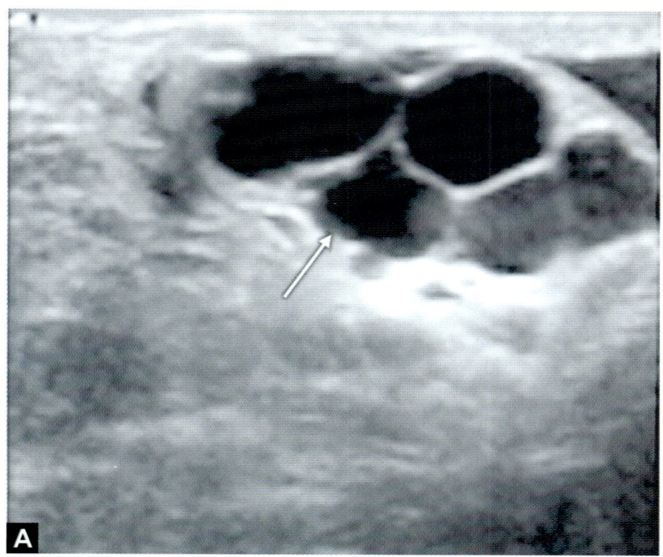

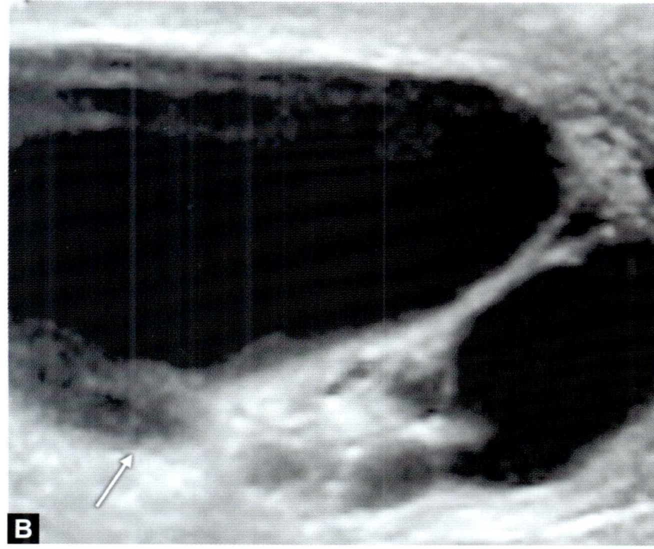

Figs. 12.31A and B: Oblique scan of scrotum showing bilateral epididymal cysts (arrow) in a case of distal vesical obstruction.

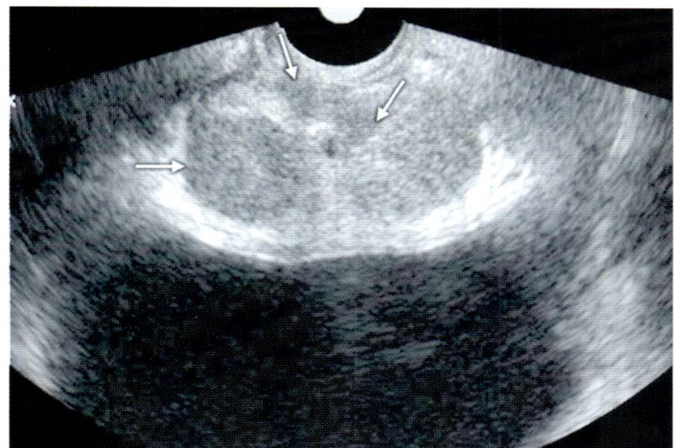

Fig. 12.32: Axial section of the prostate showing focal areas of decreased echogenicity (arrows) in tuberculosis.

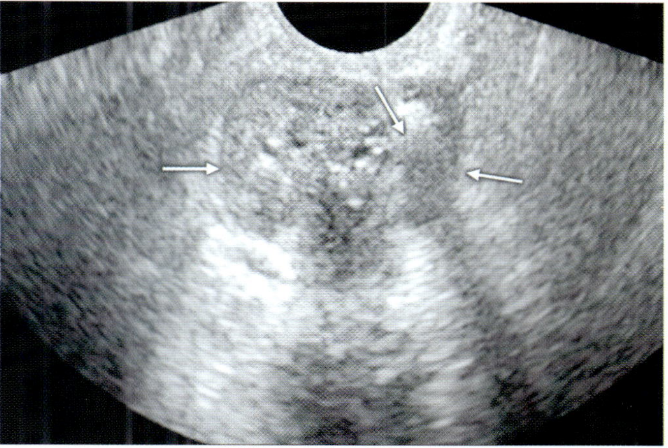

Fig. 12.33: Healing of granulomas results in dystrophic calcifications (arrow) in the prostate (arrowheads) shown in this image.

infertility or correcting a fistula and less so dealing with the underlying tuberculosis.[45]

Epididymal and Testicular Tuberculosis

Tuberculosis of the epididymis results from retrograde extension of infection from the prostate and the seminal vesicles or from hematogenous spread. Less frequently, it may be transmitted sexually or due to intravesical bacille Calmette-Guerin therapy for superficial bladder cancer.[44,46-52] Classically, the infection is said to affect the tail of the epididymis first, either because the tail has greater blood supply or because it is the first portion to be involved when there is reflux along the vas deferens.[50,53,54] However, more recently, Chung et al.[48] have suggested that the infection may in fact more frequently involve the entire epididymis or its head.

The testis may become involved secondarily by direct extension, but hematogenous spread to the testis is rarely possible.[49,53,55-57] Seventy percent of patients with tuberculous epididymitis have a previous history of tuberculosis[47,58,59] and although earlier reports suggested a greater incidence of bilateral involvement, recent reports have documented a higher proportion of unilateral disease.[48,50,54,60]

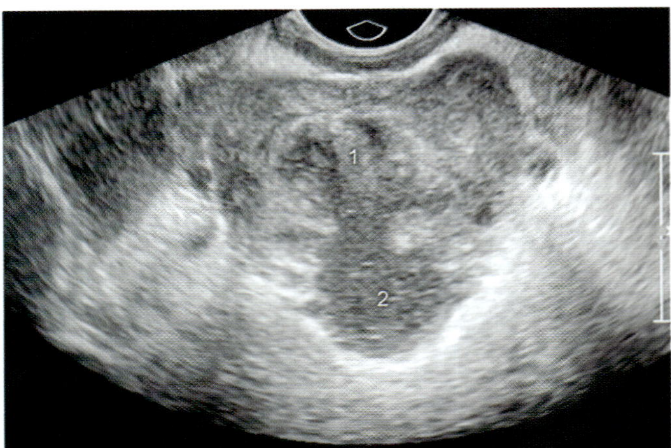

Fig. 12.34: (A) Axial and (B) longitudinal scans of the prostate showing an abscess (1) which extends outside the gland (2).

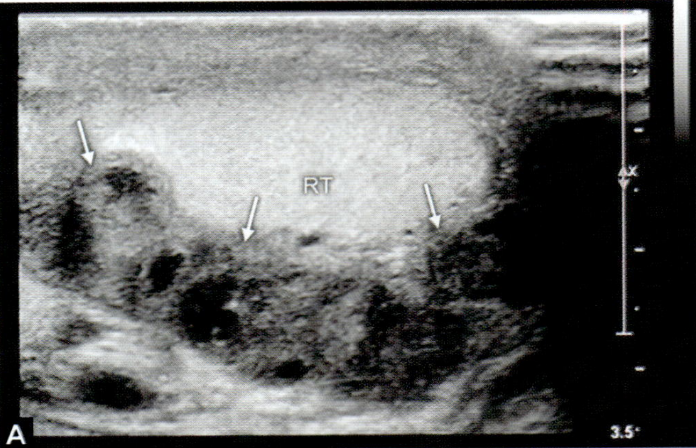

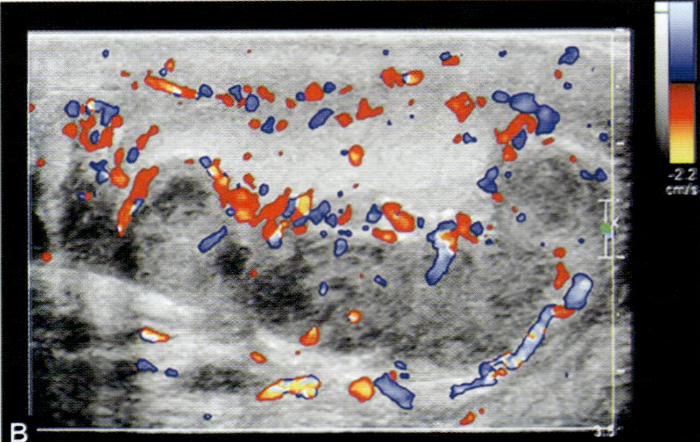

Figs. 12.35A and B: (A) Tuberculous epididymitis appearing as a diffusely enlarged heterogeneously hypoechoic epididymis (arrows); (B) color Doppler image showing the flow in the periphery and absence of the flow in the focal lesions (*Abbreviation:* RT, right testis).

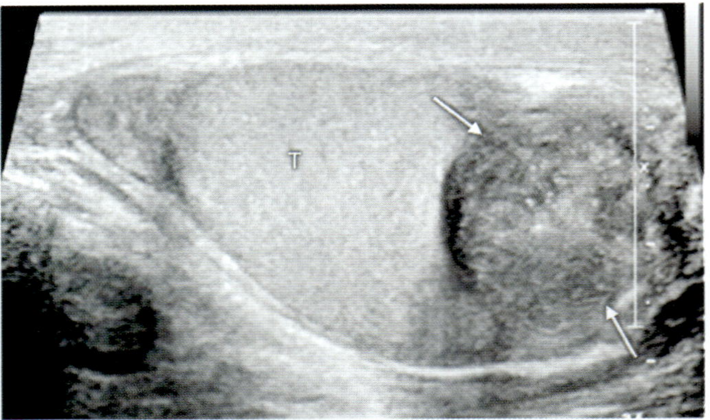

Fig. 12.36: Focal heterogeneous mass in tail of epididymis (arrows) in tuberculosis (*Abbreviation:* T, testis).

The most common symptoms of scrotal tuberculosis are of pain and swelling. Some cases are insidious and chronic, with painless or only slightly painful, epididymal swelling[46,49,56,61] but rarely, there may be a more acute presentation.[62,63] Though constitutional symptoms are rare,[60] they may occur in the presence of an abscess or sinus formation which also indicate advanced and more wide spread disease.[64]

Pathologically, there is necrosis of the tubules followed by caseation and fibrosis. There will be lesions in various stages of development, i.e. exudative, granulomatous and those healing with fibrosis[48,60,65] with calcification occurring later. When the tunica vaginalis is invaded, a hydrocele may often develop.

Ultrasound of the scrotum shows marked heterogeneity, and correlates well with the pathologic changes such as caseous necrosis, fibrosis, granuloma formation, and calcification.[48] Tuberculous epididymitis appears as a diffusely enlarged heterogeneously hypoechoic epididymis (Figs. 12.35A and B) or more focally with nodular heterogeneous hypoechoic lesions in epididymis (Fig. 12.36). Rarely, the epididymis is diffusely enlarged and homogeneously hypoechoic.[48,55,56,65,66] In an aggressive infection, an abscess may mimic a pyogenic infection (Fig. 12.37), and the abscess may extend into the scrotal wall (Fig. 12.38). When a scrotal sinus forms, an echopoor or fluid-filled tract may extend from the epididymis (usually the tail) into the scrotal wall reaching up toward the skin surface.[48,64] The scrotal skin may become thickened, a hydrocele may form, or the patient may develop calcification of the epididymis (Fig. 12.39) and tunica vaginalis.[48,54,56] Color Doppler US will demonstrate a few vessels in the periphery

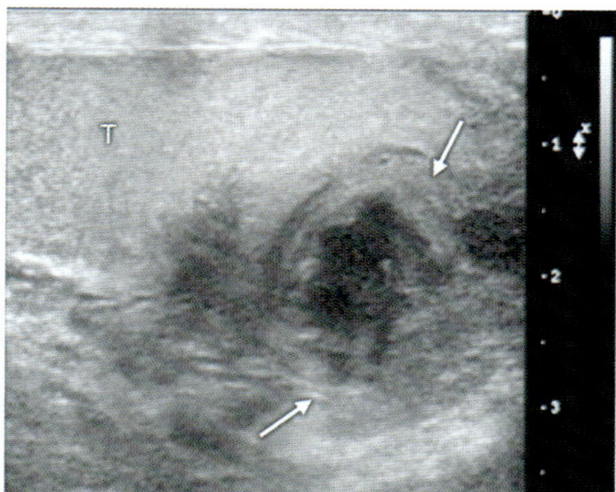

Fig. 12.37: Gray-scale image of a tuberculous abscess (arrows) in the tail of epididymis (*Abbreviation:* T, testis).

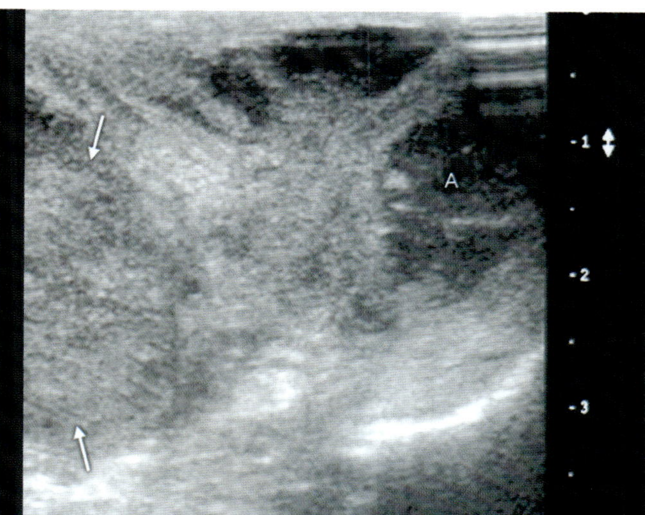

Fig. 12.38: Gray-scale image of a tuberculous abscess (arrows) in the tail of epididymis extending into the scrotal wall (A).

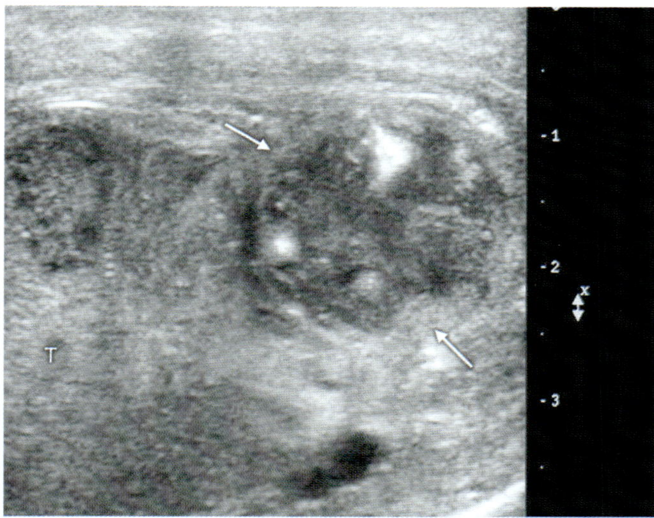

Fig. 12.39: A focal nodular heterogeneous lesion (arrows) in the tail of the epididymis with calcifications (*Abbreviation:* T, testis).

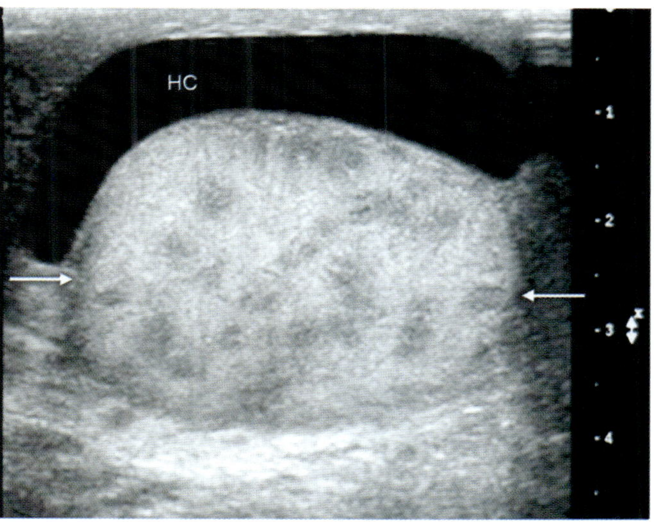

Fig. 12.40: An enlarged testis (arrows) with multiple small hypoechoic nodules. There is also hydrocele (HC).

of the epididymis with absence of flow in the focal lesions (Fig. 12.35B).[67,68] In tuberculous orchitis, a common appearance is an enlarged testis with multiple small, hypoechoic nodules (Fig. 12.40)[48,53] or rarely, diffuse enlargement of the testis with a homogeneous or heterogeneous hypoechoic texture (Fig. 12.41).[54,55,69] Another feature is a blurred separation between the testis and epididymis (Fig. 12.41). The differential diagnosis for scrotal tuberculosis includes an acute nonspecific infection and tumors,[56,69-71] the presence of both epididymal and testicular lesions is suggestive of an infection. In cases of nonspecific infection, the clinical picture is of an acute process and involvement is diffused and homogeneous as opposed to tuberculosis, which characteristically has a more chronic nature with focal heterogeneous lesions. Occasionally, the differentiation may be difficult but the presence of a sinus tract, the lack of response to antimicrobial agents and any evidence of tuberculosis in the rest of the genitourinary system might help to differentiate the conditions.[48] When a solitary lesion is found in the testis, it has to be differentiated from a tumor by histological analysis.[72]

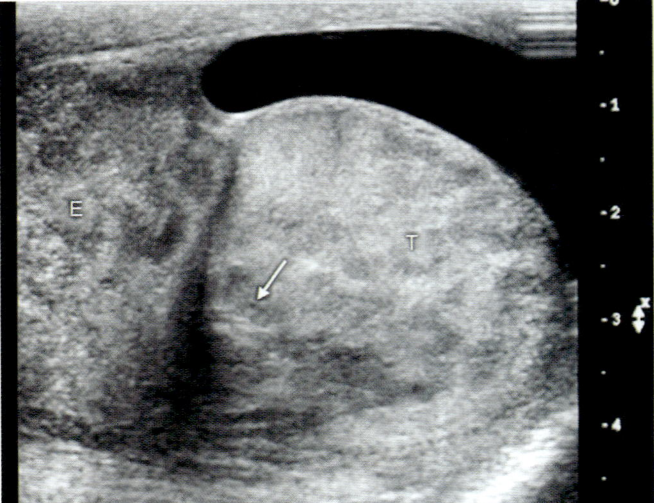

Fig. 12.41: Diffusely enlarged testis (T) with heterogeneous hypoechoic texture with a blurred interface (arrow) between the testis and the epididymis (E).

Tuberculosis of Seminal Vesicles and Vasa Deferentia

The tuberculous involvement of the seminal vesicles is the rarest form of extrapulmonary tuberculosis.[73] It occurs by hematogenous spread or by secondary involvement from prostatic infection. The course is insidious and patients are usually asymptomatic with eventual development of fibrosis and calcification causing infertility. The disease is usually bilateral and spreads contiguously to involve the vasa deferentia in which case, the patient may present initially with a low-volume ejaculate and later with infertility and a finding of aspermia. Transrectal ultrasonography reveals small solid seminal vesicles with or without calcifications (Figs. 12.42A and B). There may be single or multiple hypoechoic masses in the vas within the spermatic cord (Fig. 12.43) and possible calcification of the vas deferens (Figs. 12.44A and B). Fibrotic, atrophic seminal vesicles with aspermia have been considered a diagnostic feature of

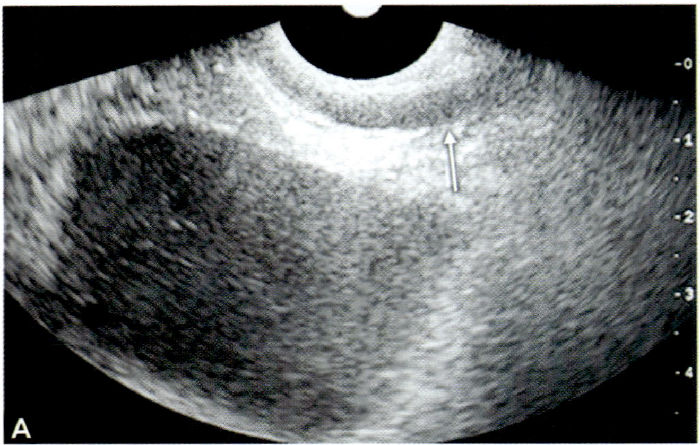

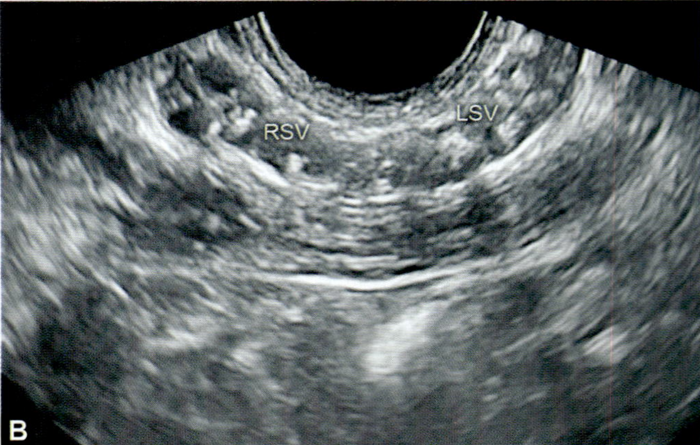

Figs. 12.42A and B: (A) Transrectal ultrasonography (TRUS) image showing a small, thin, and solid seminal vesicle (arrow); (B) extensive calcifications in both seminal vesicles (RSV and LSV) (*Abbreviations:* RSV, right seminal vesicle; LSV, left seminal vesicle).

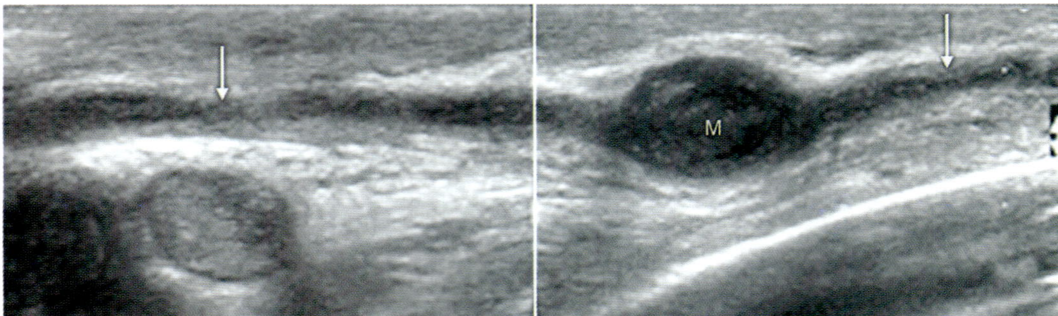

Fig. 12.43: A hypoechoic mass (M) of the vas deferens (arrows) in the spermatic cord due to tuberculosis.

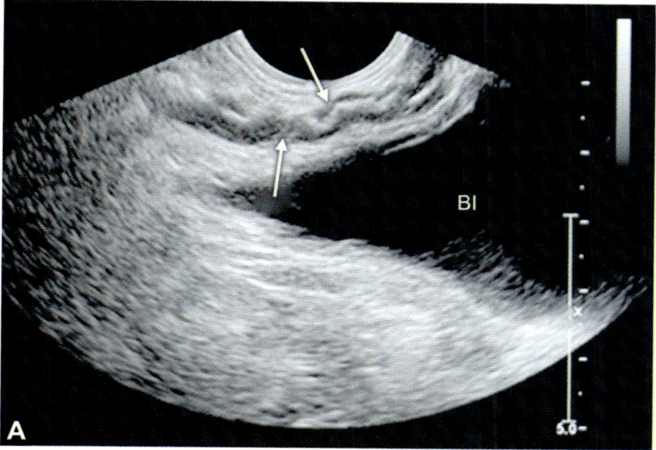

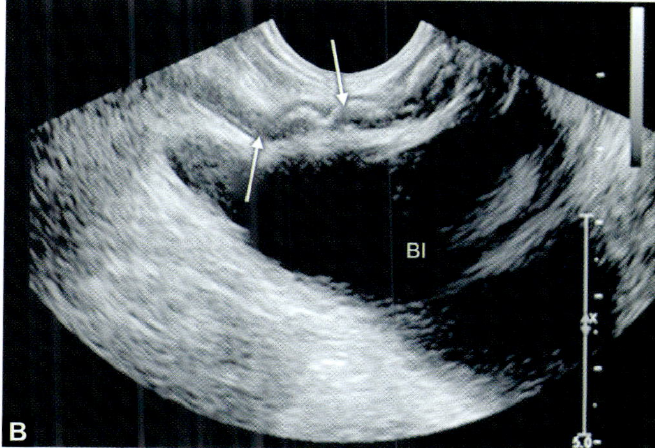

Figs. 12.44A and B: Transrectal ultrasonography (TRUS) images showing calcifications (arrows) in the vasa deferentia (arrowheads) (*Abbreviation:* BL, urinary bladder).

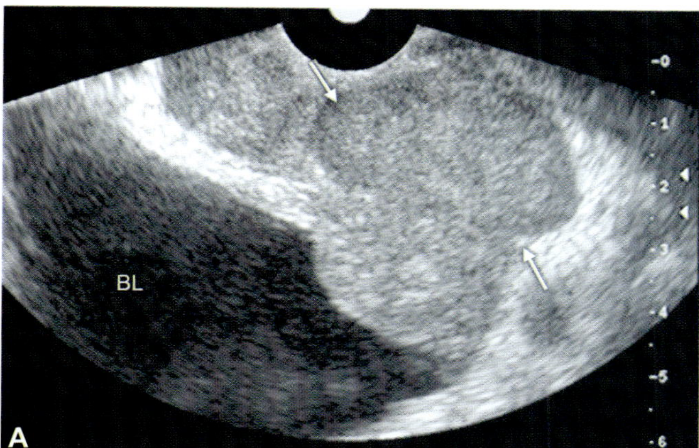

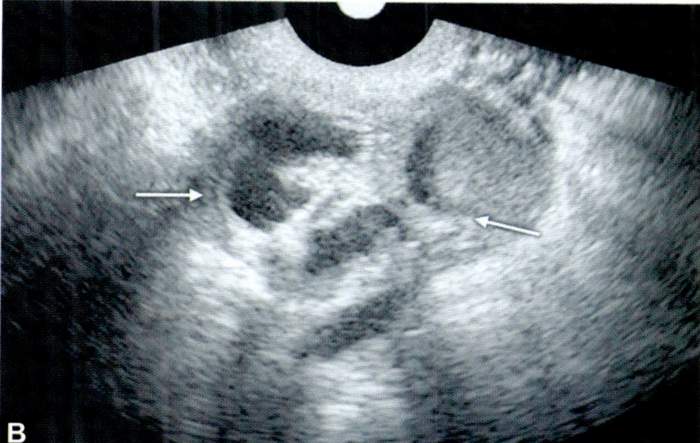

Figs. 12.45A and B: Two sections of the seminal vesicle and prostate showing an irregular solid and cystic mass (arrows) suggestive of an abscess in the seminal vesicle involving the prostate and indenting on the urinary bladder (BL).

tuberculosis and these patients need not be further evaluated and are treated with assisted reproduction.[74] The only differential diagnosis is congenital absence of the vas deferens, which will show an absent seminal vesicle and vas deferens on TRUS.[75] Rarely when there is severe infection, particularly in immunocompromised patients, an abscess of the seminal vesicle may be seen which usually also involves the prostate (Figs. 12.45A and B). These patients may present with fever and irritative voiding symptoms and in such patients, TRUS will reveal an abscess of the seminal vesicle, which is seen as an enlarged seminal vesicle with fluid and debris-filled areas within. There may be involvement of the prostate and loss of the interface between the seminal vesicle and the prostate and possibly thickening of the adjacent wall of the urinary bladder.[76] The findings mimic a pyogenic abscess and an US-guided aspiration will give proof of the underlying diagnosis of tuberculosis.

Stricture Urethra

The cause of obstruction to delivery of sperms may be a stricture of the urethra. The patient will usually have urinary symptoms. Ultrasound gel urethrogram is an excellent method to study the urethra. Sterile US gel is pushed into the urethra with a blunt cannula at the meatus. The gel distended urethra is well seen on sonography. The luminal narrowing caused by the stricture is well seen (Fig. 12.46). The length and the amount of narrowing can be measured.

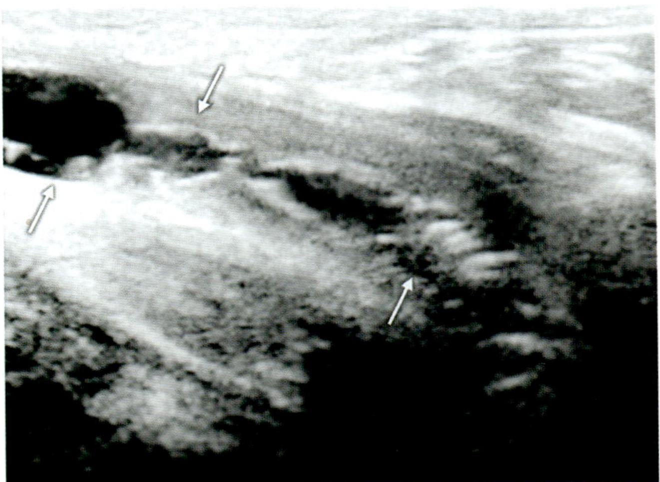

Fig. 12.46: Gel urethrogram showing the stricture (arrow) of urethra (arrowheads).

ROLE OF ULTRASOUND IN ASSISTED REPRODUCTION

Testicular volume measured by USG can predict the outcome of testicular biopsies for sperm retrieval as chances of successful sperm retrieval are significantly higher in patients with testicular volume more than 12 cc. Ultrasound-guided testicular sperm aspiration (USTSA) is more accurate and it has less complications when compared to blind testicular sperm aspiration (TSA) especially in NOA. Intraoperative sonography with power Doppler imaging enabled good visualization of the testicular parenchyma, easy sampling and avoidance of prominent vessels. In patients with EDO, sperms can be aspirated from the seminal vesicles under TRUS guidance. Transrectal ultrasonography is also helpful intraoperatively for identification of obstructing cyst and also to determine the depth of resection of ejaculatory duct for treatment of EDO.

KEY POINTS

- Transrectal ultrasonography is a very important, sensitive technique for evaluation of distal male genital tract
- Undescended testis should be diagnosed as early as possible to prevent germ cell damage
- Tracking the cord technique is a promising new technique to locate NPT
- Any patient with varicocele has to be examined in resting state and with Valsalva maneuver both in supine and erect position
- The impact of varicocele and its treatment is still a matter of debate and surgery is indicated for a young male with abnormal semen when the female is normal
- Any patient with OA to be evaluated completely by scrotal US and TRUS to determine the level and cause of obstruction
- Eighty-two percent of patients with CBAVD have at least one mutation within cystic fibrosis gene
- Agenesis of vas and seminal vesicle is associated with renal anomalies
- Ejaculatory duct obstruction causes dilatation of seminal vesicles, dilatation of tubules in epididymis, and ectasia of rete testis
- Diagnosis of a cyst causing obstruction of ejaculatory ducts can be resected with good results
- Ultrasound-guided testicular sperm aspiration may be more accurate than blind TSA

ACKNOWLEDGMENTS

The authors thank Dr Sathiya Senthil for her assistance in copy editing, and Mr Srambical Sreedharan, electronic data processing (EDP) for technical assistance, in the preparation of this chapter. The authors also thank all the clinical colleagues for their cooperation.

REFERENCES

1. Edey AJ, Sidhu PS. Male infertility: role of imaging in the diagnosis and management. Imaging. 2008;20:139-46.
2. Sidhu PS. Diseases of the testis and epididymis. In: Baxter GM, Sidhu PS (Eds). Ultrasound of the Urogenital System, 1st edition. Stuttgart, Germany: Thieme; 2006. pp. 153-80.
3. Nöske HD, Weidner W. Varicocele—a historical perspective. World J Urol. 1999;17(3):151-7.
4. Marmar JL. The pathophysiology of varicoceles in the light of current molecular and genetic information. Hum Reprod Update. 2001;7(5):461-72.
5. Naughton CK, Nangia AK, Agarwal A. Pathophysiology of varicoceles in male infertility. Hum Reprod Update. 2001;7(5):473-81.
6. Witt MA, Lipshultz LI. Varicocele: a progressive or static lesion? Urology. 1993;42(5):541-3.
7. Schoor RA, Elhanbly SM, Niederberger C. The pathophysiology of varicocele-associated male infertility. Curr Urol Rep. 2001;2(6):432-6.
8. Benoff S, Gilbert BR. Varicocele and male infertility: part I. Preface. Hum Reprod Update. 2001;7(1):47-54.
9. Benoff S, Marmar JL, Hurley IR. Molecular and other predictors for infertility in patients with varicoceles. Front Biosci. 2009;14:3641-72.

10. Dubin L, Amelar RD. Varicocele size and results of varicocelectomy in selected subfertile men with varicocele. Fertil Steril. 1970;21(8):606-9.
11. Beddy P, Geoghegan T, Browne RF, et al. Testicular varicoceles. Clin Radiol. 2005;60(12):1248-55.
12. Cornud F, Belin X, Amar E, et al. Varicocele: strategies in diagnosis and treatment. Eur Radiol. 1999;9(3):536-45.
13. Barozzi L, De Gaetano A, Derchi L. In: Guido Gnocchi (Ed). Color Doppler Uro- Genitale. 1996.
14. Isidori AM, Lenzi A. In: Genua SRL (Ed). Scrotal Ultrasound: Morphological and Functional Atlas. Forum Service; 2008.
15. Elder JS. The undescended testis. Hormonal and surgical management. Surg Clin North Am. 1988;68(5):983-1005.
16. MacKinnon AE. The undescended testis. Indian J Pediatr. 2005;72(5):429-32.
17. Cain MP, Garra B, Gibbons MD. Scrotal-inguinal ultrasonography: a technique for identifying the nonpalpable inguinal testis without laparoscopy. J Urol. 1996;156(2 Pt 2):791-4.
18. Nijs SM, Eijsbouts SW, Madern GC, et al. Nonpalpable testes: is there a relationship between ultrasonographic and operative findings? Pediatr Radiol. 2007;37(4):374-9.
19. Vijayaraghavan SB. Sonographic localization of nonpalpable testis: tracking the cord technique. Indian J Radiol Imaging. 2011;21(2):134-41.
20. Hutcheson JC, Snyder HM, Zuniga ZV, et al. Ectopic and undescended testes: 2 variants of a single congenital anomaly? J Urol. 2000;163(3):961-3.
21. Rao PL, Gupta V, Kumar V. Anterior abdominal wall—an unusual site for ectopic testis. Pediatr Surg Int. 2005;21(8):687-8.
22. Rusnack SL, Wu HY, Huff DS, et al. The ascending testis and the testis undescended since birth share the same histopathology. J Urol. 2002;168(6):2590-1.
23. Schuppe HC, Pilatz A, Hossain H, et al. Orchitis and male infertility. Urologe A. 2010;49(5):629-35.
24. Subramanyam BR, Horii SC, Hilton S. Diffuse testicular disease: sonographic features and significance. AJR Am J Roentgenol. 1985;145(6):1221-4.
25. Nagamine WH, Mehta SV, Vade A. Testicular adrenal rest tumors in a patient with congenital adrenal hyperplasia: sonographic and magnetic resonance imaging findings. J Ultrasound Med. 2005;24(12):1717-20.
26. Howlett DC, Jones AJ, Saunders AJ. Case of the month. Painless testicular nodularity in a young man. Br J Radiol. 1997;70(839):1195-6.
27. Doria-Rose VP, Biggs ML, Weiss NS. Subfertility and the risk of testicular germ cell tumors (United States). Cancer Causes Control. 2005;16(6):651-6.
28. Skakkebaek NE, Jorgensen N. Testicular dysgenesis and fertility. Andrologia. 2005;37(6):217-8.
29. Raman JD, Nobert CF, Goldstein M. Increased incidence of testicular cancer in men presenting with infertility and abnormal semen analysis. J Urol. 2005;174(5):1819-22.
30. Petersen PM, Skakkebaek NE, Vistisen K, et al. Semen quality and reproductive hormones before orchiectomy in men with testicular cancer. J Clin Oncol. 1999;17(3):941-7.
31. Moon MH, Kim SH, Cho JY, et al. Scrotal US for evaluation of infertile men with azoospermia. Radiology. 2006;239(1):168-73.
32. Kuligowska E, Fenlon HM. Transrectal US in male infertility: spectrum of findings and role in patient care. Radiology. 1998;207(1):173-81.
33. Donat R, McNeill AS, Fitzpatrick DR, et al. The incidence of cystic fibrosis gene mutations in patients with congenital bilateral absence of the vas deferens in Scotland. Br J Urol. 1997;79(1):74-7.
34. Gazvani R, Lewis-Jones DI. Cystic fibrosis mutation screening before assisted reproduction. Int J Androl. 2004;27(1):1-4.
35. Cornud F, Amar E, Hamida K, et al. Imaging in male hypofertility and impotence. BJU Int. 2000;86(Suppl 1): 153-63.
36. Hendry WF. Disorders of ejaculation: congenital, acquired and functional. Br J Urol. 1998;82(3):331-41.
37. Ammar T, Sidhu PS, Wilkins CJ. Male infertility: the role of imaging in diagnosis and management. Br J Radiol. 2012;85(Spec No 1):S59-68.
38. Jarow JP, Espeland MA, Lipshultz LI. Evaluation of the azoospermic patient. J Urol. 1989;142(1):62-5.
39. Galosi AB, Montironi R, Fabiani A, et al. Cystic lesions of the prostate gland: an ultrasound classification with pathological correlation. J Urol. 2009;181(2):647-57.
40. Vijayaraghavan SB. Ultrasonography of genitourinary tuberculosis. In: Sidhu PS, Joshi M (Eds). Genitourinary Ultrasound. New York: WB Saunders Company; 2010. pp. 367-78.
41. Kapoor R, Ansari MS, Mandhani A, et al. Clinical presentation and diagnostic approach in cases of genitourinary tuberculosis. Indian J Urol. 2008;24(3):401-5.
42. Hamrick-Turner J, Abbitt PL, Ros PR. Tuberculosis of the lower genitourinary tract: findings on sonography and MR. AJR Am J Roentgenol. 1992;158(4):919.
43. Wolf LE. Tuberculous abscess of the prostate in AIDS. Ann Intern Med. 1996;125(2):156.
44. Tikkakoski T, Karstrup S, Lohela P, et al. Tuberculosis of the lower genitourinary tract: ultrasonography as an aid to diagnosis and treatment. J Clin Ultrasound. 1993;21(4): 269-71.
45. Kumar R. Reproductive tract tuberculosis and male infertility. Indian J Urol. 2008;24(3):392-5.
46. Wolf JS, McAninch JW. Tuberculous epididymo-orchitis: diagnosis by fine needle aspiration. J Urol. 1991;145(4): 836-8.
47. Riehle RA, Jayaraman K. Tuberculosis of testis. Urology. 1982;20(1):43-6.
48. Chung JJ, Kim MJ, Lee T, et al. Sonographic findings in tuberculous epididymitis and epididymo-orchitis. J Clin Ultrasound. 1997;25(7):390-4.
49. Koyama Y, Iigaya T, Saito S. Tuberculous epididymo-orchitis. Urology. 1988;31(5):419-21.
50. Gow JG. Genitourinary tuberculosis. In: Walsh P, Gittes RF, Perlmutter AD (Eds). Campbell's Urology, 5th edition. Philadelphia: WB Saunders; 1986.

51. Smith DR. Specific infections of the urinary tract. In: Smith DR (Ed). General Urology, 10th edition. Los Altos, California: Lange Medical Publications; 1981.
52. Muttarak M, Lojanapiwat B, Chaiwun B, et al. Preoperative diagnosis of bilateral tuberculous epididymo-orchitis following intravesical Bacillus Calmette-Guérin therapy for superficial bladder carcinoma. Australas Radiol. 2002;46(2):183-5.
53. Drudi FM, Laghi A, Iannicelli E, et al. Tubercular epididymitis and orchitis: US patterns. Eur Radiol. 1997;7(7):1076-8.
54. Kim SH, Pollack HM, Cho KS, et al. Tuberculous epididymitis and epididymo-orchitis: sonographic findings. J Urol. 1993;150(1):81-4.
55. Heaton ND, Hogan B, Michell M, et al. Tuberculous epididymo-orchitis: clinical and ultrasound observations. Br J Urol. 1989;64(3):305-9.
56. Muttarak M, Peh WC, Lojanapiwat B, et al. Tuberculous epididymitis and epididymo-orchitis: sonographic appearances. AJR Am J Roentgenol. 2001;176(6):1459-66.
57. Turkvatan A, Kelahmet E, Yazgan C, et al. Sonographic findings in tuberculous epididymo-orchitis. J Clin Ultrasound. 2004;32(6):302-5.
58. Ferrie BG, Rundle JS. Tuberculous epididymo-orchitis. A review of 20 cases. Br J Urol. 1983;55(4):437-9.
59. Ross JC, Gow JG, St Hill CA. Tuberculous epididymitis. A review of 170 patients. Br J Surg. 1961;48:663-6.
60. Mostofi FK, Davis CJ. Male reproductive system and prostate. In: Kissane JM (Ed). Anderson's Pathology, 9th edition. St Louis: Mosby; 1990.
61. Reeve HR, Weinerth JL, Peterson LJ. Tuberculosis of epididymis and testicle presenting as hydrocele. Urology. 1974;4(3):329-31.
62. Gorse GJ, Belshe RB. Male genital tuberculosis: a review of the literature with instructive case reports. Rev Infect Dis. 1985;7(4):511-24.
63. Wechsler H, Westfall M, Lattimer JK. The earliest signs and symptoms in 127 male patients with genitourinary tuberculosis. J Urol. 1960;83:801-3.
64. Borthwick WM. The pathogenesis of tuberculous epididymitis. Edinb Med J. 1946;53:55-70.
65. Hill GS, Billey-Kijner C. Paratesticular structures: nontumorous conditions. In: Hill GS (Ed). Uropathology. New York: Churchill Livingstone; 1989.
66. Kim SH. Genitourinary tuberculosis. In: Pollack HM, McClennan BL (Eds). Clinical Urolography, 2nd edition. Philadelphia: WB Saunders Company; 2000. pp. 1193-228.
67. Yang DM, Chang MS, Oh YH, et al. Chronic tuberculous epididymitis: color Doppler US findings with histopathologic correlation. Abdom Imaging. 2000;25(5):559-62.
68. Yang DM, Yoon MH, Kim HS, et al. Comparison of tuberculous and pyogenic epididymal abscesses: clinical, gray-scale sonographic, and color Doppler sonographic features. AJR Am J Roentgenol. 2001;177(5):1131-5.
69. Kratzik C, Hainz A, Kuber W, et al. Sonographic appearance of benign intratesticular lesions. Eur Urol. 1988;15 (3-4):196-9.
70. Hamm B. Differential diagnosis of scrotal masses by ultrasound. Eur Radiol. 1997;7(5):668-79.
71. Salmeron I, Ramirez-Escobar MA, Puertas F, et al. Granulomatous epididymo-orchitis: sonographic features and clinical outcome in brucellosis, tuberculosis and idiopathic granulomatous epididymo-orchitis. J Urol. 1998;159(6): 1954-7.
72. Dempsey J, Brooks J, Scott RL. Testicular pseudotumor caused by mycobacterium bovis epididymitis. J Clin Ultrasound. 1992;20(3):200-3.
73. Eastham JA, Spires KS, Abreo F, et al. Seminal vesicle abscess due to tuberculosis: role of tissue culture in making the diagnosis. South Med J. 1999;92(3):328-9.
74. Paick J, Kim SH, Kim SW. Ejaculatory duct obstruction in infertile men. BJU Int. 2000;85(6):720-4.
75. Kumar R, Thulkar S, Kumar V, et al. Contribution of investigations to the diagnosis of bilateral vas aplasia. ANZ J Surg. 2005;75(9):807-9.
76. Pal DK. Tubercular abscess of the seminal vesicle. Ind J Tub. 2003;50:155.

Chapter

13

Three-Dimensional Ultrasound in Subfertility

Kannamannadiar Jayaprakasan, Nick Raine-Fenning

Chapter Outline

INTRODUCTION

Conventional two-dimensional (2D) transvaginal ultrasound has been one of the key modes of investigation in subfertile women, but recent developments have seen the introduction of three-dimensional (3D) ultrasound. The role of 2D transvaginal ultrasonography as a reliable diagnostic modality in evaluation of the pelvic organs is well established.[1] However, the planes of the pelvic structures that it can generate are limited with only sagittal and transverse views being available to interpret, which makes it difficult to obtain a 3D impression of the region of interest.[2] While an experienced ultrasonographer can create their own 3D interpretation of the object of interest based on a sequence of 2D images, its objective demonstration is not possible. Furthermore, the interpretation of the ultrasound images largely depends on the original, real-time examination because of associated limitations in data storage and while 2D cineloops and video recordings can be made. These require a great deal of administrative time and necessitate large archives both physically and in terms of data memory. Three-dimensional ultrasound imaging overcomes most, if not all, of these limitations.[3]

THREE-DIMENSIONAL ULTRASOUND

Three-dimensional ultrasound or "volume sonography" involves the acquisition of a series of 2D images from a preselected region of interest.[4] These data have relative positional information within the acquired volume dataset. Three-dimensional ultrasound scanning consists of four basic steps: (1) data acquisition, (2) data storage, (3) data retrieval, volume analysis and processing, and (4) archiving of volumes.[3,5] The acquisition is usually done in duplicate with the first acquisition obtaining gray-scale information and the second, Doppler data to allow assessment of blood flow within the organs.

Data Acquisition

Three-dimensional ultrasound involves the acquisition and display of echo information from multiple 2D scan images of a volume of tissue, rather than from a single 2D slice. A solid 3D volume is reconstructed from these sets of images incorporating the positional information both in time and space using computing software. Various methods for the acquisition and subsequent display and assessment of 3D ultrasound data are available.[6]

Two methods are commonly used for the acquisition of 3D ultrasound data: manual or free hand and automated.[5] Manual acquisition of data involves the observer moving the probe over the organ of interest in order to generate images. The commonly used "automated" technique involves the use of a dedicated 3D probe, the activation of which, rotate the ultrasound beam across an operator-selected region of interest (the volume "box") to acquire a series of 2D images at predefined intervals while the probe is held stationary.[5]

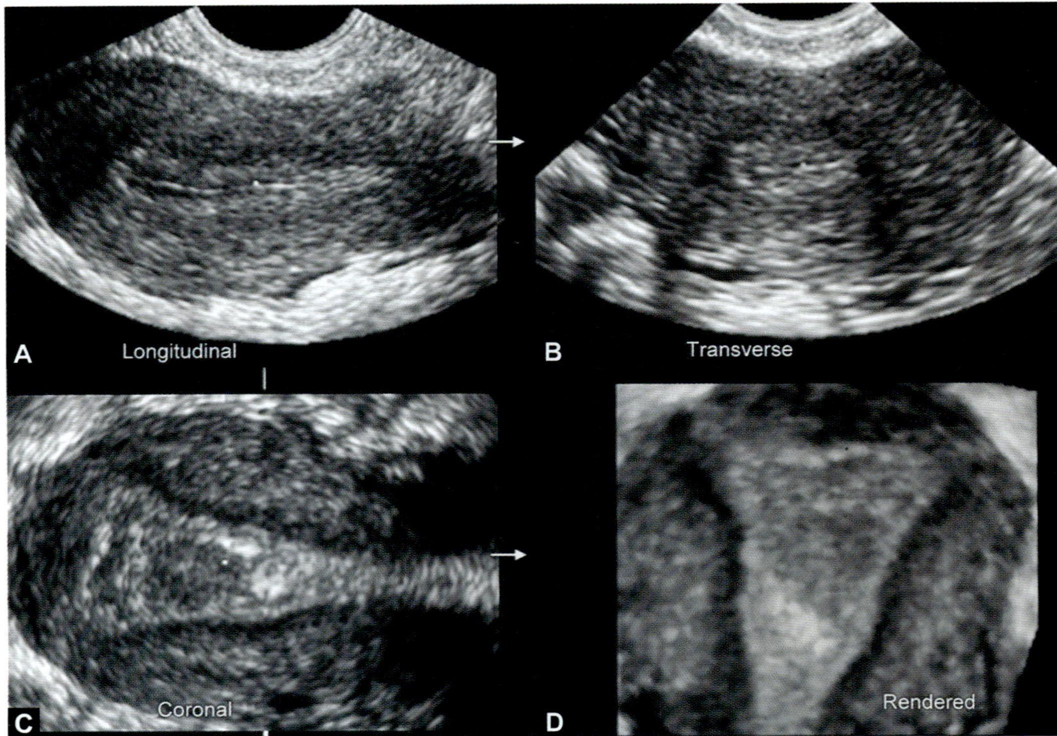

Figs. 13.1A to D: A multiplanar view of the uterus. A typical multiplanar display of a 3D ultrasound dataset of the uterus is shown. The upper left image represents (A) the longitudinal plane, the upper right image (B) the transverse plane, and the lower left image (C) the coronal plane. Lower right image is showing (D) the rendered view of the uterus in coronal plane.

The operator can determine the speed of acquisition and alter the volume box. The resolution is higher with a slower acquisition speed because the number of 2D images within the acquired volume is maximized but is more susceptible to movement artifact.[7] However, resolution is variable within the 3D volume with highest in the plane of acquisition and lowest in the reconstructed coronal plane.[5] Another major limitation is the maximum volume that can be measured due to the position and size of the transducer. The procedure is well tolerated by women as the transducer is the same size as standard transvaginal probe and transducer movement is actually reduced compared to conventional imaging, which involves a dynamic assessment of the pelvic organs.

Data Display

The acquired 3D data may be displayed in a variety of ways depending on the tissue and area of interest and analyzed in a virtual real-time manner as the user can obtain any image plane they desire. The most commonly used display in gynecology is the multiplanar view, which simultaneously shows three perpendicular planes: sagittal, transverse, and reconstructed coronal views (Figs. 13.1A to C).[8,9] An unlimited number of multiplanar displays are possible by scrolling through and/or rotating the volume to define uterine abnormalities and evaluate ovarian and endometrial morphology. The coronal plane, unique to 3D ultrasound, is perpendicular to the transducer face and facilitate the identification of surface irregularities which can then be accounted for during volume measurement.[1] Other ways of displaying the volume data includes image rendering (Fig. 13.1D) which enhances the contrast between any two areas by recreating an impression of depth.[2] These techniques are less important in the field of gynecology than obstetrics where they have been more frequently reported.[9] A rendering modality, "inversion mode" has also been described in which the gray scale of the volume voxels is inverted to demonstrate the fluid-filled anechoic structures as hyperechoic images (Fig. 13.2). This modality provides an added value to establish the diagnosis of a variety of gynecological conditions like hydrosalpinx.[10] Another useful feature of 3D display is the cineloop in which the rendered volume is rotated up to

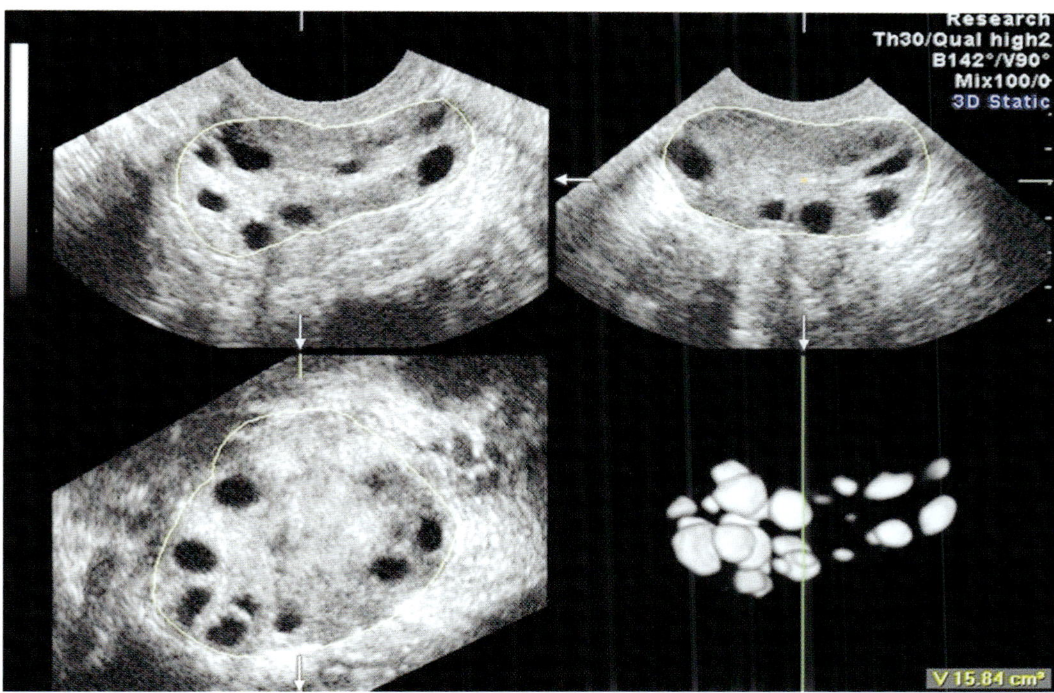

Fig. 13.2: Inversion mode of an ovary: Anechoic follicles within the ovary are inverted to hyperechoic structures as seen in the lower right image.

180° allowing the observer to view the structure from different angles.[11] Tomographic ultrasound imaging (TUI) is another displaying modality in which the volume dataset is divided into multiple slices, simultaneously displayed on the ultrasound screen (Fig. 13.3). The number and the width of the slices displayed can be manipulated on the machine to optimize the display of the anatomical details of the region of interest.

Data Analysis

An important advantage of 3D imaging is its capability of accurately measuring the volume of a structure of interest, even if it is irregular in shape. While volume may be estimated from measurements made with conventional 2D ultrasound, such measurements use various formulae based on certain geometric assumptions which may introduce significant errors in volume estimation.[12] Simultaneous display of the three mutually related orthogonal planes of a structure at a defined point using 3D ultrasound may facilitate more accurate measurement of volume than 2D ultrasound although it still involves a degree of geometric assumption.[13] While there are two basic methods ("full planar" or "contour" method and rotational method) employed to calculate volume from a 3D dataset, the currently used method is "rotational" method possible through Virtual Organ Computer-Aided Analysis (VOCAL), which generates a 3D model of the object of interest[14] (Fig. 13.4). The technique involves manual delineation of the object of interest in the multiplanar display that shows the three perpendicular planes characteristic of 3D ultrasound. The volume measurements using the 3D rotational methods have been shown to be more reproducible than 2D measurements.[15,16]

Three-dimensional ultrasound can also be used to acquire vascular information through the simultaneous application of power Doppler ultrasound. Conventional color Doppler is not suited to 3D imaging due to the continual changes in color induced by variations in blood flow velocity and direction.[17] Power Doppler imaging is a variant of color Doppler that utilizes the amplitude of the Doppler signal to display the total integrated Doppler power from a Doppler-shifted ultrasound signal in color rather than the mean Doppler frequency shift.[18] Power Doppler produces a more stable image that facilitates data acquisition and assessment particularly of longer vascular segments, which are displayed continuously on screen.[19] This information is acquired as the ultrasound beam is swept through an angle determined by the observer dependent on the size and position of the object of interest. The power

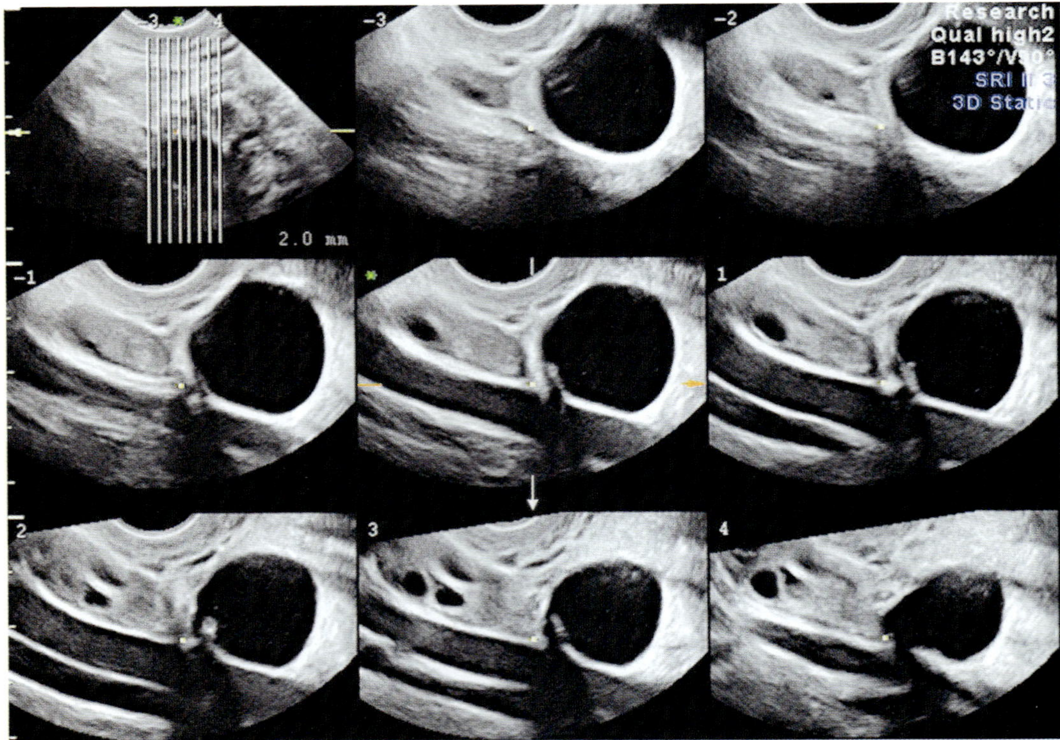

Fig. 13.3: Tomographic ultrasound images of an ovary and paraovarian cyst.

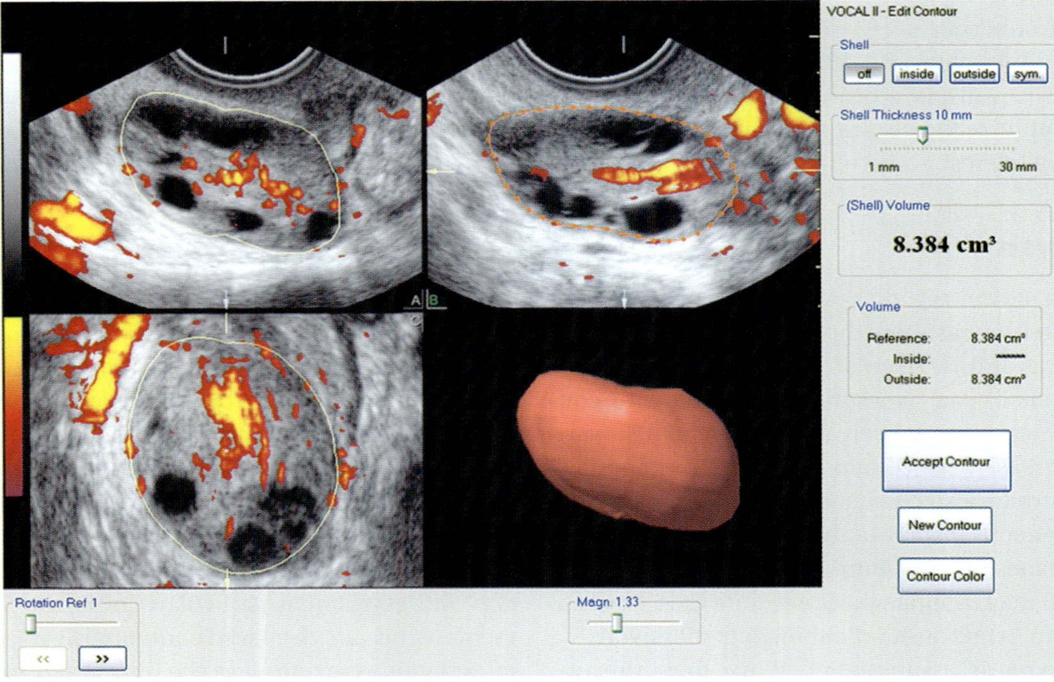

Fig. 13.4: Volume calculation of an ovary using virtual organ computer-aided analysis (VOCAL).

Doppler signal may then be quantified by one of several currently available software programs.

The vast majority of the medical literature and almost all gynecology applications report the use of the "histogram" facility within four-dimensional (4D) view software (GE medical systems). This calculates three indices of vascularity based on the power Doppler signal intensity and the distribution of the color voxels within the defined volume, where a voxel refers to a volume element or 3D pixel. The vascularization index (VI) reflects the ratio of power Doppler information within the total dataset relative to both color and gray information, the flow index (FI) represents the mean power Doppler signal intensity, and the vascularization flow index (VFI) represents a combination of the two (Fig. 13.5).[20] The VI is presented as a percentage while the FI and VFI may range between 0 and 100. They are generally quoted without units.

Recently introduced softwares [e.g. sonography-based automated volume calculation (SonoAVC); GE medical systems] integrated within the 3D ultrasound machines have allowed automated volume calculation of fluid-filled structures. Automatic data analysis has the potential to remove any observer bias and to reduce the time needed for measurements and has been shown to be valid and reliable.[21-23] SonoAVC identifies and quantifies hypoechoic regions within a 3D dataset. SonoAVC is an ideal tool to study follicular development within the ovary (Fig. 13.6) and provides automatic estimation of their absolute dimensions, mean diameter, and volume. Each individual volume is given a specific color and the automated measurements of its mean diameter (relaxed sphere diameter), its maximum dimensions (x, y, and z diameters), and its volume are displayed by these colors in descending order of size. An unlimited number of volumes can theoretically be quantified which makes it an ideal tool for assessment of the ovaries in women undergoing controlled ovarian stimulation. There are limitations to SonoAVC; however, it is important to recognize them. Some follicles are not identified following the initial automatic assessment, some follicles are identified incorrectly, and in most cases there is some extraovarian artifact. There are several options for postprocessing that require manual or automatic modification of the initial output. Manual techniques may be used for single follicles but the automated options are applied to the dataset as a whole. SonoAVC can be used to quantify and track ovarian cysts

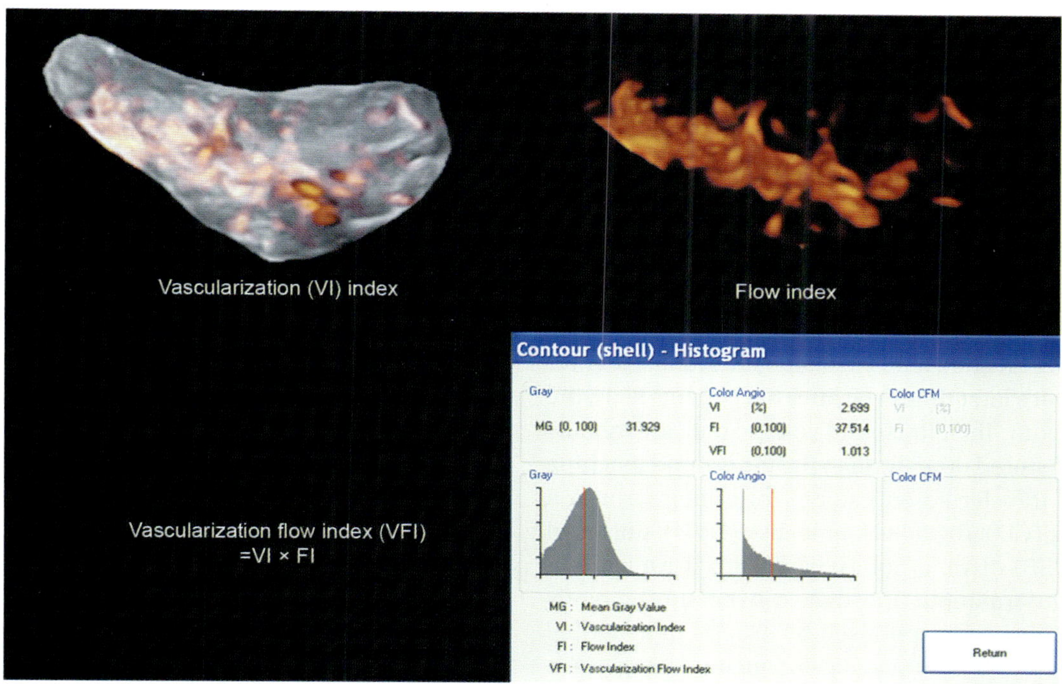

Fig. 13.5: Vascular quantification using VOCAL and histogram facility demonstrating three different vascularity indices (lower right image). The VI reflects the ratio of power Doppler information within the total dataset relative to both color and gray information, the FI represents the mean power Doppler signal intensity and the VFI represents a combination of the two. (*Abbrivation:* FI; flow index; VFI, vascularization flow index; VOCAL, Virtual Organ Computer-Aided Analysis; VI, vascularization index)

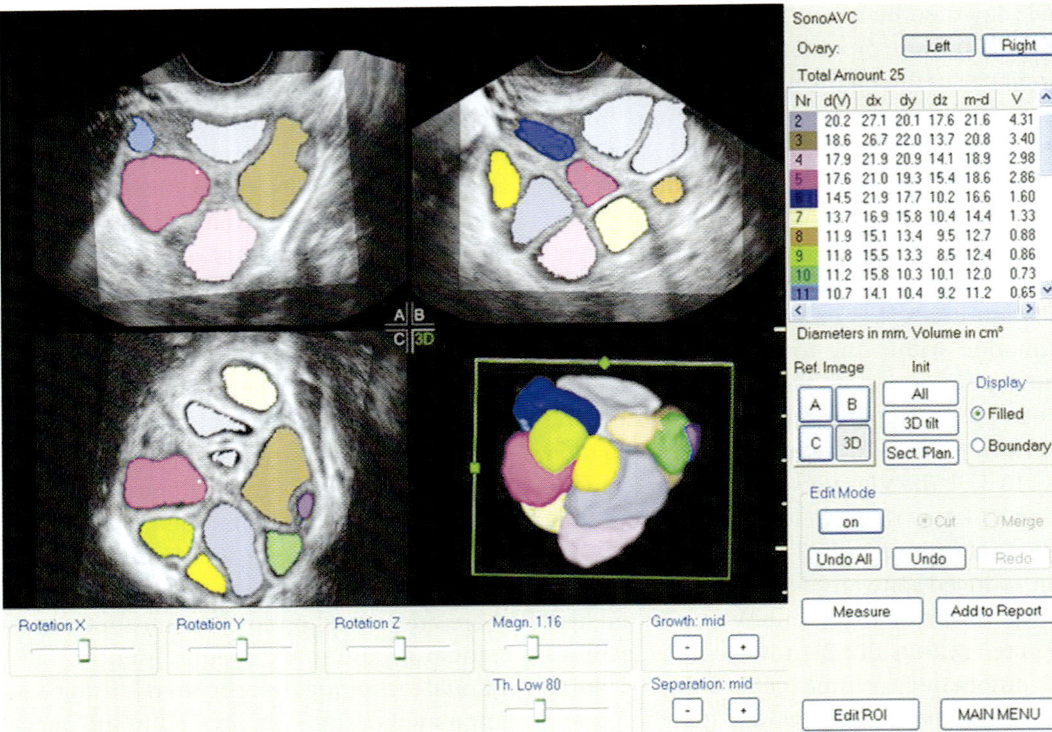

Fig. 13.6: Automated evaluation of a stimulated ovary using SonoAVC demonstrating the number of follicles, relaxed sphere diameter, and x, y, and z diameters of each follicles.

and to count the number of antral follicles within a normal or a polycystic ovary, although the software performs less well with smaller follicles, for which there is a need for more extensive postprocessing.

Data Storage and Archiving

The digital technology central to its development also means that 3D imaging lends itself to data storage and reexamination at a later time even after the patients leave the ultrasound room. The ultrasound volume data are initially acquired and stored directly on to the ultrasound machine and then be transferred and stored for a long term in a compact disk (CD), digital versatile disk (DVD), universal serial bus (USB) drive, or an external hard drive without any loss of information. The data can be subsequently analyzed offline and reappraised by experts in a "virtual real-time consultation." The data storage not only permits a prolonged assessment of the data if necessary but also allows long-term data storage for medicolegal purposes.

Advocates of 3D ultrasound[24] suggest that the features specific to 3D ultrasound offer the user several advantages in comparison to 2D ultrasound (Box 13.1). Many clinicians remain unconvinced by its reputed advantages and 3D ultrasound is not without disadvantages (Box 13.2). These mainly relate to the cost implications and training

Box 13.1: Potential advantages of 3D ultrasound

- Multiple data display modalities
- Improved anatomical and vascular information
- Improved assessment of complex anatomic anomalies
- A better specificity in regard to the confirmation of normality
- Standardization of the ultrasound examination procedure
- Storage of digital datasets for subsequent offline analysis
- Postacquisition processing is possible
- Accurate and reproducible measurement of organ dimensions, volumes, and vascularity
- Automated volume measurement of fluid-filled structures is possible
- Reduced scanning times with cost-effective use of equipment and ultrasonographer time
- Telemedicine and tertiary consultation

Box 13.2: Disadvantages of 3D ultrasound

- A dependence on 2D image clarity for the definition of organ interfaces
- Attenuation of 2D ultrasound means that image quality differs with depth within any 3D volume
- Prone to acquisition artifact due to physiological movements, such as respiration, cardiac or vascular pulsation, or inadvertent patient movement
- May need increased total time due to additional post-acquisition processing
- Cost implications in purchasing equipment

requirements. Three-dimensional ultrasound does require specific equipment but this is becoming widely available and is incorporated in most new systems. It is the additional training that has probably limited its development more although there are many courses available offering theoretical and hands on training.

APPLICATION OF THREE-DIMENSIONAL ULTRASOUND IN SUBFERTILITY

A baseline ultrasound assessment of the pelvis is regularly performed by most fertility units to screen for any pelvic pathologies that are known to have a negative effect on fertility and early pregnancy. The other key areas that the pretreatment assessment facilitates include the prediction of the woman's ovarian reserve, identification of ovarian position with respect to accessibility for oocyte retrieval, and evaluation of the chance of implantation of an embryo (endometrial receptivity). Furthermore, ultrasound allows for the direct monitoring of response to controlled ovarian stimulation, and facilitates oocyte retrieval and embryo transfer (ET). While 2D ultrasound is absolutely adequate for all the aforementioned indications, 3D ultrasound can be used as an adjunct to this and can be performed after a baseline assessment has been concluded. This chapter focuses on the general role of 3D imaging in the field of reproductive medicine while application of 3D ultrasound for various pathologies and interventions has been detailed in previous chapters.

The Uterus

The Normal Uterus

When visualized in the coronal plane, the uterine fundus appears to be flat or slightly upwardly convex (Figs. 13.1C and D). The endometrial appearance varies according to the stage of the menstrual cycle but generally has a homogenous echotexture and an increased echogenicity when compared with the myometrium. It is important that the uterus is visualized in the mid coronal plane and that the fundus is clearly visualized to ensure that uterine anomalies are not missed and that an entirely normal uterus is not mistaken for an abnormal one. The cervix which appears as a tubular echogenic structure is also best visualized in the coronal view. However, it is important to remember that the view through the center of the cervical canal may require the demonstration of a different coronal plane to that providing the mid coronal view of the uterus according to the degree of version and flexion of the uterus.

Congenital Uterine Anomalies

Congenital uterine anomalies are associated with an increased risk of abnormal pregnancy outcome,[25-27] which is improved after hysteroscopic septoplasty.[28] This is undoubtedly the area where 3D ultrasound has contributed the most and has become the investigation of choice in units where available. Jurkovic et al. compared the use of 3D ultrasound to detect congenital uterine anomalies against hysterosalpingography and 2D ultrasound in 61 patients with a history of infertility and recurrent miscarriage.[29] They identified that while 3D ultrasound and hysterosalpingography, which was considered the gold standard tool for the investigation of uterine anomalies at the time, came to the same conclusion regarding the normality of the uterus, 2D ultrasound was less specific and resulted in more false positive findings. Raga et al. and Wu et al. reported similar results shortly afterward suggesting 3D ultrasound offered a 100% specificity for the exclusion of uterine anomalies and was able to differentiate between the different anomalies.[30,31] The main benefit of 3D ultrasound for the assessment of uterine anomalies is that it allows us to image the uterine fundus and serosal outline simultaneously in the coronal plane, which is difficult and frequently impossible, to obtain with conventional 2D ultrasound. This view allows the user to easily identify that the uterus is abnormal and then classify the abnormality (Fig. 13.7). Three-dimensional ultrasound is now the gold standard tool for the assessment of uterine anomalies as it is less invasive than hysterosalpingography but just as sensitive and facilitates the differentiation of the type of anomaly.

3D ultrasound is time efficient, cost-effective, readily available, objective, highly reproducible and can be used

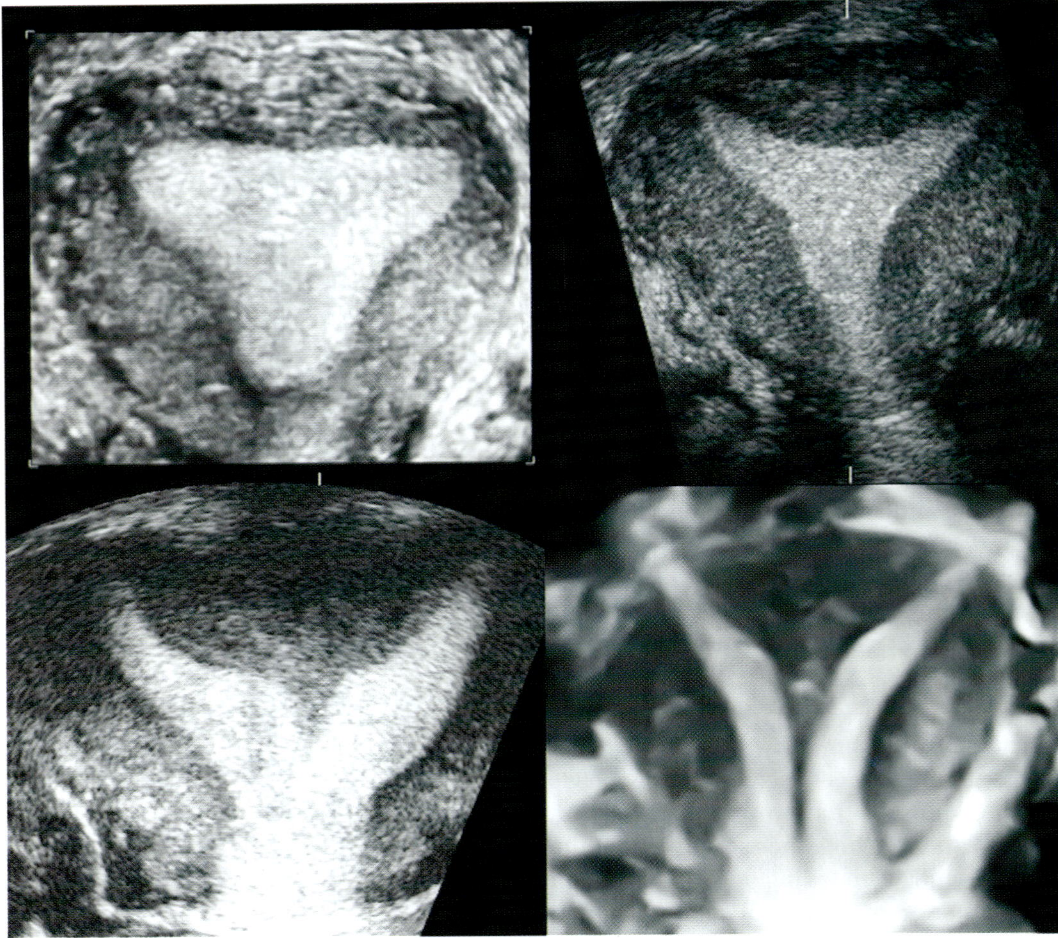

Fig. 13.7: Coronal plane, unique to 3D ultrasound, of uterus demonstrating different uterine shapes: Normal uterus (top left), arcuate uterus (top right), partial subseptate uterus (lower left), and complete septate uterus (lower right).

at the patient's bedside alongside a self-explanatory classification system, such as that of ESHRE-European Society for Gynaecological Endoscopy (ESGE). Furthermore, it can be used in conjunction with hysteroscopic surgery, to plan and guide the procedure by assessing the depth of the septal resection.[32]

Fibroids: Three-dimensional ultrasound has recently been used to map the exact location of fibroids in relation to the endometrial cavity and surrounding structures (Fig. 13.8). This is extremely important in triaging patients for surgery which is dependent on the exact position of the fibroid and the extent of its endometrial involvement. An improvement in the diagnostic specificity of ultrasound with 3D imaging has been shown by Sylvestre et al. in their study of 209 subfertile patients thought to have an intrauterine lesion on transvaginal 2D ultrasound or hysterosalpingography.[33] Using saline infusion sonography with 2D and then 3D ultrasound, 92 patients were subsequently identified as having a variety of intrauterine lesions suggesting a sensitivity and specificity of 97% and 11% for 2D ultrasound, 87% and 45% for 3D ultrasound, and 98% and 100% for 2D saline infusion sonography. Of 59 patients that had undergone hysteroscopy, the sensitivity and positive predictive value of saline infusion sonography were 98% and 95% when performed in combination with 2D ultrasound and 100% and 92% with 3D ultrasound, respectively. The study clearly demonstrates how simple contrast media potentially increase the specificity of 2D ultrasound as 55% (116 of 209) of patients were found to have normal cavities following the infusion of saline. This was largely due to the correct localization of leiomyomas as intramural rather than submucosal (54 of 101).

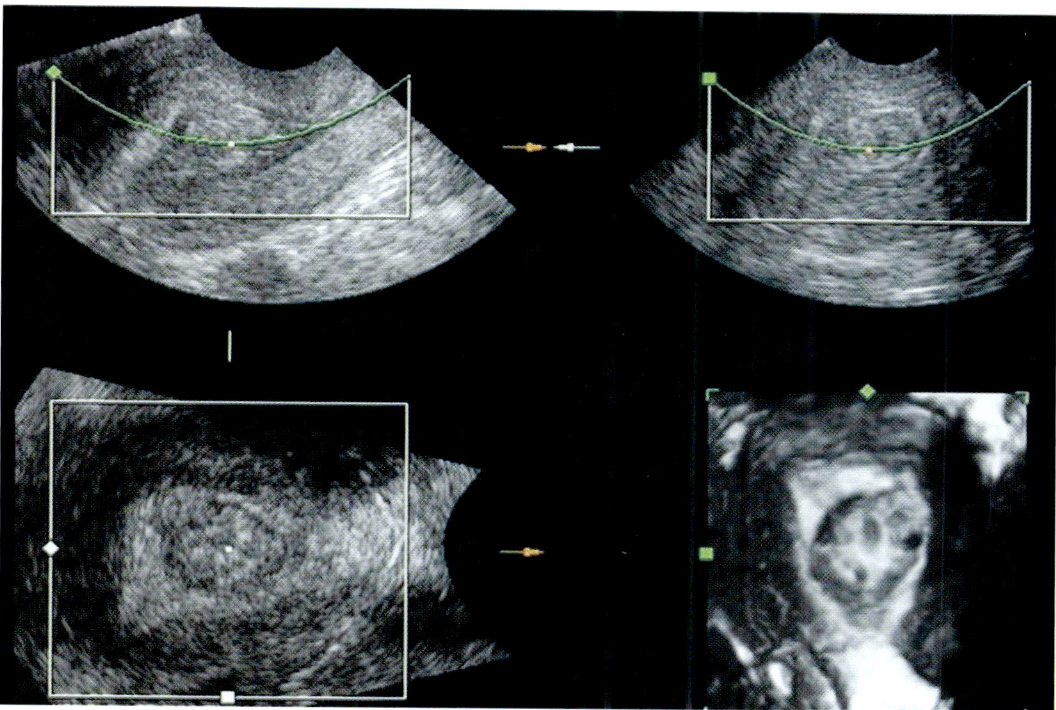

Fig. 13.8: Multiplanar view of an intracavitary fibroid with rendered view shown in the lower right image.

Adenomyosis: The diagnosis of adenomyosis is often made retrospectively following histopathological examination of the uterus after hysterectomy. Ultrasound is useful however and shows disruption of the myometrial-endometrial border and an irregular, thickened junctional zone in many cases [*see* Fig. 3.14B (Chapter 3)]. However, magnetic resonance imaging appears to have a higher sensitivity and specificity (70–82% sensitivity and 84–92% specificity) than 3D ultrasound (53–70% sensitivity and 65–97% specificity).[34]

Endometrial polyps: An accurate diagnosis as to whether or not a patient has an endometrial polyp is crucial when planning further management, and may determine whether outpatient or inpatient hysteroscopy is more appropriate dependent on the size of the polyp and its pedicle (Fig. 13.9). This has the potential to improve the use of resources and could be cost-effective. Some studies have shown that by using 3D ultrasound, with or without the instillation of saline, the accuracy of diagnosis is greater than that of 2D ultrasound. La-Torre et al. studied the specificity of 2D ultrasound against 3D ultrasound in 23 women with endometrial polyps.[35] They concluded that 2D ultrasound had a specificity of 69%, 3D a specificity of 88%, and 3D sonohysterography a specificity of 100%.

However, Ayida et al., who performed a similar study, found that 2D and 3D ultrasound were comparable when used in conjunction with saline sonohysterography.[36]

Studies have shown that the uterine cavity, endometrial lining, and myometrium are the best visualized using sonohysterography[37] and that these images are further improved by the use of 3D ultrasound.[38,39] Three-dimensional ultrasound allows the images to be captured as the saline is introduced and these can then be reviewed after the procedure even if the saline leaks out quickly afterward (Fig. 13.10). One such study[39] looked at 36 women with postmenopausal bleeding who underwent 3D sonohysterography. The results were compared against 2D ultrasound alone, 2D sonohysterography and hysteroscopy with histological correlation. The results revealed that 3D sonohysterography provided the most useful images of the uterine cavity and endometrial thickness and that these correlated well with the hysteroscopic findings.

The Ovary

Polycystic Ovarian Syndrome

The criteria used to define the polycystic ovary are the presence of 12 or more follicles measuring 2–9 mm or an

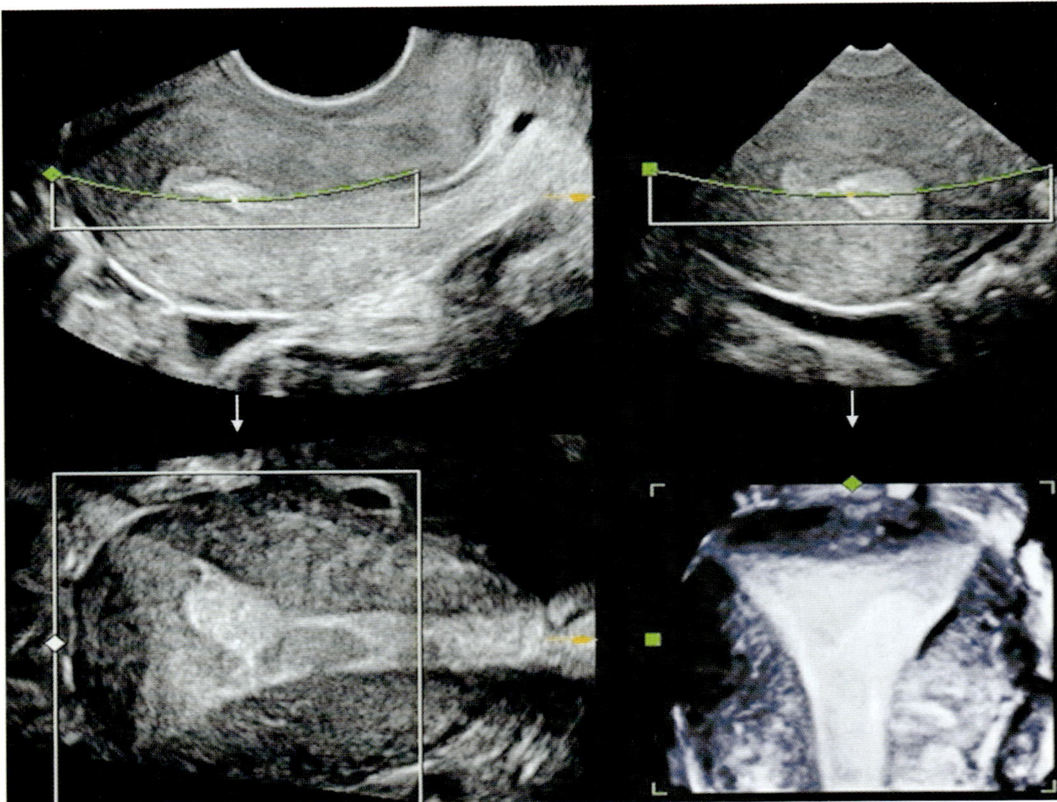

Fig. 13.9: Polyp: A 3D multiplanar view of a broad-based endometrial polyp.

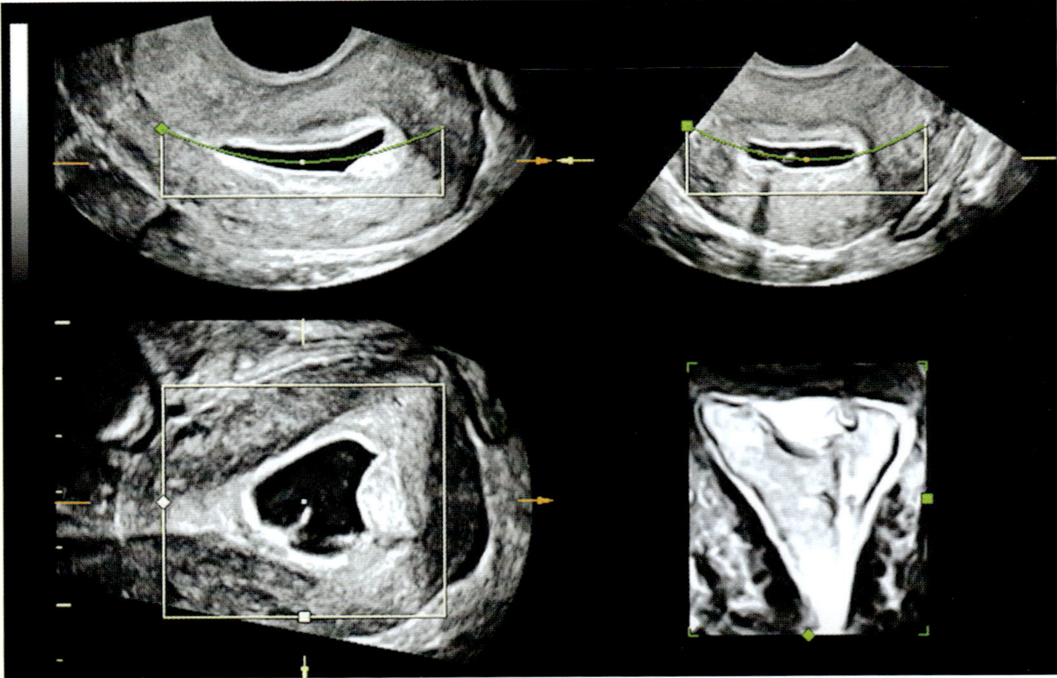

Fig. 13.10: Three-dimensional saline infusion sonohysterography: A 3D acquisition was undertaken during the instillation of saline. A small broad-based polyp is seen attached to the fundus.

increased ovarian volume (>10 cm^3).[40] Stromal vascularity and blood flow velocities are higher in women with polycystic ovaries[41,42] and it has been suggested that this may be one of the reasons why women with polycystic ovarian syndrome have a tendency toward ovarian hyperstimulation. Kyei-Mensah et al.[43] used 3D ultrasound to compare polycystic ovaries against normal ovaries and demonstrated that there was an increased stromal volume in women with polycystic ovaries. However, using a similar approach, Nardo et al. were unable to demonstrate any relationship between serum follicle-stimulating hormone (FSH), luteinizing hormone (LH), or testosterone and ovarian stromal volume in 23 infertile women with clomiphene citrate-resistant polycystic ovary syndrome (PCOS) at the same stage of the menstrual cycle.[44] Three-dimensional imaging can calculate ovarian volumes more accurately than measurements based on 2D estimations,[45] and facilitates detailed follicle counts should, arguably, mean it may become the ultrasound technique of choice for the diagnosis in the future.

Ovarian Cysts

Ovarian cysts are commonly diagnosed with transvaginal ultrasound, which offers a sensitivity of 88–100% and specificity of 62–96% to discriminate between benign and malignant adnexal masses.[34] The commonly encountered benign ovarian cysts are confidently diagnosed using ultrasound as they demonstrate characteristic sonographic appearance.[46]

Functional or simple ovarian cysts are usually smaller with a diameter of 6 cm or less and are sonolucent (Fig. 13.11). They are usually follicular cysts, unilocular with a thin, smooth outer and inner wall. Hemorrhagic cysts typically contain spiders-weblike material that represents layers of fibrin. Blood clots may be seen and can be confused with papillary projections. Ultrasound characteristics of a dermoid cyst are highly variable, ranging from predominantly cystic to uniformly dense. Most dermoid cysts are easily identifiable sonographically owing to their fat and hair content. The distinctive feature is the presence

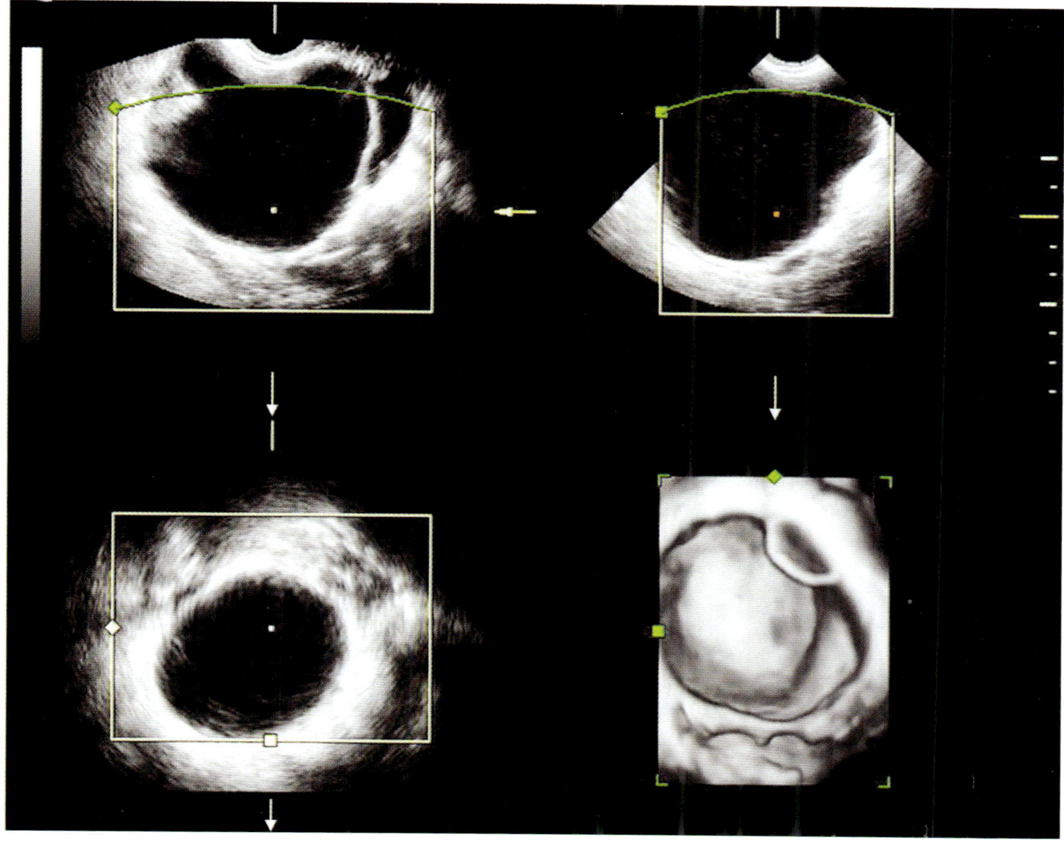

Fig. 13.11: Three-dimensional multiplanar view of a simple ovarian cyst.

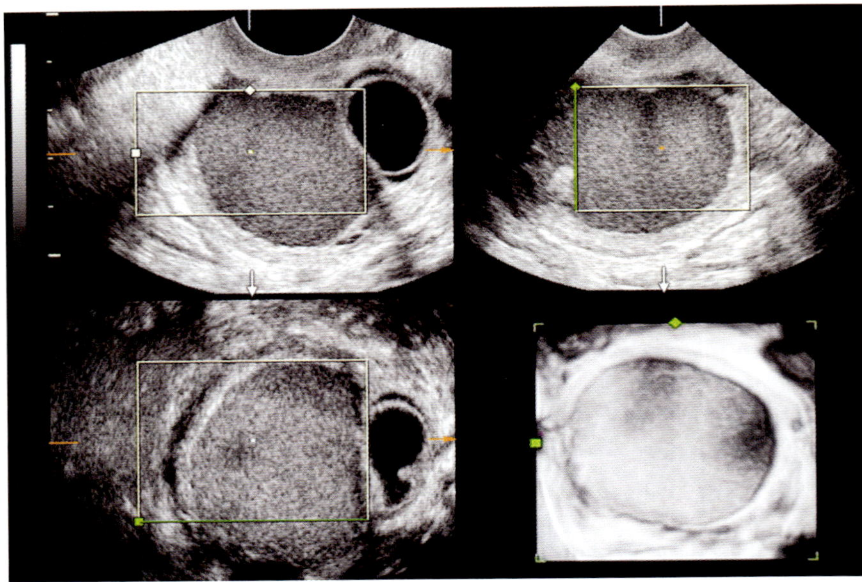

Fig. 13.12: Three-dimensional multiplanar view of an ovarian endometrioma.

of a discrete highly echogenic focus, with posterior shadowing (Rokitansky protuberance). Other characteristics considered pathognomonic are fine, echogenic bands representing hair within the cystic area and the presence of a fat-fluid level. The most consistent ultrasonographic feature of endometrioma (Fig. 13.12) has been the typical "ground glass" appearance, characterized by diffuse low-level internal echoes within the cyst. They have thick walls, and some of them show septations. One or more "solid masses" are occasionally seen to protrude from the cyst wall into the cyst lumen, which is described as "wall nodularity." Although 3D techniques has the potential to improve the diagnostic accuracy of ultrasound for differentiating these benign ovarian cysts as it offers an improved spatial orientation through provision of different image displays such as multiplanar view, TUI, and different rendering modalities, this needs to be tested in prospective studies.

Ovarian Reserve

Ovarian reserve, defined by the size and quality of the remaining ovarian follicular pool at any given time, reflects the fertility potential of a woman.[47] It is important to assess ovarian reserve accurately prior to commencing assisted reproduction treatment as it allows specialists to individualize patient treatment. There are essentially three parameters to assess when using ultrasound to assess ovarian reserve: (1) antral follicle count, (2) ovarian volume, and (3) stromal blood flow. These have been detailed in Chapter 6.

Ovarian volume can be calculated more reliably and accurately using 3D ultrasound data.[15] If the volume is less than 3 cm^3 then a poor response is likely but if it is more than 10 cm^3 the ovary can be considered polycystic, the patient is at an increased risk of ovarian hyperstimulation syndrome. Studies using 3D ultrasound to investigate the relationship between ovarian volume and in vitro fertilization (IVF) outcomes have, however, generated different results and suggests volume may not be an important predictor. Schild et al.[48] assessed ovarian volume following downregulation but prior to ovarian stimulation in 152 cycles of IVF. There was no correlation between ovarian volume and IVF outcome and somewhat unexpectedly a trend toward smaller ovarian measurements in the conception group, albeit an insignificant one, was noted. Similar results were noted by Ng et al. (2006)[49] who also concluded that ovarian volume does not appear to be a significant predictor of ovarian response.

Studies assessing antral follicle counts have been more encouraging than those assessing ovarian volume measurements, as they appear to demonstrate a more positive correlation with IVF outcomes. Transvaginal ultrasound can be used to assess the number of antral follicles measuring between 2 and 10 mm in diameter during the early follicular phase of the menstrual cycle. A poor response to ovarian stimulation is likely if there are less than ten follicles in total[50] whereas ovarian hyperstimulation syndrome is more prevalent in women with more than 12 follicles in either ovary.[51] Although the reproducibility of antral follicle count measurement is improved with 3D ultrasound when compared to 2D ultrasound,[52] the prediction of ovarian response during assisted reproduction treatment is not enhanced with the use of 3D techniques.[50]

The additional use of power Doppler does not appear to improve the prediction of ovarian response above that of antral follicle counts.[49,53] Ovarian blood flow quantified using quantitative 3D power Doppler angiography was similar between the normal responders (control group) and the aberrant responders (study groups) and did not appear to have any predictive value in prospective observation studied.[54,55]

Endometrial Receptivity

Successful implantation following ET primarily depends on the quality and competence of the embryo but is also affected by the endometrium and its ability to accept the developing blastocyst ("endometrial receptivity") and is unlikely to occur in an endometrium measuring less than 5 mm in diameter.[56] Studies by Schild et al.[57] and Yaman et al.[58] showed no significant differences between endometrial thickness and volume measurements in patients who conceived compared to those who did not, but did suggest a minimal volume of 2.0–2.5 cm^3 was required for implantation to occur. This concept is supported by Raga et al.[59] who assessed endometrial volume in 72 women on the day of ET and noted that no pregnancies occurred in patients with an endometrial volume below 1 cm^3 and that implantation rates were significantly lower when the endometrial volume was less than 2 cm^3. It is uncertain if volume measurements provide more predictive information than standard 2D measures of endometrial thickness as this has not been thoroughly assessed in randomized, blinded trials.

Various studies have evaluated predictive ability of power Doppler indices on endometrial receptivity. A more detailed and global assessment of the vascularity and blood flow within the endometrium and subendometrial region can be made using quantitative 3D power Doppler angiography.[60] Measurement of the endometrial and subendometrial VI, FI, and VFI have all been used to predict receptivity. Kupesic et al. used 3D to assess endometrial vascularity in 89 patients on the day of ET and reported a significantly higher endometrial FI, but not VI and VFI, in successful conception cycles.[61] Wu et al. also found 3D power Doppler angiography to be an important determinant of endometrial receptivity but on the day of human chorionic gonadotropin (hCG) administration in 54 patients undergoing their first IVF cycle.[62] In this study, the subendometrial VFI proved to be the best predictor of conception being superior to the VI, FI, and endometrial volume in receiver operating characteristics curve analysis. Interestingly, 3D ultrasound may also be used to examine endometrial vascularity and determine endometrial receptivity prior to ovarian stimulation. Schild et al. reported significantly lower indices of subendometrial vascularity at downregulation in 15 patients that subsequently conceived than in 60 nonconception cycles with the FI the strongest predictive factor of IVF success.[63] This may reflect the hormonal sensitivity of the endometrium in that women responding well to pituitary desensitization may be expected to also respond well to controlled ovarian stimulation.

The majority of these studies have only assessed a single time point and not considered the cyclical variation known to occur throughout the menstrual cycle and during controlled ovarian stimulation, which itself may have a negative effect on endometrial development.[63] Raine-Fenning et al. demonstrated cyclical changes in endometrial and subendometrial vascularity characterized by a preovulatory peak and a postovulatory fall maximal at the time of the peri-implantation window.[64] A similar pattern was observed in women with unexplained subfertility but these women had significantly lower preovulatory values leading the authors to speculate that the change in blood flow may be a more important determinant of endometrial receptivity than any absolute value and any given time point.[65] Ng et al. reported a lower endometrial VI and VFI on the day of oocyte retrieval in women who conceived following IVF than in a comparable nonpregnant group while the endometrial FI and subendometrial VI, FI, and VFI were all similar.[66] The predictive value of these 3D vascular indices for endometrial receptivity was poor, however, with an area under the curve close to 0.5 for all the indices. Contrary to this, a more recent study reported a significant predictive power for the indices particularly in cases where lower-quality embryos or a single embryo are transferred during IVF treatment for all three 3D power Doppler vascular indices on the day of oocyte retrieval.[67] However, in cases where multiple good-quality embryos were transferred, the vascular indices were similar between pregnant and nonpregnant groups. This finding is in agreement with that of Ng et al. who noted similar endometrial vascularity in a good prognosis group defined as those under 35 years of age who had more than two good-quality embryos to choose from for ET.[68] These findings may simply reflect the degree of estrogenization which is known to drive angiogenesis and likely to be higher in women responding well to gonadotropin. The current data do suggest, however, that endometrial perfusion may be an important factor when the transfer of lower-quality embryos or a single embryo is performed, but not with transfer of multiple good-quality embryos.

Tubal Assessment

Assessment of tubes using 3D ultrasound [3D hysterosalpingo contrast sonography (HyCoSy)] has been detailed in Chapter 5. The contrast is injected as in conventional HyCoSy and 3D power Doppler helps to visualize the whole tube with spill [*see* Fig. 5.11 (Chapter 5)]. This technique has shown to be superior to conventional HyCoSy. Three-dimensional HyCoSy technique allows simultaneous visualization of the uterine cavity and whole tube.

Follicular Monitoring

Ultrasonography is regarded as a safe, accurate, and efficient method of monitoring follicular development in response to ovarian stimulation and is an essential part of assisted reproduction treatment. Follicular monitoring using both 2D and 3D ultrasound is detailed in Chapter 9. Application of 3D ultrasound with automated assessment during follicle monitoring during IVF (Fig. 13.6) may improve workflow and measurement reproducibility.[21,23] However, the clinical outcome has not been improved with the use of automated follicle tracking to time the hCG trigger for oocyte maturation and egg collection in a randomized controlled trial.[69]

Ultrasound-Guided Procedures

Ultrasound is used to direct the transvaginal collection of oocytes and the subsequent transfer of embryos into the uterus (*see* Chapter 10). There are no reported advantages in application of 3D ultrasound for egg collection and in fact it is technically more challenging to do the procedure with real-time 3D/4D ultrasound than with conventional 2D ultrasound. While ET using 2D ultrasound is straightforward and relatively easy, recent reports on utilizing 3D ultrasound is reported to improve visualization and greater accuracy in the placement of embryos within the uterine cavity.[70,71] Identifying the point of maximum implantation potential (MIP) which is an intersection of two lines that are drawn parallel to both cornua on a mid coronal section of uterus [*see* Fig. 9.26 (Chapter 9)], and performing ET at the MIP may potentially improve IVF outcome. However, considering lack of universal availability of 3D ultrasound machine and limited evidence base on its advantage, 3D/4D ultrasound-guided ET cannot be recommended for routine use.

CONCLUSION

Three-dimensional ultrasound imaging is increasingly used as a day-to-day imaging modality in reproductive medicine. Three-dimensional ultrasound should not be considered as a direct replacement for conventional 2D ultrasound but rather as an enhancement of present technology. Three-dimensional imaging has several obvious benefits that relate to an improved spatial orientation and the demonstration of additional image planes such as the coronal plane. Similarities can be drawn with the additional information gained from the use of computerized tomography and magnetic resonance imaging. Three-dimensional ultrasonography has become a moderately easy technique to learn but experience in 2D ultrasonography is essential to obtain the images required for 3D visualization. However, other than its application in the assessment and differentiation of uterine anomalies, there is very little evidence that 3D ultrasound results in clinically relevant benefit or negate the need for further investigation in a fertility unit.

KEY POINTS

- Three-dimensional ultrasound involves the acquisition of a series of 2D images from a preselected region of interest
- Three-dimensional ultrasound scanning consists of four basic steps; data acquisition, data storage, data retrieval, volume analysis and processing, and archiving of volumes
- The acquired 3D data may be displayed in a variety of image modalities such as multiplanar view, various rendering options, and TUI
- The coronal plane, perpendicular to the transducer face, is unique to 3D ultrasound

- Measurement of volume and vascularity indices using 3D ultrasound is more objective and reproducible than with 2D ultrasound
- Three-dimensional ultrasound and associated software (Sono-AVC) allow automated volume calculation of fluid-filled structures
- Three-dimensional ultrasound has the benefit of offering reduced scanning time, storage of images for re-evaluation, and teleconsultation
- Many clinicians remain unconvinced by its reputed advantages and have concerns regarding the cost implications and training requirements
- Other than its application in the assessment and differentiation of uterine anomalies, there is very little evidence that 3D ultrasound results in clinically relevant benefit or negate the need for further investigation in a fertility unit

REFERENCES

1. Maymon R, Herman A, Ariely S, et al. Three-dimensional vaginal sonography in obstetrics and gynaecology. Hum Reprod Update. 2000;6(5):475-84.
2. Nelson TR, Pretorius DH. Three-dimensional ultrasound imaging. Ultrasound Med Biol. 1998;24(9):1243-70.
3. Merz E. Three-dimensional transvaginal ultrasound in gynecological diagnosis. Ultrasound Obstet Gynecol. 1999;14(2):81-6.
4. Benacerraf BR, Benson CB, Abuhamad AZ, et al. Three- and 4-dimensional ultrasound in obstetrics and gynecology: proceedings of the American Institute of Ultrasound in Medicine Consensus Conference. J Ultrasound Med. 2005;24(12):1587-97.
5. Bega G, Lev-Toaff AS, O'Kane P, et al. Three-dimensional ultrasonography in gynecology: technical aspects and clinical applications. J Ultrasound Med. 2003;22(11):1249-69.
6. Whittingham TA. Medical diagnostic applications and sources. Prog Biophys Mol Biol. 2007;93(1-3):84-110.
7. Riccabona M, Nelson TR, Pretorius DH, et al. Distance and volume measurement using three-dimensional ultrasonography. J Ultrasound Med. 1995;14(12):881-6.
8. Merz E, Benoit B, Blaas HG, et al. Standardization of three-dimensional images in obstetrics and gynecology: consensus statement. Ultrasound Obstet Gynecol. 2007;29(6):697-703.
9. Jurkovic D. Three-dimensional ultrasound in gynecology: a critical evaluation. Ultrasound Obstet Gynecol. 2002;19(2): 109-17.
10. Benacerraf BR. Inversion mode display of 3D sonography: applications in obstetric and gynecologic imaging. AJR Am J Roentgenol. 2006;187(4):965-71.
11. Timor-Tritsch IE, Monteagudo A, Tsymbal T, et al. Three-dimensional inversion rendering: a new sonographic technique and its use in gynecology. J Ultrasound Med. 2005;24(5):681-8.
12. Gilja OH, Hausken T, Berstad A, et al. Measurements of organ volume by ultrasonography. Proc Inst Mech Eng H. 1999;213(3):247-59.
13. Brunner M, Obruca A, Bauer P, et al. Clinical application of volume estimation based on three-dimensional ultrasonography. Ultrasound Obstet Gynecol. 1995;6(5): 358-61.
14. Bordes A, Bory AM, Benchaïb M, et al. Reproducibility of transvaginal three-dimensional endometrial volume measurements with virtual organ computer-aided analysis (VOCAL) during ovarian stimulation. Ultrasound Obstet Gynecol. 2002;19(1):76-80.
15. Raine-Fenning NJ, Campbell BK, Clewes JS, et al. The interobserver reliability of ovarian volume measurement is improved with three-dimensional ultrasound, but dependent upon technique. Ultrasound Med Biol. 2003;29(12):1685-90.
16. Yaman C, Sommergruber M, Ebner T, et al. Reproducibility of transvaginal three-dimensional endometrial volume measurements during ovarian stimulation. Hum Reprod. 1999;14(10):2604-8.
17. Downey DB, Fenster A. Vascular imaging with a three-dimensional power Doppler system. AJR Am J Roentgenol. 1995;165(3):665-8.
18. Rubin JM, Adler RS, Fowlkes JB, et al. Fractional moving blood volume: estimation with power Doppler US. Radiology. 1995;197(1):183-90.
19. Ohishi H, Hirai T, Yamada R, et al. Three-dimensional power Doppler sonography of tumor vascularity. J Ultrasound Med. 1998;17(10):619-22.
20. Pairleitner H, Steiner H, Hasenoehrl G, et al. Three-dimensional power Doppler sonography: imaging and quantifying blood flow and vascularization. Ultrasound Obstet Gynecol. 1999;14(2):139-43.
21. Raine-Fenning N, Jayaprakasan K, Clewes J. Automated follicle tracking facilitates standardization and may improve work flow. Ultrasound Obstet Gynecol. 2007;30(7):1015-8.
22. Raine-Fenning N, Jayaprakasan K, Clewes J, et al. SonoAVC: a novel method of automatic volume calculation. Ultrasound Obstet Gynecol. 2008;31(6):691-6.
23. Raine-Fenning N, Jayaprakasan K, Deb S, et al. Automated follicle tracking improves measurement reliability in patients undergoing ovarian stimulation. Reprod Biomed Online. 2009;18(5):658-63.
24. Pretorius DH, Nelson TR. Three-dimensional ultrasound. Ultrasound Obstet Gynecol. 1995;5(4):219-21.
25. Kupesic S. Clinical implications of sonographic detection of uterine anomalies for reproductive outcome. Ultrasound Obstet Gynecol. 2001;18(4):387-400.
26. Jayaprakasan K, Chan YY, Sur S, et al. Prevalence of uterine anomalies and their impact on early pregnancy in women conceiving after assisted reproduction treatment. Ultrasound Obstet Gynecol. 2011;37(6):727-32.
27. Chan YY, Jayaprakasan K, Tan A, et al. Reproductive outcomes in women with congenital uterine anomalies:

a systematic review. Ultrasound Obstet Gynecol. 2011;38(4):371-82.
28. Homer HA, Li TC, Cooke ID. The septate uterus: a review of management and reproductive outcome. Fertil Steril. 2000;73(1):1-14.
29. Jurkovic D, Geipel A, Gruboeck K, et al. Three-dimensional ultrasound for the assessment of uterine anatomy and detection of congenital anomalies: a comparison with hysterosalpingography and two-dimensional sonography. Ultrasound Obstet Gynecol. 1995;5(4):233-7.
30. Raga F, Bonilla-Musoles F, Blanes J, et al. Congenital Mullerian anomalies: diagnostic accuracy of three-dimensional ultrasound. Fertil Steril. 1996;65(3):523-8.
31. Wu MH, Hsu CC, Huang KE. Detection of congenital Mullerian duct anomalies using three-dimensional ultrasound. J Clin Ultrasound. 1997;25(9):487-92.
32. Saravelos SH, Jayaprakasan K, Ojha K, Li TC. Assessment of the uterus with three-dimensional ultrasound in women undergoing ART. Hum Reprod Update. 2017;23(2):188-210.
33. Sylvestre C, Child TJ, Tulandi T, et al. A prospective study to evaluate the efficacy of two- and three-dimensional sonohysterography in women with intrauterine lesions. Fertil Steril. 2003;79(5):1222-5.
34. Walker K, Jayaprakasan K, Raine-Fenning NJ. Ultrasound in benign gynaecology. Obstetrics, Gynaecology & Reproductive Medicine. 2007;17(2):33-44.
35. La Torre R, De Felice C, De Angelis C, et al. Transvaginal sonographic evaluation of endometrial polyps: a comparison with two-dimensional and three-dimensional contrast sonography. Clin Exp Obstet Gynecol. 1999;26 (3-4):171-3.
36. Ayida G, Kennedy S, Barlow D, et al. Contrast sonography for uterine cavity assessment: a comparison of conventional two-dimensional with three-dimensional transvaginal ultrasound; a pilot study. Fertil Steril. 1996;66(5):848-50.
37. Bronz L, Suter T, Rusca T. The value of transvaginal sonography with and without saline instillation in the diagnosis of uterine pathology in pre- and postmenopausal women with abnormal bleeding or suspect sonographic findings. Ultrasound Obstet Gynecol. 1997;9(1):53-8.
38. Lev-Toaff AS, Pinheiro LW, Bega G, et al. Three-dimensional multiplanar sonohysterography: comparison with conventional two-dimensional sonohysterography and X-ray hysterosalpingography. J Ultrasound Med. 2001;20(4):295-306.
39. Bonilla-Musoles F, Raga F, Osborne NG, et al. Three-dimensional hysterosonography for the study of endometrial tumors: comparison with conventional transvaginal sonography, hysterosalpingography, and hysteroscopy. Gynecol Oncol. 1997;65(2):245-52.
40. Balen AH, Laven JS, Tan SL, et al. Ultrasound assessment of the polycystic ovary: international consensus definitions. Hum Reprod Update. 2003;9(6):505-14.
41. Agrawal R, Conway G, Sladkevicius P, et al. Serum vascular endothelial growth factor and Doppler blood flow velocities in in vitro fertilization: relevance to ovarian hyperstimulation syndrome and polycystic ovaries. Fertil Steril. 1998;70(4):651-8.
42. Pan HA, Wu MH, Cheng YC, et al. Quantification of Doppler signal in polycystic ovary syndrome using three-dimensional power Doppler ultrasonography: a possible new marker for diagnosis. Hum Reprod. 2002;17(1):201-6.
43. Kyei-Mensah AA, LinTan S, Zaidi J, et al. Relationship of ovarian stromal volume to serum androgen concentrations in patients with polycystic ovary syndrome. Hum Reprod. 1998;13(6):1437-41.
44. Nardo LG, Buckett WM, White D, et al. Three-dimensional assessment of ultrasound features in women with clomiphene citrate-resistant polycystic ovarian syndrome (PCOS): ovarian stromal volume does not correlate with biochemical indices. Hum Reprod. 2002;17(4):1052-5.
45. Wu MH, Pan HA, Chang FM. Three-dimensional and power Doppler ultrasonography in infertility and reproductive endocrinology. Taiwan J Obstet Gynecol. 2007;46(3):209-14.
46. Jermy K, Luise C, Bourne T. The characterization of common ovarian cysts in premenopausal women. Ultrasound Obstet Gynecol. 2001;17(2):140-4.
47. Broekmans FJ, Kwee J, Hendriks DJ, et al. A systematic review of tests predicting ovarian reserve and IVF outcome. Hum Reprod Update. 2006;12(6):685-718.
48. Schild RL, Knobloch C, Dorn C, et al. The role of ovarian volume in an in vitro fertilization programme as assessed by 3D ultrasound. Arch Gynecol Obstet. 2001;265(2):67-72.
49. Ng EH, Tang OS, Chan CC, et al. Ovarian stromal vascularity is not predictive of ovarian response and pregnancy. Reprod Biomed Online. 2006;12(1):43-9.
50. Jayaprakasan K, Hilwah N, Kendall NR, et al. Does 3D ultrasound offer any advantage in the pretreatment assessment of ovarian reserve and prediction of outcome after assisted reproduction treatment? Hum Reprod. 2007;22(7):1932-41.
51. Delvigne A, Rozenberg S. Epidemiology and prevention of ovarian hyperstimulation syndrome (OHSS): a review. Hum Reprod Update. 2002;8(6):559-77.
52. Jayaprakasan K, Campbell BK, Clewes JS, et al. Three-dimensional ultrasound improves the interobserver reliability of antral follicle counts and facilitates increased clinical work flow. Ultrasound Obstet Gynecol. 2008;31(4):439-44.
53. Kupesic S, Kurjak A, Bjelos D, et al. Three-dimensional ultrasonographic ovarian measurements and in vitro fertilization outcome are related to age. Fertil Steril. 2003;79(1):190-7.
54. Jayaprakasan K, Al-Hasie H, Jayaprakasan R, et al. The three-dimensional ultrasonographic ovarian vascularity of women developing poor ovarian response during assisted reproduction treatment and its predictive value. Fertil Steril. 2009;92(6):1862-9.
55. Jayaprakasan K, Jayaprakasan R, Al-Hasie HA, et al. Can quantitative three-dimensional power Doppler angiography be used to predict ovarian hyperstimulation syndrome? Ultrasound Obstet Gynecol. 2009;33(5):583-91.

56. Friedler S, Schenker JG, Herman A, et al. The role of ultrasonography in the evaluation of endometrial receptivity following assisted reproductive treatments: a critical review. Hum Reprod Update. 1996;2(4):323-35.
57. Schild RL, Indefrei D, Eschweiler S, et al. Three-dimensional endometrial volume calculation and pregnancy rate in an in-vitro fertilization programme. Hum Reprod. 1999;14(5):1255-8.
58. Yaman C, Ebner T, Sommergruber M, et al. Role of three-dimensional ultrasonographic measurement of endometrium volume as a predictor of pregnancy outcome in an IVF-ET program: a preliminary study. Fertil Steril. 2000;74(4):797-801.
59. Raga F, Bonilla-Musoles F, Casañ EM, et al. Assessment of endometrial volume by three-dimensional ultrasound prior to embryo transfer: clues to endometrial receptivity. Hum Reprod. 1999;14(11):2851-4.
60. Raine-Fenning NJ, Campbell BK, Clewes JS, et al. The reliability of virtual organ computer-aided analysis (VOCAL) for the semiquantification of ovarian, endometrial and subendometrial perfusion. Ultrasound Obstet Gynecol. 2003;22(6):633-9.
61. Kupesic S, Bekavac I, Bjelos D, et al. Assessment of endometrial receptivity by transvaginal color Doppler and three-dimensional power Doppler ultrasonography in patients undergoing in vitro fertilization procedures. J Ultrasound Med. 2001;20(2):125-34.
62. Wu HM, Chiang CH, Huang HY, et al. Detection of the subendometrial vascularization flow index by three-dimensional ultrasound may be useful for predicting the pregnancy rate for patients undergoing in vitro fertilization-embryo transfer. Fertil Steril. 2003;79(3):507-11.
63. Schild RL, Holthaus S, d'Alquen J, et al. Quantitative assessment of subendometrial blood flow by three-dimensional-ultrasound is an important predictive factor of implantation in an in-vitro fertilization programme. Hum Reprod. 2000;15(1):89-94.
64. Raine-Fenning NJ, Campbell BK, Kendall NR, et al. Quantifying the changes in endometrial vascularity throughout the normal menstrual cycle with three-dimensional power Doppler angiography. Hum Reprod. 2004;19(2):330-8.
65. Raine-Fenning NJ, Campbell BK, Kendall NR, et al. Endometrial and subendometrial perfusion are impaired in women with unexplained subfertility. Hum Reprod. 2004;19(11):2605-14.
66. Ng EH, Chan CC, Tang OS, et al. The role of endometrial and subendometrial blood flows measured by three-dimensional power Doppler ultrasound in the prediction of pregnancy during IVF treatment. Hum Reprod. 2006;21(1):164-70.
67. Mercé LT, Barco MJ, Bau S, et al. Are endometrial parameters by three-dimensional ultrasound and power Doppler angiography related to in vitro fertilization/ embryo transfer outcome? Fertil Steril. 2008;89(1): 111-7.
68. Ng EH, Chan CC, Tang OS, et al. The role of endometrial blood flow measured by three-dimensional power Doppler ultrasound in the prediction of pregnancy during in vitro fertilization treatment. Eur J Obstet Gynecol Reprod Biol. 2007;135(1):8-16.
69. Raine-Fenning N, Deb S, Jayaprakasan K, et al. Timing of oocyte maturation and egg collection during controlled ovarian stimulation: a randomized controlled trial evaluating manual and automated measurements of follicle diameter. Fertil Steril. 2010;94(1):184-8.
70. Gergely RZ, DeUgarte CM, Danzer H, et al. Three-dimensional/ four-dimensional ultrasound-guided embryo transfer using the maximal implantation potential point. Fertil Steril. 2005;84(2):500-3.
71. Fang L, Sun Y, Su Y, et al. Advantages of 3-dimensional sonography in embryo transfer. J Ultrasound Med. 2009;28(5):573-8.

INDEX

Page numbers followed by *b* refer to box, *f* refer to figure and *t* refer to table.

O

P

R

S

T

U

V

W